BOOST YOUR SCORES

START SMART • STAY COMPETITIVE • FINISH STRONG

D1581038

USMLE | CONSULT
STEPS ① ② ③

SAVE 30%

GOLJAN REVIEWED AND APPROVED!

USMLE Consult Step 1 Question Bank

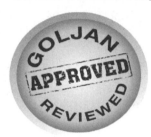

- More than 2,500 questions **written and reviewed by Drs. Edward Goljan and John Pelley**, among many other top Elsevier authors
- **Questions written at varying levels of difficulty** to mirror the NBME's exam blueprint
- **High-yield hits—** bonus remediation content-from names you trust, like Goljan, Brochert, Robbins, Drake and Costanzo
- Test **customization**, with detailed, **instant results analysis**

- Bonus access to the Scorrelator, an advanced assessment tool that generates a score indicative of what you can expect on the actual USMLE Step 1 or COMLEX Level I exams

Robbins Pathology Question Bank

- 500 questions focused on pathology
- High-yield hits with **bonus content from Robbins & Cotran Pathologic Basis of Disease**

Additional Review Plans Available at usmleconsult.com

- BUY TOGETHER AND SAVE! Step 1 Question Bank + Robbins Pathology Question Bank
- BEST VALUE! **Step 1 Premium Review** Step 1 Q-Bank, Robbins Q-bank, Scorrelator, and online access to a Go Paperless eBook at Student Consult
- **Step 2 CK Question Bank and Step 2 Premium Review**
- **Step 3 CCS Case Bank + Step 3 Question Bank and Step 3 Premium Review**

Order securely at www.usmleconsult.com

Activate discount code

MOORERR30

at checkout to redeem savings

ELSEVIER

©Elsevier 2010-2014. Offer valid at usmleconsult.com only.

BRITISH MEDICAL ASSOCIATION

0921765

Rapid Review Series

Series Editor
Edward F. Goljan, MD

BEHAVIORAL SCIENCE, SECOND EDITION
Vivian M. Stevens, PhD; Susan K. Redwood, PhD; Jackie L. Neel, DO;
Richard H. Bost, PhD; Nancy W. Van Winkle, PhD;
Michael H. Pollak, PhD

BIOCHEMISTRY, THIRD EDITION
John W. Pelley, PhD; Edward F. Goljan, MD

GROSS AND DEVELOPMENTAL ANATOMY, THIRD EDITION
N. Anthony Moore, PhD; William A. Roy, PhD, PT

HISTOLOGY AND CELL BIOLOGY, SECOND EDITION
E. Robert Burns, PhD; M. Donald Cave, PhD

MICROBIOLOGY AND IMMUNOLOGY, THIRD EDITION
Ken S. Rosenthal, PhD; Michael J. Tan, MD

NEUROSCIENCE
James A. Weyhenmeyer, PhD; Eve A. Gallman, PhD

PATHOLOGY, THIRD EDITION
Edward F. Goljan, MD

PHARMACOLOGY, THIRD EDITION
Thomas L. Pazdernik, PhD; Laszlo Kerecsen, MD

PHYSIOLOGY
Thomas A. Brown, MD

LABORATORY TESTING IN CLINICAL MEDICINE
Edward F. Goljan, MD; Karlis Sloka, DO

USMLE STEP 2
Michael W. Lawlor, MD, PhD

USMLE STEP 3
David Rolston, MD; Craig Nielsen, MD

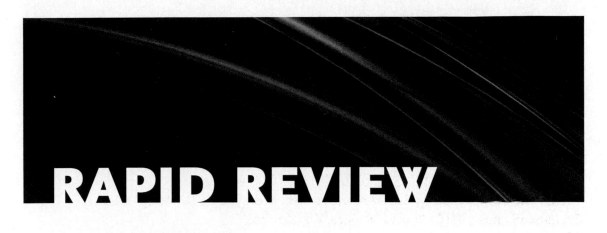

RAPID REVIEW

GROSS AND DEVELOPMENTAL ANATOMY

THIRD EDITION

N. Anthony Moore, PhD
Professor of Anatomy
University of Mississippi Medical Center
Jackson, Mississippi

William A. Roy, PT, PhD
Professor of Basic Sciences
Touro University Nevada
Henderson, Nevada

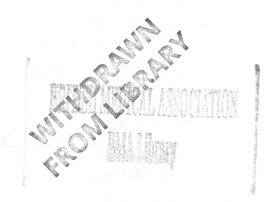
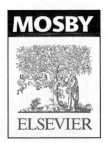

MOSBY

ELSEVIER

1600 John F. Kennedy Blvd.
Ste 1800
Philadelphia, PA 19103-2899

RAPID REVIEW GROSS AND DEVELOPMENTAL ANATOMY, Third Edition

Copyright © 2010, 2007, 2003 by Mosby, Inc., an affiliate of Elsevier Inc.   ISBN-13: 978-0-323-07294-6

Notice

Library of Congress Cataloging-in-Publication Data
Moore, N. Anthony.
  Rapid review gross and developmental anatomy / N. Anthony Moore, William A. Roy.—3rd ed.
    p. ; cm.—(Rapid review series)
  Rev. ed. of: Gross and developmental anatomy / N. Anthony Moore, William A. Roy. 2nd ed. c2007.
  ISBN 978-0-323-07294-6
    1. Human anatomy.   2. Human anatomy–Examinations, questions, etc. I. Roy, William A.   II. Moore,
N. Anthony Gross and developmental anatomy.   III. Title.   IV. Series: Rapid review series.
    [DNLM: 1. Anatomy–Outlines. QS 18.2 M823r 2011]
    QM23.2.M675 2011
    612–dc22

                                                                                          2010002962

Acquisitions Editor: James Merritt
Developmental Editor: Christine Abshire
Publishing Services Manager: Hemamalini Rajendrababu
Project Manager: Nayagi Athmanathan
Design Direction: Steven Stave

Printed in China

Last digit is the print number: 9 8 7 6 5 4 3 2 1

To my friend and mentor Duane Haines for his unfailing support and counsel.

—NAM

To my postdoctoral mentors, Maurits Persson and the late Jan Langman, for their guidance and encouragement.

—WAR

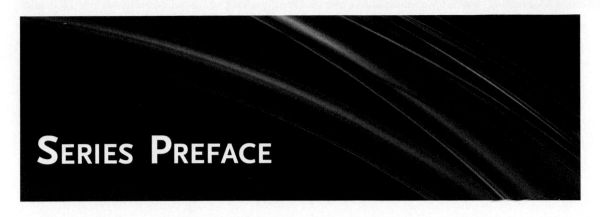

SERIES PREFACE

The First and Second Editions of the *Rapid Review Series* have received high critical acclaim from students studying for the United States Medical Licensing Examination (USMLE) Step 1 and consistently high ratings in *First Aid for the USMLE Step 1*. The new editions will continue to be invaluable resources for time-pressed students. As a result of reader feedback, we have improved upon an already successful formula. We have created a learning system, including a print and electronic package, that is easier to use and more concise than other review products on the market.

SPECIAL FEATURES

Book

- **Outline format:** Concise, high-yield subject matter is presented in a study-friendly format.
- **High-yield margin notes:** Key content that is most likely to appear on the exam is reinforced in the margin notes.
- **Visual elements:** Full-color figures are utilized to enhance your study and recognition of key concepts. Abundant two-color schematics and summary tables enhance your study experience.
- **Two-color design:** Colored text and headings make studying more efficient and pleasing.

New! Online Study and Testing Tool

- A minimum of **350 USMLE Step 1–type MCQs:** Clinically oriented, multiple-choice questions that mimic the current USMLE format, including high-yield images and complete rationales for all answer options.
- **Online benefits:** New review and testing tool delivered via the USMLE Consult platform, the most realistic USMLE review product on the market. Online feedback includes results analyzed to the subtopic level (discipline and organ system).
- **Test mode:** Create a test from a random mix of questions or by subject or keyword using the timed **test mode**. USMLE Consult simulates the actual test-taking experience using NBME's FRED interface, including style and level of difficulty of the questions and timing information. Detailed feedback and analysis shows your strengths and weaknesses and allows for more focused study.
- **Practice mode:** Create a test from randomized question sets or by subject or keyword for a dynamic study session. The **practice mode** features unlimited attempts at each question, instant feedback, complete rationales for all answer options, and a detailed progress report.
- **Online access:** Online access allows you to study from an Internet-enabled computer wherever and whenever it is convenient. This access is activated through registration on www.studentconsult.com with the pin code printed inside the front cover.

Student Consult

- **Full online access:** You can access the complete text and illustrations of this book on www.studentconsult.com.
- **Save content to your PDA:** Through our unique Pocket Consult platform, you can clip selected text and illustrations and save them to your PDA for study on the fly!
- **Free content:** An interactive community center with a wealth of additional valuable resources is available.

PREFACE TO THE THIRD EDITION

The United States Medical Licensing Examination Step 1 incorporates the major themes and essential concepts of gross and developmental anatomy into relevant clinical vignettes. *Rapid Review Gross and Developmental Anatomy* is designed to help you review these themes and concepts while articulating their clinical relevance.

- High-yield margin notes recall topics of clinical significance that likely will be tested on Step 1.
- Clinical correlations appear in pink boxes directly within the outline to emphasize the clinical application of the preceding concept.
- Development and developmental defects are integrated into the outline.
- Netter images, diagnostic images, and simple line drawings facilitate recall of essential gross anatomy and development.
- Comprehensive tables summarize essential clinically oriented information.
- Web questions emulate the USMLE Step 1 format. Complete discussions of each answer and distractors facilitate your review.

We hope that you will find this integrated approach helps you to prepare for your USMLE Step 1 examination. Good luck!

N. Anthony Moore, PhD
William A. Roy, PT, PhD

ACKNOWLEDGMENT OF REVIEWERS

The publisher expresses sincere thanks to the medical students and faculty who provided many useful comments and suggestions for improving both the text and the questions in previous editions. Our publishing program will continue to benefit from the combined insight and experience provided by your reviews. For always encouraging us to focus on our target, the USMLE Step 1, we thank the following:

Ellen K. Carlson, University of Iowa College of Medicine

John D. Cowden, Yale University School of Medicine

Mark D. Fisher, University of Virginia School of Medicine

Charles E. Galaviz, University of Iowa College of Medicine

Brian Harrison, University of Illinois Chicago School of Medicine

Gregory L. Lacy, Tulane University School of Medicine

Erica L. Magers, Michigan State University College of Human Medicine

Mrugeshkumar K. Shah, MD, MPH, Harvard Medical School/Spaulding Rehabilitation Hospital

Lara Wittine, University of Iowa College of Medicine

Julie E. Zurakowski, Northeastern Ohio Universities College of Medicine

ACKNOWLEDGMENTS

The authors thank Edward Goljan, Series Editor, for constructive suggestions and some clinical correlations in this edition; Christine Abshire, Developmental Editor, for her hard work, attention to detail, and patience; and James Merritt, Senior Acquisitions Editor, for arranging the inclusion of color images from the Netter collection. This volume builds upon work done by the editors of earlier editions: Susan Kelly, Katie DeFrancesco, and Therese Grundl. Some of Matt Chansky's original illustrations have been retained, and we appreciate the permission to include new figures from other Elsevier publications.

We thank Duane Haines, Professor and Chairman of Anatomy, University of Mississippi Medical Center, for his encouragement and for creating an academic environment conducive to scholarly activity. I (WAR) also thank Mitchell Forman, Dean and Professor, and Ronald Hedger, Medical Director of Student Health Services and Associate Professor, Touro University Nevada College of Osteopathic Medicine, for helpful discussions and for patiently answering my questions about assorted diseases and injuries.

Finally, we gratefully acknowledge the contributions of the many student physicians whose constructive criticisms, both formal and informal, have greatly increased this book's value as preparation for the USMLE Step 1 and COMLEX Level 1.

N. Anthony Moore, PhD
William A. Roy, PT, PhD

Contents

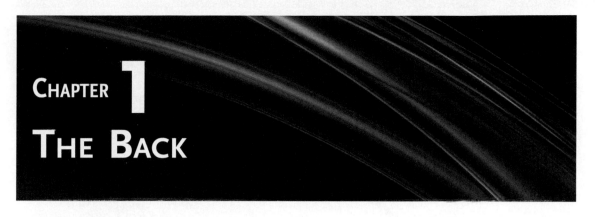

CHAPTER 1

THE BACK

I. Typical Vertebra
- **Body, vertebral arch, processes** for muscular attachment and articulation with adjacent vertebrae, and **vertebral foramen (Figure 1-1)**

A. **The Body**
Anterior weightbearing cylinder

B. **Vertebral Arch**
1. Overview
   a. U-shaped component attached to posterior aspect of body
   b. Provides attachment for spinous, transverse, and articular processes
2. **Pedicle** has superior and inferior vertebral notches.
3. **Lamina** fuses in posterior midline with opposite lamina.

C. **Transverse Processes**

D. **Articular Processes**
1. **Superior** and **inferior articular processes** project from junction of pedicle and lamina separated by **pars interarticularis**
2. Form synovial **zygapophysial (facet) joints** with articular processes of adjacent vertebrae

> Zygapophysial joints are synovial joints that may develop osteoarthritis with age or trauma.

E. **Vertebral Foramen**
1. Space enclosed by vertebral arch and body
2. Collectively form **vertebral canal** for **spinal cord** and meninges

F. **Intervertebral Foramina**
1. Formed between **inferior** and **superior vertebral notches** in **pedicles** of adjacent vertebrae
2. Transmit **spinal nerves** and related blood vessels

> Compressing spinal nerve in intervertebral foramen may cause radiculopathy

Any **space-occupying lesion** in an **intervertebral foramen** may compress the spinal nerve or its roots and produce **back pain** that may radiate into an extremity. Motor nerve fibers may become involved, resulting in **loss of strength.**

II. Vertebral Column
- Comprises 33 vertebrae in normal adult: 7 cervical, 12 thoracic, 5 lumbar, 5 sacral, 4 coccygeal

> 7 cervical, 12 thoracic, 5 lumbar, 5 sacral, and 4 coccygeal vertebrae

A. **Cervical Vertebrae (see Figure 1-1; Table 1-1)**
1. Typical cervical vertebrae: C3-C6
   a. **Spinous processes** allow neck extension because they are short.
   b. **Articular processes** with nearly horizontal facets allow relatively free movement in all directions at the expense of stability.
   c. **Transverse foramen** in each transverse process allows passage of **vertebral artery** and vein.
2. **C1 (atlas) (Figure 1-2; see Table 1-1)**
   a. Midline **anterior tubercle on anterior arch** and **posterior tubercle on posterior arch**
   b. **Sulcus for vertebral artery** on **posterior arch** on each side
3. **C2 (axis) (Figure 1-3; see Table 1-1)**

> The vertebral artery ascends transverse foramina of vertebrae C1-6.

The **dens** (odontoid process) and **body of the axis** develop from separate ossification centers. The ossification centers may **fail to fuse,** and this anomaly must be distinguished from an **odontoid fracture** in patients with cervical trauma. The dens also may be **congenitally absent.**

> The dens may be congenitally absent or fail to fuse with the body of the axis.

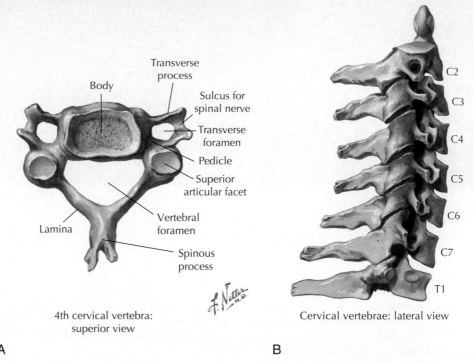

Body

Transverse process

Sulcus for spinal nerve

Transverse foramen

Pedicle

Superior articular facet

Vertebral foramen

Lamina

Spinous process

4th cervical vertebra: superior view

C2
C3
C4
C5
C6
C7
T1

Cervical vertebrae: lateral view

A   B

1-1: Typical cervical vertebrae. **A,** Superior view of a typical cervical vertebra. **B,** Lateral view of articulated cervical vertebrae. *(From Greene, W B: Netter's Orthopaedics. Philadelphia, Saunders, 2006, Figure 13-4.)*

TABLE 1-1. FEATURES OF VERTEBRAE

VERTEBRA	BODY	SPINOUS PROCESS	TRANSVERSE PROCESS	ARTICULAR PROCESSES
C1 (atlas)	None; anterior and posterior arches with paired lateral masses	None; tubercle on posterior arch	Long and stout; transverse foramen	Articulate with skull at atlanto-occipital joints and with axis at atlantoaxial joints
C2 (axis)	Dens projects superiorly from its body	Short; often bifid	Short; transverse foramen	Facets lie in horizontal plane (superior to inferior)
C3-C6	Small and broad transversely	Short; often bifid	Small and short; transverse foramen	Facets lie in horizontal plane (superior to inferior)
C7 (vertebra prominens)		Long	Small or absent transverse foramen	
Thoracic vertebrae	Cylindrical and heart-shaped; costal facets for heads of ribs	Long; angled inferiorly	Large; articular facet for articulation with tubercle of rib	Facets lie in frontal plane (anterior to posterior)
Lumbar vertebrae	Relatively large, wide, and kidney-shaped	Short, thick, quadrangular; project posteriorly	Thin; relatively long	Facets lie in sagittal plane (left to right)

1-2: Atlas (C1) from superior view. *(From Greene, W B: Netter's Orthopaedics. Philadelphia, Saunders, 2006, Figure 13-4.)*

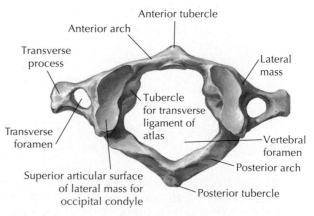

Anterior tubercle

Anterior arch

Transverse process

Lateral mass

Tubercle for transverse ligament of atlas

Transverse foramen

Vertebral foramen

Posterior arch

Posterior tubercle

Superior articular surface of lateral mass for occipital condyle

Atlas (C1): superior view

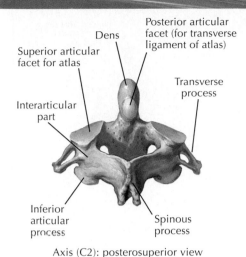

Axis (C2): posterosuperior view

A

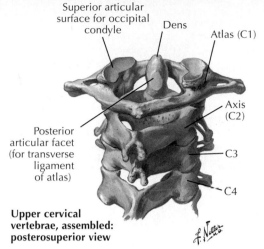

Upper cervical vertebrae, assembled: posterosuperior view

B

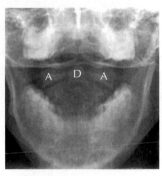

Radiograph of atlantoaxial joints (open mouth odontoid view)

A Lateral masses of atlas (C1 vertebra)
D Dens of axis (C2 vertebra)

C

1-3: Axis (C2) and atlantoaxial joints. **A,** Posterosuperior view of axis. **B,** Posterosuperior view of articulated atlas and axis. Posterior articular facet of dens is for articulation with transverse ligament of atlas at median atlantoaxial joint. **C,** Open mouth radiograph of atlantoaxial joints. *(From Netter, F H: Atlas of Human Anatomy, 4th ed. Philadelphia, Saunders, 2006, Plate 17.)*

4. **C7**
   a. Called **vertebra prominens** because of its **long spinous process,** which helps in **counting vertebrae.**
   b. **Small transverse foramen** does *not* contain vertebral artery.

> **Dislocations** may cause cervical vertebra to move out of alignment because **articular surfaces lie in nearly a horizontal plane** and are less stable. Although the **spinal cord** may be compressed, it may escape severe injury because of the large vertebral canal. Nevertheless, all movement of patients suspected of having a **neck injury** should be minimized until the cervical spine is properly stabilized. Injury to the cervical spinal cord may not appear on a radiograph.
>
> **Failure of segmentation of cervical vertebrae** results in congenital fusion, causing **Klippel-Feil syndrome,** which is characterized by a short, stiff neck.

Vertebra prominens is helpful in counting vertebrae.

Dislocations without fracture occur only in cervical spine.

Klippel-Feil syndrome is congenital fusion of cervical vertebrae.

B. **Thoracic Vertebrae (Figure 1-4; see Table 1-1)**
   • **Articular processes** are oriented to favor lateral bending and rotation, although range of movement is limited by the rib cage, thin intervertebral discs, and overlapping spinous processes.
   1. **Typical thoracic vertebrae: T2-T9**
      a. **Costal demifacets** on the **body** articulate with the head of the corresponding rib and the inferior rib.
      b. **Costal facet** on **transverse process** articulates with tubercle of corresponding rib
   2. **T1 and T10-T12**
      a. **Complete facet** on the body articulates with the entire head of the corresponding rib.
      b. Inferior **demifacet** on body of T1 articulates with superior part of head of rib 2

> **Traumatic injury to the thoracic vertebrae** may produce **dislocation with fracture** because articular facet joints are arranged vertically. An **aortic aneurysm** may cause left-sided **erosion to bodies of T5-T8** as seen on a radiograph.

An aneurysm of the descending thoracic aorta may erode bodies of vertebrae T5-8 on the left side.

C. **Lumbar Vertebrae (Figures 1-5 and 1-6; see Table 1-1)**
   • **Articular processes** with facets oriented to favor flexion and extension

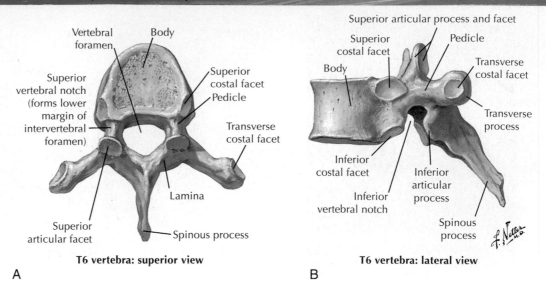

T6 vertebra: superior view

A

T6 vertebra: lateral view

B

1-4: Typical thoracic vertebra. **A,** Superior view. **B,** Lateral view. *(From Netter, F H: Atlas of Human Anatomy, 4th ed. Philadelphia, Saunders, 2006, Plate 154.)*

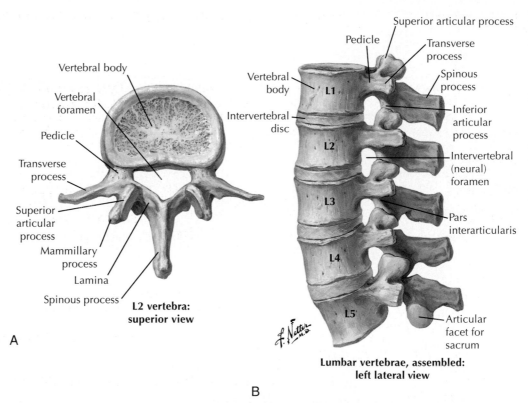

L2 vertebra: superior view

A

Lumbar vertebrae, assembled: left lateral view

B

1-5: Lumbar vertebrae. **A,** Superior view of a typical lumbar vertebra. **B,** Lateral view of articulated lumbar vertebrae. Intervertebral foramina transmit spinal nerves. *(From Netter, F H: Atlas of Human Anatomy, 4th ed. Philadelphia, Saunders, 2006, Plate 155.)*

Spondylolysis is a fracture of pars interarticularis that may cause spondylolisthesis.

Traumatic injury to lumbar vertebrae may produce **dislocation with fracture** because articular surfaces are arranged vertically.

Stress fractures of the pars interarticularis occur frequently in lumbar vertebrae **(spondylolysis),** with the posterior part of the vertebral arch separating from the anterior part to cause **back pain.** It occurs commonly in **L5** in adolescent athletes involved in sports that require **repeated spinal hyperextension.** The vertebral column is not misaligned in unilateral fractures, which show up in oblique lumbar radiographs as a **collar on the neck of the "Scottie dog" (Figure 1-6).**

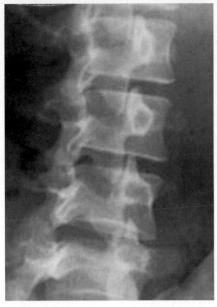
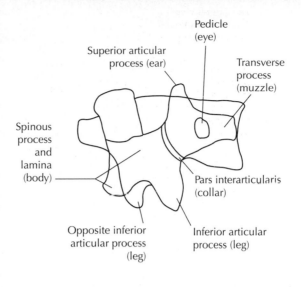

Spinous process and lamina (body)

Superior articular process (ear)

Pedicle (eye)

Transverse process (muzzle)

Pars interarticularis (collar)

Opposite inferior articular process (leg)

Inferior articular process (leg)

A   B

1-6: A, Oblique radiograph of lumbar spine showing characteristic "Scottie dog" form **(B).** The appearance of a collar indicates a fracture of the pars interarticularis.

In **spondylolisthesis,** a vertebral body is displaced forward on the vertebral body immediately below. It occurs frequently at the **L5/S1 level** and is often secondary to **bilateral pars interarticularis fractures.** Alignment of the vertebral column is compromised, and the **cauda equina** may be affected. Patients with spondylolisthesis may encounter **difficulty during childbirth** because of the resulting narrowed pelvic inlet.

Spondylolisthesis may interfere with childbirth.

Degenerative changes in the **lumbar spine** and **ligamenta flava** may cause narrowing of the spinal canal **(spinal stenosis).** The resulting compression of neural structures produces **pain on walking or standing** that is relieved by bending forward or sitting **(neurogenic claudication).** This differs from **vascular claudication** of the lower extremities that is relieved by standing still.

Neurogenic claudication from lumbar spinal stenosis differs from vascular claudication in being unrelieved by standing still.

   D. Sacrum
   1. Wedge-shaped bone formed by fusion of **five sacral vertebrae**
   2. Articulates superiorly with L5 at **lumbosacral joint** and laterally with hip bones at **sacroiliac joints**
   3. Four pairs of **anterior sacral foramina** for anterior rami and four pairs of **posterior sacral foramina** for posterior rami of spinal nerves S1-S4
   4. **Sacral canal** contains dural sac down to lower border of S2.
   5. **Sacral hiatus** in place of spine and laminae of S5 (and sometimes S4) with **sacral cornua** located laterally

When administering **caudal epidural anesthesia, sacral cornua** are used as landmarks to locate the **sacral hiatus.**

Sacral cornua are landmarks for caudal epidural anesthesia.

   E. Coccyx
   • Triangular bone formed from fusion of **four coccygeal vertebrae;** often C1 is not fused.
III. Joints and Ligaments of Vertebral Column
   A. Joints between Vertebrae
   1. **Intervertebral discs (Figure 1-7)**
      a. **Fibrocartilaginous joints** between bodies of adjacent vertebrae except C1/C2, sacrum, and coccyx

There is no intervertebral disc between vertebrae C1/C2.

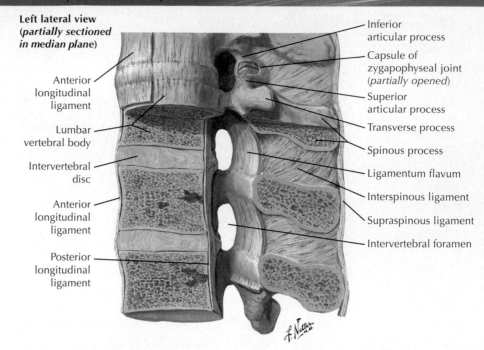

Left lateral view (*partially sectioned in median plane*)

Anterior longitudinal ligament

Lumbar vertebral body

Intervertebral disc

Anterior longitudinal ligament

Posterior longitudinal ligament

Inferior articular process

Capsule of zygapophyseal joint (*partially opened*)

Superior articular process

Transverse process

Spinous process

Ligamentum flavum

Interspinous ligament

Supraspinous ligament

Intervertebral foramen

1-7: Ligaments connecting vertebrae. (*From Netter, F H: Atlas of Human Anatomy, 4th ed. Philadelphia, Saunders, 2006, Plate 158.*)

    b. Separated from each vertebral body by thin plate of **hyaline cartilage**
    c. Permit little movement between adjacent vertebrae but cumulatively allow considerable flexibility of column
    d. Function as **shock absorbers**
       (1) **Anulus fibrosus**
          (a) **Fibrocartilaginous** portion of disc surrounding nucleus pulposus; **thinner posteriorly**
          (b) Firmly attached to **anterior and posterior longitudinal ligaments**
       (2) **Nucleus pulposus**
          (a) Incompressible gelatinous center of intervertebral disc located closer to its posterior surface
          (b) Produces shock-absorbing quality of disc
          (c) Loses water temporarily during daily activities and permanently with age as it gradually becomes replaced by fibrocartilage

The nucleus pulposus loses water temporarily each day and permanently with age.

An intervertebral disc usually herniates posterolaterally just lateral to posterior longitudinal ligament.

Intervertebral discs herniate most commonly at L4/L5 and L5/S1 and compress traversing nerve root.

> **Rupture of the nucleus pulposus** through the **anulus fibrosus** causes a **herniated intervertebral disc.** Herniated discs usually occur in lumbar (L4/L5 or L5/S1) or cervical regions (C5/C6 or C6/C7) of individuals younger than age 50 and may impinge on **spinal nerves** or their roots. Herniations may follow degenerative changes in the anulus fibrosus or be caused by sudden compression of the nucleus pulposus. Herniated lumbar discs usually involve the nerve root descending to exit the intervertebral foramen inferior to the vertebra below **(traversing root)** rather than the nerve root leaving the vertebral canal at the level of the disc **(exiting root) (Figure 1-8).**

1-8: Herniated lumbar intervertebral disc. Herniation usually occurs posterolaterally and affects traversing root, not exiting root (i.e., herniation at L4-L5 affects L5 root, whereas herniation at L5-S1 affects S1 root).

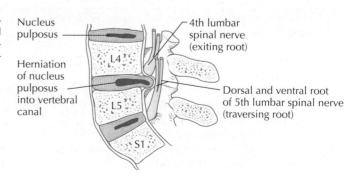

Nucleus pulposus

Herniation of nucleus pulposus into vertebral canal

4th lumbar spinal nerve (exiting root)

Dorsal and ventral root of 5th lumbar spinal nerve (traversing root)

L4

L5

S1

2. **Facet joints (zygapophysial/zygapophyseal joints)**
   a. **Synovial joints** between **superior and inferior articular facets** of adjacent vertebrae
   b. Provide varying amounts of flexion, extension, rotation, or lateral bending depending on vertebral level

Facet joints diseased by **osteoarthritis** (degenerative joint disease) border the intervertebral foramen, and **osteophytes** may impinge on an adjacent spinal nerve, causing severe pain. Lumbar zygapophysial joints may be **denervated** by surgical or percutaneous radiofrequency neurotomy **(percutaneous rhizolysis)** to relieve low back pain. Each joint is innervated by medial branches of two adjacent posterior rami, and both branches must be sectioned.

Osteoarthritis is degenerative joint disease from aging or trauma.

Osteophyte on zygapophysial joint may compress spinal nerve

B. Ligaments Connecting Vertebrae (Table 1-2; see Figure 1-7)

Because its presence reinforces the intervertebral disc in the posterior midline, the **posterior longitudinal ligament** reduces the incidence of **disc herniations** that may compress the **spinal cord** and **cauda equina.**

The cervical spinal cord may be injured without x-ray evidence of vertebral damage.

The **cervical spinal cord may be injured** by transient inward bulging of the **ligamentum flavum** during sudden forced hyperextension. A radiograph may not show vertebral damage.

Whiplash (cervical extension sprain) is forceful hyperextension of the cervical spine that stretches the **anterior longitudinal ligament** and adjacent structures. **Rear-end automobile collisions** often cause whiplash, and symptoms include neck pain, headache, and pain and numbness radiating into the upper extremities.

Rear-end automobile collision causes whiplash injury.

C. Craniocervical Joints and Ligaments
1. **Atlantooccipital joint (Figure 1-9)**
   a. Paired **synovial joint** between **occipital condyle** and **superior articular facet** of **atlas**
   b. Allows **flexion/extension** of head (nodding head "yes") and some lateral flexion but **no rotation**
   c. **Posterior atlantooccipital membrane** penetrated by **vertebral artery** and **suboccipital nerve**
2. **Atlantoaxial joint (see Figure 1-9)**
   a. Paired **lateral atlantoaxial joints** and **median atlantoaxial joint** with dens held against **anterior arch of atlas** by **transverse ligament of atlas**
   b. Allows **rotation of head** (shaking head "no") but not flexion, extension, or lateral bending

Atlantooccipital joints: nodding head "yes." Atlantoaxial joints: shaking head "no"

Atlantoaxial dislocation or subluxation (partial dislocation) may injure the **spinal cord** and medulla. Subluxation can occur after **rupture of the transverse ligament of the atlas** caused by congenital weakness, trauma, or **rheumatoid arthritis (Figure 1-10).** A weak or absent transverse ligament occurs in 15% to 20% of **Down syndrome** patients. Subluxation due to rupture of the transverse ligament of the atlas may be apparent on a lateral x-ray only if the spine is flexed.

The transverse ligament of atlas may rupture in rheumatoid arthritis and Down syndrome patients.

TABLE 1-2. LIGAMENTS OF VERTEBRAL COLUMN

LIGAMENT	ATTACHMENT	COMMENTS
Supraspinous	Connects tips of spinous processes	Limits flexion of vertebral column; expanded in cervical region as ligamentum nuchae
Interspinous	Connects spinous processes of adjacent vertebrae	Limits flexion of vertebral column
Anterior longitudinal	Attached to anterior surface of vertebral bodies and intervertebral discs	Limits extension of vertebral column; supports anulus fibrosus and may be strained or torn in whiplash
Posterior longitudinal	Attached to posterior surface of vertebral bodies and intervertebral discs and lies within vertebral canal	Limits flexion of vertebral column; supports anulus fibrosus and directs herniation of intervertebral disc posterolaterally
Ligamentum flavum	Paired ligament that connects laminae of adjacent vertebrae	Limits flexion of vertebral column; yellowish due to elastic tissue

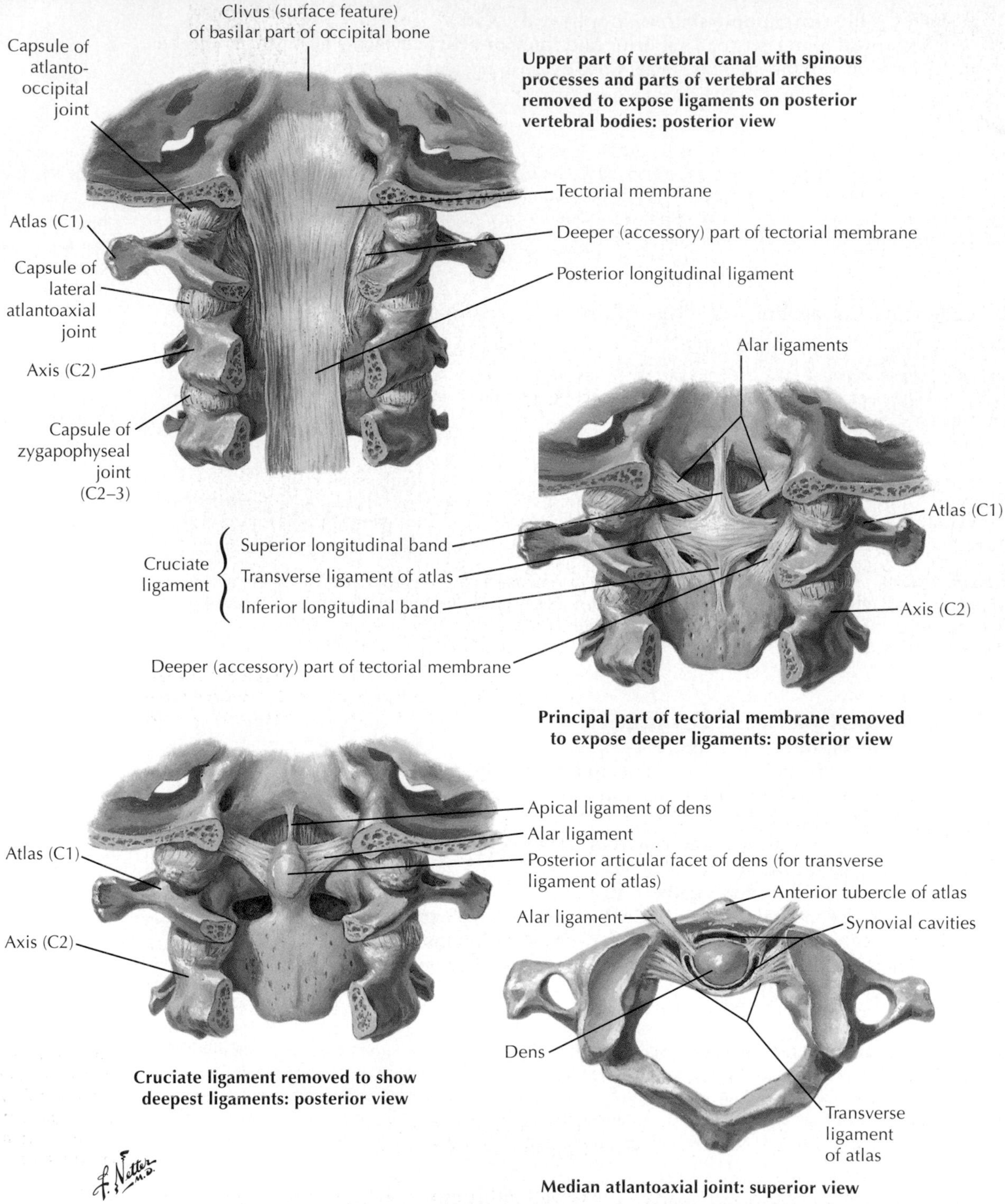

Clivus (surface feature) of basilar part of occipital bone

Capsule of atlanto-occipital joint

Atlas (C1)

Capsule of lateral atlantoaxial joint

Axis (C2)

Capsule of zygapophyseal joint (C2–3)

Upper part of vertebral canal with spinous processes and parts of vertebral arches removed to expose ligaments on posterior vertebral bodies: posterior view

Tectorial membrane

Deeper (accessory) part of tectorial membrane

Posterior longitudinal ligament

Alar ligaments

Atlas (C1)

Axis (C2)

Cruciate ligament
- Superior longitudinal band
- Transverse ligament of atlas
- Inferior longitudinal band

Deeper (accessory) part of tectorial membrane

Principal part of tectorial membrane removed to expose deeper ligaments: posterior view

Atlas (C1)

Axis (C2)

Cruciate ligament removed to show deepest ligaments: posterior view

Apical ligament of dens

Alar ligament

Posterior articular facet of dens (for transverse ligament of atlas)

Anterior tubercle of atlas

Alar ligament

Synovial cavities

Dens

Transverse ligament of atlas

Median atlantoaxial joint: superior view

1-9: Internal craniocervical ligaments connecting skull and vertebral column. Atlas and axis are separately attached to skull base to ensure maximum stability. Strong transverse ligament of atlas (horizontal part of cruciate ligament) binds dens in place to protect posteriorly related spinal cord. *(From Netter, F H: Atlas of Human Anatomy, 4th ed. Philadelphia, Saunders, 2006, Plate 22.)*

Osteophytes on uncovertebral joints may cause neck pain.

3. **Uncovertebral joints (of Luschka)**
    a. Jointlike structures that can develop postnatally in cervical spine between lips of bodies of adjacent vertebrae
    b. **Osteophyte** formation here may cause **neck pain.**
4. **Cruciate ligament (Table 1-3; see Figure 1-9)**
    - Consists of **transverse ligament of atlas** with superior and inferior extensions

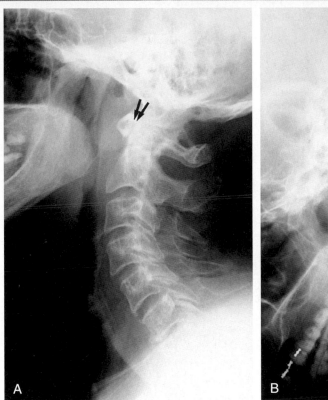 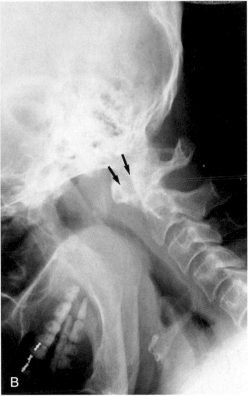

1-10: Lateral x-rays of the cervical spine in a rheumatoid arthritis patient with a ruptured transverse ligament of the atlas. **A,** Little space is apparent between the anterior arch of the atlas and the dens in neck extension *(arrows)*. **B,** Increased space is seen between the anterior arch and dens in flexion *(arrows)*. *(From Mettler, F A: Essentials of Radiology, 2nd ed. Philadelphia, Saunders, 2004, Figure 8-9.)*

TABLE 1-3. CRANIOCERVICAL LIGAMENTS

LIGAMENT	ATTACHMENT	COMMENTS
Tectorial membrane	Continuation of posterior longitudinal ligament from body of axis to anterior margin of foramen magnum	Covers dens and transverse ligament of atlas posteriorly
Apical ligament	Extends from apex of dens to anterior margin of foramen magnum	
Alar ligament	Stout paired ligament connecting side of dens to medial aspect of occipital condyle	Limits rotation at atlantoaxial joints
Cruciate ligament	Expansion of transverse ligament of atlas	Binds dens tightly against anterior arch of atlas

D. Curvatures of Vertebral Column
  1. **Normal curvatures (Figure 1-11)**
    a. Primary curves
      (1) **Concave anteriorly** (same direction as fetal curvature)
      (2) Retained in **thoracic** and **sacral** regions of adult
    b. Secondary curves
      • Become **convex anteriorly** in **cervical** and **lumbar** regions when infant begins to hold head up and to stand, respectively
  2. **Abnormal curvatures (Figure 1-12)**
    a. **Scoliosis**
      (1) Any **lateral curvature** of spine
      (2) May be thoracic, lumbar, or thoracolumbar and is designated **right or left** according to convex side of major curve

> Normal adult vertebral column is concave anteriorly in thoracic and sacral regions, convex anteriorly in cervical and lumbar regions.

> Scoliosis is a lateral curvature of the thoracolumbar spine.

Scoliosis may be **nonstructural and reversible** (e.g., discrepancy in length of lower limbs) or **structural and irreversible** (e.g., idiopathic or neuropathic). **Idiopathic** right thoracic scoliosis in **adolescent females** is the most common form, and additional spinal curves that place the eyes in a horizontal plane may develop to compensate. A **rib hump** appears on the convex side during forward bending in structural scoliosis due to the posterior displacement of ribs from **vertebral rotation.** Congenital scoliosis may result from failure of one side of a vertebral body to form **(hemivertebra)** or **asymmetric fusion** of vertebrae.

> Idiopathic scoliosis in adolescent females is the most common form.

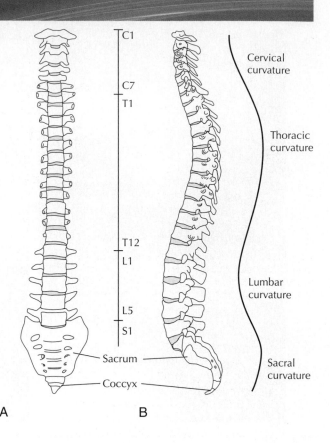

1-11: Normal curvatures of vertebral column. **A,** Anterior view. **B,** Lateral view.

C1
C7
T1
T12
L1
L5
S1
Sacrum
Coccyx

Cervical curvature
Thoracic curvature
Lumbar curvature
Sacral curvature

A   B

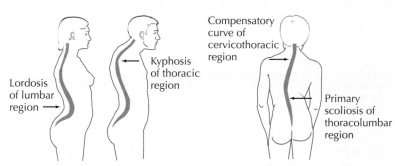

1-12: Abnormal curvatures of vertebral column.

Lordosis of lumbar region →

Kyphosis of thoracic region

Compensatory curve of cervicothoracic region

Primary scoliosis of thoracolumbar region

  b. **Kyphosis**
    • Abnormal curvature that is **convex posteriorly**

Kyphosis is increased thoracic spine curvature that is common in postmenopausal women.

> In **osteoporosis, kyphosis of the thoracic spine** may occur after **compression fractures** produce a wedge-shaped deformity of vertebral bodies. Although most common in **postmenopausal women,** kyphosis can occur in elderly men. An **adolescent form of kyphosis** (Scheuermann's disease) results from disturbances in hyaline cartilage growth plates of thoracic vertebral bodies. Bracing may limit progression of the adolescent form. Kyphosis and scoliosis may occur together **(kyphoscoliosis).**

  c. **Lordosis**
    (1) Abnormal curvature that is **convex anteriorly**
    (2) **Normal compensation of lumbar spine** during **pregnancy** but may develop with **obesity** in both males and females

Lordosis is increased anterior convexity of lumbar spine and is normal late in pregnancy.

IV. **The Development of the Vertebral Column (Figure 1-13)**
  A. **Origin from Somites**
    1. Mesenchymal cells from **sclerotome of somites** form condensations around the neural tube and notochord.

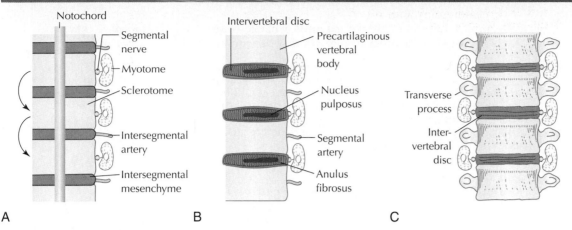

1-13: Development of vertebral column. **A,** Caudal and cranial halves of adjacent sclerotomes fuse to form vertebral bodies (*arrows*). **B,** Note position of segmental neurovascular structures and myotomes relative to developing vertebral bodies. Intervertebral discs develop in middle of original sclerotomes. **C,** Muscles that develop from myotomes bridge intervertebral discs and move adjacent vertebrae.

2. Condensation and proliferation of caudal half of one sclerotome join cranial half of next sclerotome to form a **vertebral body**
3. **Anulus fibrosus** of intervertebral disc is formed from mesenchymal cells of **sclerotome** that fill space between adjacent vertebral bodies as they form

B. **Contribution from Notochord**
   - **Notochord** persists within each intervertebral disc and undergoes mucoid degeneration to form **nucleus pulposus.**

V. **Congenital Abnormalities of Vertebral Column and Spinal Cord (Figure 1-14)**
   A. **Spina Bifida Occulta**
      1. Results from vertebral arch failing to fuse in midline
      2. Frequently occurs at L5 or S1 and may be marked by a **tuft of hair** and/or **pigmented skin**
      3. *Not* associated with any neurological deficit
   B. **Spina Bifida Cystica**
      1. Overview
         a. Protrusion of meninges and/or spinal cord through defect in vertebral arches
         b. Occurs in about 1:1000 births
         c. Often detected through high levels of **alpha-fetoprotein** in maternal serum or amniotic fluid
         d. May have reduced incidence with vitamin and **folic acid supplements** before conception and increased incidence with anticonvulsant **valproic acid** during week 4
      2. **Spinal meningocele**
         a. Protrusion of **meninges** through a defect in vertebral arches
         b. May be associated with neurological deficits

Vertebral bodies develop from the caudal half of one sclerotome and the cranial half of the succeeding sclerotome.

The nucleus pulposus is a remnant of the embryonic notochord.

Spina bifida occulta is usually asymptomatic and detectable only by x-ray.

Neural tube defects cause high alpha-fetoprotein levels in maternal serum and amniotic fluid.

Neural tube defects may be preventable by folic acid supplements before and during pregnancy.

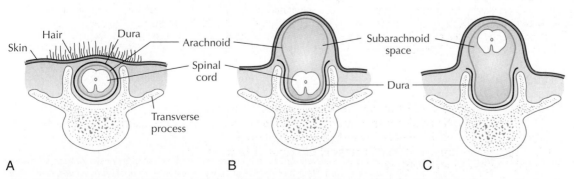

1-14: Transverse sections showing types of spina bifida. Each defect includes a failure of formation of the vertebral arch. **A,** Spina bifida occulta. **B,** Meningocele. **C,** Meningomyelocele.

3. **Meningomyelocele**
   a. Protrusion of **spinal cord and/or nerve roots** in meningeal sac
   b. Causes **neurological deficits** that depend on level and extent of lesion

Meningomyelocele is congenital protrusion of spinal cord and nerve roots through vertebral defect with neurological damage.

> If only nerve roots are involved in spina bifida with meningomyelocele, resultant paralysis is flaccid (lower motor neuron lesion), but spinal cord damage results in spastic paralysis (upper motor neuron lesion); mixed types of paralysis may occur. Hydrocephalus commonly develops due to herniation of the brainstem and cerebellar tonsils through the foramen magnum (Arnold-Chiari malformation). The exposed meninges and spinal cord are vulnerable to infection.

VI. **The Muscles of the Back**
   A. **Development of the Back Muscles (Figure 1-15)**
      1. **Differentiating somites** give rise to segmental **myotomes;** each myotome splits into the dorsal **epimere** and ventral **hypomere.**
      2. **Epimere** gives rise to **epaxial muscles,** which are **intrinsic back muscles** innervated by the **posterior rami** of spinal nerves.
      3. **Hypomere** gives rise to **hypaxial** muscles that are innervated by the **anterior rami** of spinal nerves.
      4. **Limb muscles** that arise from **hypomere** migrate into limb buds and are therefore innervated by **anterior rami** of spinal nerves

Posterior rami innervate intrinsic back muscles. Anterior rami innervate all other muscles of trunk and extremities.

      5. **Superficial muscles of back** are actually muscles of **upper limb** that develop from limb bud mesoderm and migrate into back, carrying with them their nerve supply from **anterior rami**
   B. **Other Features**
      1. **Triangle of auscultation**
         a. Bounded medially by **trapezius,** laterally by **scapula** and **rhomboid major,** and inferiorly by **latissimus dorsi**
         b. Allows **lung sounds** to be clearly heard at sixth intercostal space because no muscle intervenes between skin and rib cage when shoulders are pulled forward

Triangle of auscultation allows posterior access to sixth intercostal space.

      2. **Thoracolumbar fascia**
         a. Forms investing sleeve that encloses **intrinsic back muscles** by attaching anteriorly to **transverse processes** of lumbar vertebrae and posteriorly to **spinous processes** of lumbar and lower thoracic vertebrae
         b. Fuses with aponeuroses of **internal abdominal oblique, transversus abdominis,** and **latissimus dorsi**

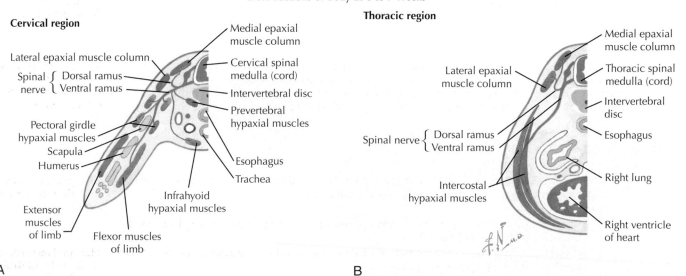

Cross Sections of Body at 6 to 7 Weeks

Cervical region

Lateral epaxial muscle column
Spinal { Dorsal ramus
nerve { Ventral ramus
Pectoral girdle hypaxial muscles
Scapula
Humerus
Extensor muscles of limb
Flexor muscles of limb
Infrahyoid hypaxial muscles
Medial epaxial muscle column
Cervical spinal medulla (cord)
Intervertebral disc
Prevertebral hypaxial muscles
Esophagus
Trachea

Thoracic region

Lateral epaxial muscle column
Spinal nerve { Dorsal ramus
{ Ventral ramus
Intercostal hypaxial muscles
Medial epaxial muscle column
Thoracic spinal medulla (cord)
Intervertebral disc
Esophagus
Right lung
Right ventricle of heart

A   B

1-15: Development of muscles of limb **(A)** and trunk **(B)**. Intrinsic back muscles are derived from epimere and are innervated by posterior (dorsal) rami of spinal nerves. Muscles of limbs and of anterior and lateral body wall develop from hypomere and are supplied by anterior (ventral) rami. *(From Netter, F H: The Netter Collection of Medical Illustrations, Vol. 8: Musculoskeletal System, Part 1: Anatomy, Physiology, and Metabolic Disorders. Philadelphia, Saunders Elsevier, 1987, p. 142, Section II, Plate 18.)*

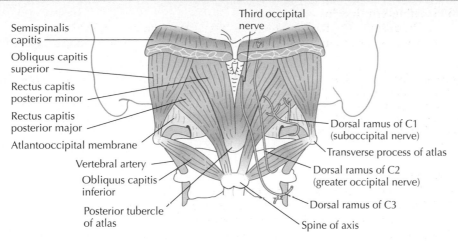

Semispinalis capitis

Obliquus capitis superior

Rectus capitis posterior minor

Rectus capitis posterior major

Atlantooccipital membrane

Vertebral artery

Obliquus capitis inferior

Posterior tubercle of atlas

Third occipital nerve

Dorsal ramus of C1 (suboccipital nerve)

Transverse process of atlas

Dorsal ramus of C2 (greater occipital nerve)

Dorsal ramus of C3

Spine of axis

1-16: Relationships of the suboccipital triangle, posterior view. In the triangle, the vertebral artery lies on the posterior arch of the atlas and then pierces the atlantooccipital membrane to enter the foramen magnum. The suboccipital nerve (posterior ramus of C1) emerges between the posterior arch and the vertebral artery to supply suboccipital muscles. The greater occipital nerve (posterior ramus of C2) passes inferior to the obliquus capitis inferior muscle and pierces the semispinalis capitis muscle to supply the posterior scalp.

C. **Suboccipital Region (Figure 1-16)**
1. **Suboccipital triangle**
   - Bounded medially by **rectus capitis posterior major,** inferiorly by **obliquus capitis inferior,** and laterally by **obliquus capitis** superior muscles
2. **Arteries and nerves of suboccipital region**
   a. **Vertebral artery** branches from subclavian, ascends through transverse foramina of vertebrae C1-C6, and runs transversely across posterior arch of atlas under posterior atlantooccipital membrane.
   b. **Suboccipital nerve,** posterior ramus of C1, passes between vertebral artery and posterior arch of atlas to supply suboccipital muscles
   c. **Greater occipital nerve,** posterior ramus of C2, emerges inferior to **obliquus capitis inferior muscle** and ascends to supply overlying muscles and scalp
   d. **Third occipital nerve,** posterior ramus of C3, supplies scalp over occiput

Because of the course of the **vertebral artery** through transverse foramina of cervical vertebrae, individuals with **atherosclerosis** may become dizzy and experience other symptoms of **brainstem ischemia** when the neck is rotated.

Atherosclerotic vertebral artery may result in brainstem ischemia during neck rotation.

If the left subclavian artery or the brachiocephalic trunk is stenosed or occluded proximal to the origin of the vertebral artery, exercising the upper extremity may reverse blood flow through the vertebral and basilar arteries, causing **subclavian steal syndrome.** The transient neurologic symptoms are related to **brainstem** and **posterior cerebral ischemia** (e.g., dizziness, unsteadiness, visual changes).

Subclavian steal syndrome is reversed blood flow through vertebral artery with upper extremity exertion.

VII. **The Meninges and the Spinal Cord**
A. **Meninges (Figure 1-17)**
   - Three connective tissue membranes that enclose spinal cord within **vertebral canal** and are continuous with cranial meninges around brain
1. **Dura mater**
   a. Tough, fibrous outer layer that forms a closed sac around **brain** and **spinal cord,** ending inferiorly at **S2 vertebra**
   b. Continuous with **meningeal layer of dura** inside skull but separated from walls of vertebral canal by **epidural space**
   c. Follows spinal nerve roots and is continuous with **epineurium** of spinal nerve
2. **Arachnoid mater**
   a. Delicate **intermediate** layer applied to inner surface of **dura mater**
   b. Sends fine **arachnoid trabeculae** across **subarachnoid space** to pia mater

Meninges are dura mater, arachnoid mater, and pia mater.

Adult spinal cord ends at vertebra L1/L2 but dural sac ends at S2

1-17: Transverse section through the vertebral column. Note that the dura mater and the arachnoid mater are *not* separated by space. The arachnoid mater is joined to the pia by thin trabeculae with intervening space filled by cerebrospinal fluid (CSF). The spinal cord is thus surrounded by and suspended in a fluid-filled space.

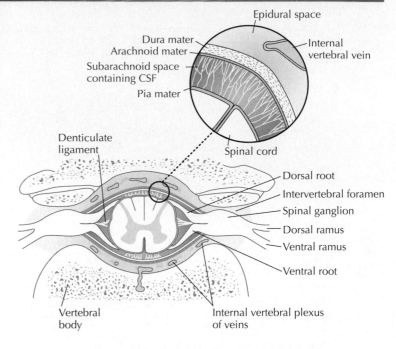

3. **Pia mater**
   - Fine vascular layer inseparable from surface of **spinal cord**

Meningitis is inflammation of meninges usually due to self-limiting viral or life-threatening bacterial infection.

Meningitis is characterized by severe headache, fever, and stiff neck. **Viral meningitis** is usually benign and self-limiting.

Bacterial meningitis is diagnosed by analysis of CSF collected by lumbar puncture.

Bacterial meningitis is serious and may be fatal, even with treatment. Diagnosis is confirmed by analyzing **cerebrospinal fluid** from lumbar puncture. Flexion of the neck of a supine patient will stretch inflamed meninges, producing characteristic pain and possibly eliciting involuntary hip and knee flexion **(Brudzinski's sign)** that minimizes tension on meninges. **Kernig's sign** is similar pain elicited by raising one lower limb while the knee is kept fully extended (straight leg raise). Pain can be relieved by flexing the knee and reducing tension on the meninges. **Pneumococcal meningitis** is the most common and most serious form of bacterial meningitis in adults.

B. **Features Related to Meninges (see Figure 1-17)**
   1. **Epidural space**
      a. Lies between **dural sac** and walls of vertebral canal
      b. Contains **epidural fat** and **internal vertebral venous plexus**
   2. **Subdural space**
      a. **Artifact** of pathology and not a true space
      b. Formed by physical separation of dura mater from arachnoid mater by hemorrhage **(subdural hematoma)** or CSF collection **(subdural hygroma)**
   3. **Subarachnoid space**
      a. Lies between **arachnoid mater** and **pia mater** and extends inferiorly to **S2 vertebra**
      b. Contains **cerebrospinal fluid** that protects spinal cord and removes catabolites from neuronal activity
      c. Below spinal cord forms **lumbar cistern,** which contains cauda equina

Subdural space is pathological artifact created by collection of blood or CSF

Lumbar puncture should not be performed in patient with intracranial mass

Lumbar puncture is usually performed between vertebrae L3/L4 or L4/L5.

When performing a **lumbar puncture,** the needle enters the subarachnoid space to **extract cerebrospinal fluid** (spinal tap) or to **inject anesthetic** (spinal block) **or contrast material (Figure 1-18).** The needle is usually inserted between **L3/L4 or L4/L5.** Remember that the spinal cord may end as low as L3 in adults and does end at L3 in infants. Before the procedure, the patient should be examined for signs of **increased intracranial pressure** (e.g., papilledema) because cerebellar tonsils may herniate through the foramen magnum due to a **space-occupying mass.**

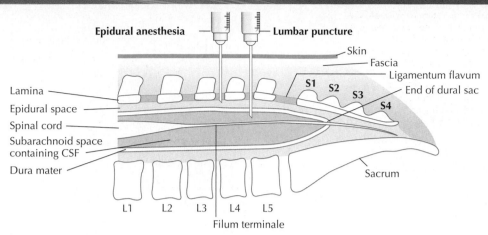

1-18: Sagittal section of the vertebral canal illustrating needle placement for epidural anesthesia and lumbar puncture. To reach the subarachnoid space, the needle must successively penetrate the skin, fascia, supraspinous ligament, interspinous ligament, ligamentum flavum, epidural space, dura, and arachnoid mater.

In **epidural anesthesia,** the needle is placed into the epidural space to inject anesthetic around roots of the lower lumbar and sacral spinal nerves without entering the subarachnoid space **(see Figure 1-18).**

> Epidural anesthesia: injection into epidural space. Spinal block: injection into subarachnoid space

4. **Denticulate ligaments**
   a. Flattened fibrous bands of **pia mater** from sides of spinal cord between posterior and anterior nerve rootlets
   b. Have toothlike projections that pierce arachnoid mater to anchor spinal cord to dura
5. **Filum terminale**
   a. Threadlike inferior extension of **pia mater** from **conus medullaris** surrounded by **cauda equina** in lumbar cistern
   b. Penetrates **arachnoid mater** and **dura mater** to become enclosed by **filum of dura,** which attaches to coccyx
6. **Vertebral venous plexus (Figure 1-19)**
   a. Interconnecting system of **valveless veins** from **coccyx** to **skull** that allows blood flow in either direction
   b. Anastomoses with **segmental veins** at all levels and with **dural venous sinuses** of cranial cavity
      (1) **Internal vertebral venous plexus** lies in **epidural space** around dural sac
      (2) **External vertebral venous plexus** surrounds **outside** of vertebral column

> Denticulate ligaments and filum terminale of pia mater anchor the spinal cord in subarachnoid space.

The **vertebral venous plexus** provides a **pathway for tumor cells** to metastasize from pelvic, abdominal, and thoracic viscera to vertebrae, spinal cord, and brain. Prostate, lung, and breast cancer can spread to the brain via the plexus. **Infections of the skin of the back** may also spread to **dural venous sinuses** of the cranial cavity via the plexus.

> Vertebral venous plexus is pathway for cancer cell metastasis from pelvic, abdominal, and thoracic regions

C. **Spinal Cord**
   1. Continuous above with medulla oblongata of brainstem and ends below near **superior border of vertebra L2** in adults, but range is T12-L3
   2. Tapers at inferior end to **conus medullaris**
   3. **Cervical enlargement** is related to **brachial plexus** and innervation of **upper extremity,** and **lumbosacral enlargement** is related to **lumbosacral plexus** and innervation of **lower extremity**
   4. **Blood supply (Figure 1-20)**
      a. **Spinal arteries**
         • Comprise one **anterior spinal artery** and paired **posterior spinal arteries,** which arise from vertebral arteries or posterior inferior cerebellar arteries
      b. **Segmental arteries**
         (1) Arise from vertebral, ascending cervical, deep cervical, posterior intercostal, and lumbar segmental arteries and travel through intervertebral foramina

> Anterior and posterior spinal arteries depend on blood flow from segmental arteries.

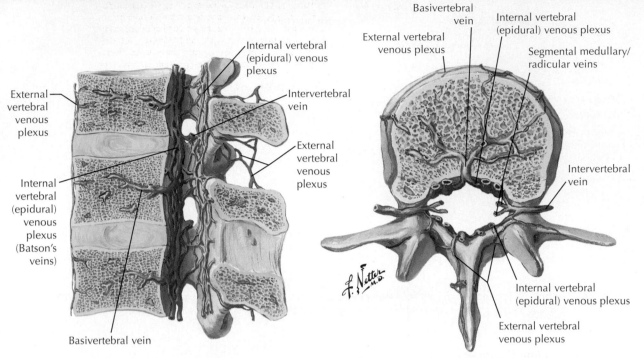

1-19: Internal vertebral venous plexus in epidural space and external vertebral plexus surrounding vertebral column communicate and drain to inferior and superior venae cavae. Internal plexus also communicates superiorly with dural venous sinuses of cranial cavity. *(From Netter, F H: Atlas of Human Anatomy, 4th ed. Philadelphia, Saunders, 2006, Plate 173.)*

      (2) Supply blood directly to spinal nerves, nerve roots, and adjacent areas of spinal cord **(radicular arteries)**
      (3) Supplement blood to spinal cord through anastomoses with anterior and posterior spinal arteries **(segmental medullary arteries)**

Loss of flow through the great anterior segmental medullary artery may cause paraplegia and sensory loss.	One segmental artery of special importance is the **great anterior segmental medullary artery** arising from a lower intercostal or upper lumbar artery. It may supply as much as the inferior two-thirds of the spinal cord, and its **occlusion** can cause **paraplegia, sensory loss** below the level of injury, and **incontinence.** The vessel may be injured during **repair of aortic aneurysms,** and it may be affected by a **tumor** involving the posterior thoracic or abdominal wall. A severe **drop in systemic blood pressure** may have the same result as occlusion.

Spinal nerves are numbered according to vertebra above except in cervical region.

5. **Spinal nerves (Figures 1-21 to 1-23)**
  a. Comprise **31 pairs** of nerves—8 cervical, 12 thoracic, 5 lumbar, 5 sacral, and 1 coccygeal—attached to corresponding **spinal cord segment**
  b. **Numbered** according to vertebra above except in cervical region
  c. Formed by union of posterior root and anterior root and divide into posterior and anterior rami
    (1) **Posterior root** (dorsal root)
      • Contains axons of **afferent** neuron cell bodies located in the **posterior root ganglion** that carry sensory information from muscle, bone, joints, and skin. Strip of skin it supplies is a **dermatome (see Figure 3-8).**

A ganglion is a collection of nerve cell bodies outside the central nervous system.

A dermatome is a strip of skin innervated by a pair of spinal nerves.

Only T1-L2 anterior nerve roots contain preganglionic sympathetic fibers.

    (2) **Anterior root** (ventral root)
      (a) Contains axons of **efferent** neuron cell bodies located in **anterior horn** gray matter of spinal cord that innervate **skeletal muscle**
      (b) At **T1-L2** level contains axons of visceral efferent **(preganglionic sympathetic)** neuron cell bodies located in **intermediolateral cell column** of spinal cord that innervate **cardiac muscle, smooth muscle,** and **glands**
    (3) **Posterior ramus**
      • Supplies **intrinsic back muscles** and overlying skin

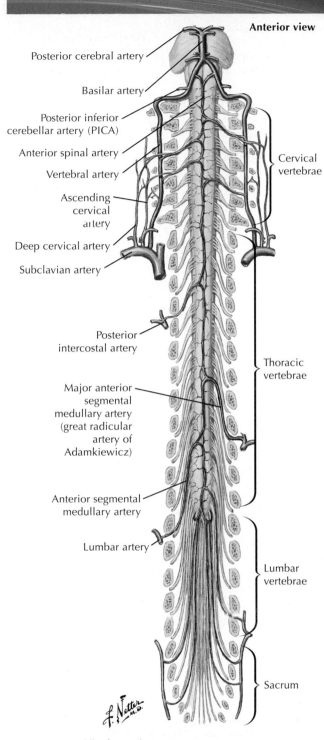

Anterior view

Posterior cerebral artery

Basilar artery

Posterior inferior cerebellar artery (PICA)

Anterior spinal artery

Vertebral artery

Ascending cervical artery

Deep cervical artery

Subclavian artery

Posterior intercostal artery

Major anterior segmental medullary artery (great radicular artery of Adamkiewicz)

Anterior segmental medullary artery

Lumbar artery

Cervical vertebrae

Thoracic vertebrae

Lumbar vertebrae

Sacrum

1-20: Anastomoses of anterior segmental medullary arteries with anterior spinal artery. Connections occur with vertebral, ascending cervical, deep cervical, posterior intercostal, and lumbar arteries. Great anterior segmental medullary artery helps supply lower ⅔ of spinal cord. *(From Netter, F H: Atlas of Human Anatomy, 4th ed. Philadelphia, Saunders, 2006, Plate 171.)*

(4) **Anterior ramus**
   • Supplies muscles and skin of anterolateral neck and trunk and all muscles and skin of upper and lower extremities
(5) **Functional components of spinal nerves (see Figures 1-22 and 1-23; Table 1-4)**
(6) **Somatic nerve plexuses**
   (a) Formed by mixing nerve fibers from **anterior rami**
   (b) Supply nerves to upper extremity **(brachial plexus)** and lower extremity **(lumbosacral plexus)**
   (c) Allow nerve fibers from several spinal cord segments to be distributed in one **peripheral nerve**
   (d) Mean that dermatomal pattern *does not* correspond to cutaneous distribution of peripheral nerves

A typical spinal nerve contains GSA, GVA, GSE, and GVE fibers.

Somatic nerve plexuses: cervical C1-C4, brachial C5-T1, lumbar L1-L4, sacral L4-S3

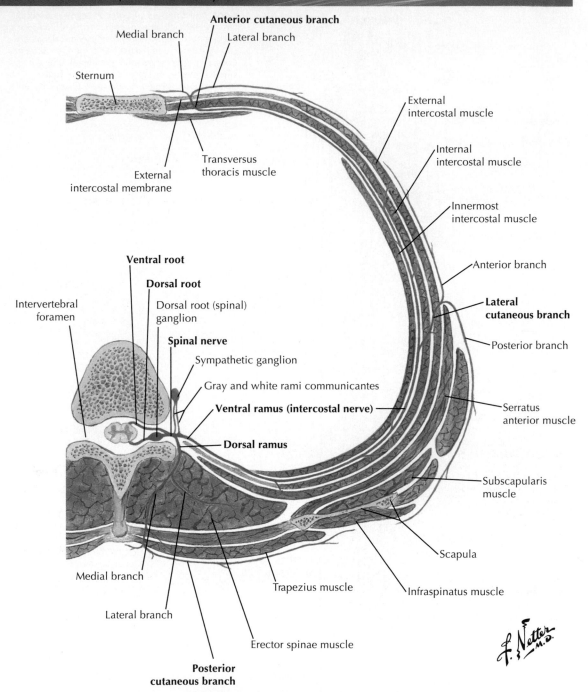

1-21: Typical thoracic spinal nerve. Note gray and white rami communicantes connecting spinal nerve to sympathetic chain ganglion. Anterior ramus of thoracic spinal nerve becomes intercostal nerve. Cutaneous branches of anterior and posterior rami supply the dermatome innervated by that spinal cord segment. *(From Netter, F H: Atlas of Human Anatomy, 4th ed. Philadelphia, Saunders, 2006, Plate 180.)*

D. Development of Spinal Cord (Figures 1-24 and 1-25)

1. **Neural tube formation** (neurulation)
   a. **Neural plate** (neuroectoderm) is induced by the **notochord** and **prechordal plate.**
   b. Developing neural tube initially remains open at the **cranial** and **caudal neuropores.**
   c. **Brain** develops from rostral swellings of neural tube after closure of cranial neuropore
   d. **Spinal cord** develops from caudal neural tube on closure of caudal neuropore

The notochord and the prechordal plate induce the neural plate to form the neural tube.

Failure of cranial neuropore closure: anencephaly. Failure of caudal neuropore closure: myeloschisis

> **Myeloschisis** (rachischisis) is an open spinal cord caused by **failure of the caudal neuropore to close at the end of week 4.** Severe neurological deficits are produced, and infection is likely. Failure of the **cranial neuropore to close on day 25** results in **anencephaly.**

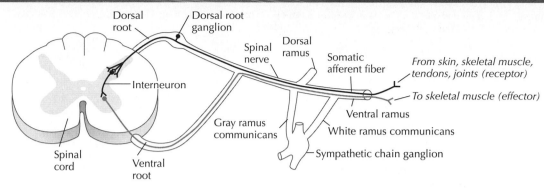

1-22: General somatic efferent (*light red*) and general somatic afferent (*dark red*) components of spinal nerve.

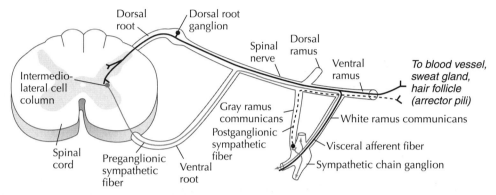

1-23: General visceral efferent (*light red*) and general visceral afferent (*dark red*) components of spinal nerve.

Table 1-4. FUNCTIONAL COMPONENTS OF SPINAL NERVES

TYPE OF NERVE FIBER	STRUCTURE(S) INNERVATED	LOCATION OF NERVE CELL BODY	COMMENTS
General somatic afferent (GSA)	Sensory from skin, muscle, bone, and joints of body wall, neck, and extremities	Posterior root ganglion	Pain, temperature, touch, and proprioception receptors
General visceral afferent (GVA)	Sensory from viscera, including circulatory system	Posterior root ganglion	Pain from internal organs may result from stretch, inflammation, spasm, or ischemia
General somatic efferent (GSE)	Motor to skeletal muscle developed from somites (lower motor neurons)	Anterior horn gray matter	Voluntary control of movement
General visceral efferent (GVE)	Motor to smooth muscle, cardiac muscle, and glands	Sympathetic chain ganglion	Involuntary; postganglionic sympathetic

2. **Neural crest**
    a. Arises from junction of neural tube and surface ectoderm
    b. Forms dorsal root ganglia, autonomic ganglia, and adrenal medulla
VIII. **The Autonomic Nervous System (Visceral Nervous System)**
    A. **Overview**
        1. Divided into sympathetic and parasympathetic nervous systems
        2. Involuntary, generally acting below consciousness to help maintain **homeostasis**
        3. Consists of two neurons in series: preganglionic neuron with cell body in central nervous system and postganglionic neuron with cell body in peripheral autonomic ganglion
    B. **Sympathetic Nervous System**
      • Controls the response to **stress** (i.e., **fight-or-flight** response)
      1. **Preganglionic sympathetic neuron (see Figure 1-23)**
        a. **Cell bodies** located only in **T1-L2 spinal cord segments**
        b. Axon may synapse on **postganglionic neuron** cell body in sympathetic chain ganglion at level of entrance into sympathetic trunk or may ascend or descend in sympathetic chain before synapsing in another ganglion

Sensory ganglia, autonomic ganglia, and adrenal medulla develop from the neural crest.

The autonomic nervous system innervates smooth muscle, cardiac muscle, and glands.

The sympathetic and parasympathetic nervous systems have preganglionic and postganglionic neurons connecting the CNS and effector.

The sympathetic nervous system is the thoracolumbar system because preganglionic neuron cell bodies are found only in T1-L2 spinal cord segments.

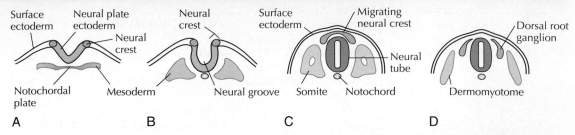

1-24: Transverse sections through embryos during successive stages of neural tube formation. **A** and **B,** Notochord induces ectoderm to form neural plate with a central neural groove and elevated lateral neural folds. **C,** Neural folds fuse in midline to form a hollow neural tube. **D,** Neural crest ectoderm separates from neural tube and surface ectoderm and begins to migrate, forming spinal posterior root ganglia and other structures.

1-25: Neural tube formation at beginning of week 4, dorsal view. **A,** Neural folds have begun to fuse in the future neck region. **B,** Fusion is complete except at cranial and caudal neuropores.

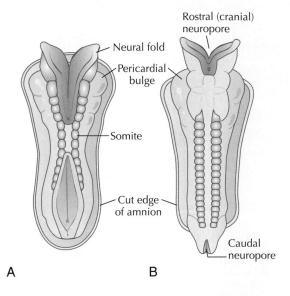

Postganglionic sympathetic neuron cell bodies are located in paravertebral or prevertebral ganglia.

c. Axon may pass into **splanchnic nerve** to reach abdominal **prevertebral ganglion** to synapse

2. **Postganglionic sympathetic neuron (see Figure 1-23)**
   a. Cell body in **paravertebral** (sympathetic chain) or **prevertebral ganglion**
   b. Axon leaves **paravertebral ganglion** through **gray ramus communicans** to join spinal nerve or through **visceral branch** to join visceral plexus
   c. Axon leaves **prevertebral ganglion** to join visceral plexus

3. **Sympathetic trunk (sympathetic chain)**
   a. Paired string like structure lying on bodies of vertebrae from base of skull to coccyx
   b. **Sympathetic (paravertebral) ganglia** formed by aggregations of **postganglionic neuron cell bodies** are swellings on the sympathetic trunk.

4. **Gray ramus communicans**
   a. Connects sympathetic ganglion to its corresponding spinal nerve
   b. Carries **postganglionic sympathetic fibers** that end on sweat glands, vascular smooth muscle, or arrector pili muscles of skin

5. **White ramus communicans**
   a. Connects each paravertebral ganglion from **T1 to L2** levels to corresponding spinal nerve

White communicating rami connect to only spinal nerves T1-L2, but gray rami connect to all spinal nerves.

   b. Carries preganglionic sympathetic fibers to sympathetic trunk for distribution to entire body, including head
   c. Contains **preganglionic sympathetic fibers** and **visceral afferent fibers**

C. **Parasympathetic Nervous System**
   1. Overview
      a. Mediates vegetative functions
      b. Innervates **visceral structures** only and is *not* distributed to body wall or extremities

Parasympathetic nerve fibers aren't present in body walls or extremities.

      c. Innervates **erectile tissue** of genitalia and **coronary arteries** but no other blood vessels

2. **Preganglionic parasympathetic neuron**
   a. Cell body in nucleus of **brainstem** or in **sacral parasympathetic nucleus** of spinal cord segments **S2-S4**
   b. Carried in **cranial nerves III, VII, IX, or X or spinal nerves S2-4**
3. **Postganglionic parasympathetic neuron**
   • Cell body in peripheral autonomic ganglion **(terminal ganglion)** lying close to or within wall of organ to be innervated

D. **General Visceral Afferent Fibers**
   1. Accompany sympathetic and parasympathetic fibers and form afferent limb of autonomic reflex arcs
   2. Follow sympathetic and parasympathetic nerve fibers to central nervous system *except* for cranial nerve III (oculomotor)
   3. Traverse **white, not gray, ramus communicans**
   4. Accompanying sympathetic nerve fibers in visceral branches (e.g., cardiac or splanchnic nerves) **carry pain** from visceral organs to spinal cord between segments T1 and L2

The parasympathetic nervous system is the craniosacral system because preganglionic neuron cell bodies are located only in the brainstem or the sacral spinal cord.

Postganglionic parasympathetic neurons are located in the terminal ganglia near or in the organ innervated.

GVA fibers accompanying sympathetic fibers carry pain from thoracic and abdominal viscera.

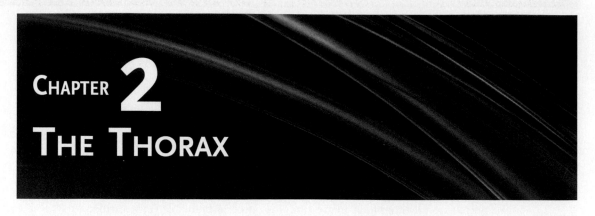

I. **The Thoracic Wall**
  A. **The Thoracic Skeleton**
    1. **Ribs (Figure 2-1, *A*)**
      a. Overview
        (1) **True ribs:** ribs 1-7 connected to sternum by costal cartilages
        (2) **False ribs:** ribs 8-12 with costal cartilages that do not reach sternum; cartilages of ribs 8-10 join cartilage immediately superior
        (3) **Floating ribs:** ribs 11 and 12, which have a free anterior end
      b. **Typical ribs: ribs 3-9**
        (1) **Head** articulates with body of corresponding vertebra and vertebra superior.
        (2) **Tubercle** articulates with transverse process of corresponding vertebra.
        (3) **Body or shaft** is twisted about its long axis, turning sharply forward at **angle.**

Ribs 1-7: true ribs. 8-12: false ribs. 11-12: floating ribs

A fracture of the well-protected rib 1 suggests severe chest trauma.

Thoracic and abdominal organ trauma may occur in children without rib fracture.

Paradoxical respiratory movements occur in flail chest.

Ribs 1 and 2 (protected by the clavicle) and ribs 11 and 12 are seldom fractured. In adults, a typical rib usually fractures near the **angle,** the point of greatest curvature. In a **severe crush injury** on one side, multiple ribs may fracture in two places. Fractured segments **(flail chest)** are sucked in during inspiration and pushed out during expiration, producing **paradoxical respiratory movements.** Associated **pulmonary contusions** contribute to respiratory insufficiency. The more flexible ribs and costal cartilages of **children** mean that blunt trauma may injure thoracic organs without fracturing ribs, masking the seriousness of the injury.

A segment of rib can be excised to gain access to the thoracic cavity **(thoracotomy)** by longitudinally splitting the **periosteum.** Osteogenic cells of the periosteum regenerate bone to fill the defect.

      c. **Atypical ribs: ribs 1, 2, 10-12**
        • Ribs 1 and 10-12 articulate with only one vertebra each.
      d. **Cervical rib**
        • Elongated transverse process of C7, often attached to first thoracic rib by a fibrous band

A cervical rib may cause thoracic outlet syndrome.

In **thoracic outlet syndrome,** the **subclavian artery** or **inferior trunk of the brachial plexus** is stretched or compressed between the anterior and middle scalene muscles, often when the arm is hanging at the side. It produces numbness and tingling in the extremity, simulating a cervical disc problem. Thoracic outlet syndrome may be due to a **cervical rib, hypertrophied scalene muscles,** or an anomalous **fibrous band.**

    2. **Sternum (Figure 2-1, *A*)**
      a. **Manubrium**
        (1) Easily palpable **jugular (suprasternal) notch** on superior border at root of neck
        (2) Articulates with clavicle, first costal cartilage, superior part of second costal cartilage, and body of sternum
      b. **Body**

Anterior view

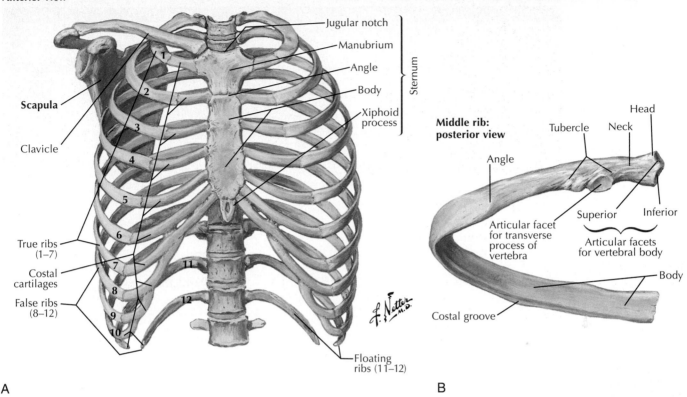

2-1: Thoracic skeleton and typical rib. **A,** Anterior view of thoracic skeleton showing relationships of ribs and costal cartilages to sternum. **B,** Posterior view of a typical rib. It consists of a head, neck, and body with a tubercle located at the junction of neck and body. *(From Netter, F H: Atlas of Human Anatomy, 4th ed. Philadelphia, Saunders, 2006, Plates 185 and 186.)*

(1) Articulates with manubrium, second through seventh costal cartilages, and xiphoid process

(2) Has **marrow cavity** used for **bone marrow biopsy**

c. **Xiphoid process**

(1) May be bifid or perforated

(2) Can be palpated in infrasternal angle at T10 vertebral level

Xiphisternal joint marks inferior border of heart and superior border of liver.

A traumatic sternal fracture requires evaluation for heart injury.

The sternum is split in the midline (**sternotomy**) and the two halves retracted for surgery on the heart (e.g., **coronary bypass surgery**) or other thoracic organs. The halves are wired back together.

Defective ossification may result in a lack of fusion of the right and left halves of the sternum, producing a **sternal cleft**. A **congenital perforation** in the body (**sternal foramen**) may be mistaken for a **bullet wound**. A **caving in** of the sternum and costal cartilages during development (**pectus excavatum or funnel chest**) may impair cardiac and respiratory function. It is the **most common congenital abnormality of the chest wall** and usually is apparent at birth but may not become pronounced until puberty. A **congenital protrusion** of the sternum and costal cartilages (**pectus carinatum or pigeon chest**) may occur alone or as part of syndrome, sometimes impairing respiration and decreasing endurance.

Pectus excavatum: funnel chest. Pectus carinatum: pigeon chest

Pectus excavatum is the most common congenital defect of the thoracic wall.

Sternal angle marks level of second costal cartilages, which is useful in counting ribs.

Sternal angle marks level of tracheal bifurcation and inferior boundary of aortic arch.

3. **Joints of thoracic wall (Table 2-1)**

The **sternal angle** is a landmark for physical diagnosis because it is a convenient starting place for **counting ribs.** It is also useful because it indicates the level of a horizontal plane marking the **bifurcation of the trachea,** the **beginning and end of the arch of the aorta,** and the **division into superior and inferior mediastinum.**

TABLE 2-1. JOINTS OF THORACIC WALL

JOINT	ARTICULATING STRUCTURES	COMMENTS
Manubriosternal	Manubrium with body of sternum	Sternal angle marks level of second costal cartilage
Costovertebral		
Joints of head of rib	Head of rib with body of corresponding vertebra and vertebra above	Ribs 1 and 10-12 articulate with only one vertebra
Costotransverse	Tubercle of rib with transverse process of corresponding vertebra	Not present with ribs 11-12
Costochondral	Rib with costal cartilage	
Sternocostal	Costal cartilages 1-7 with sternum	

2-2: Typical intercostal space. The neurovascular bundle lies between the internal intercostal and the innermost intercostal muscles near the superior border of the intercostal space.

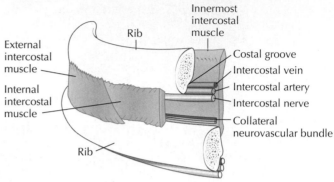

B. The Muscles of the Thoracic Wall (Figure 2-2)

Paralysis of the intercostal muscles results in intercostal tissues being sucked in during inspiration and ballooning out during expiration.

VAN = intercostal Vein, Artery, and Nerve from superior to inferior in intercostal space.

To enter the pleural cavity, a needle is inserted at the superior border of the lower rib bounding the intercostal space.

C. The Intercostal Space (see Figure 2-2)

To block an intercostal nerve, the needle is inserted near the inferior border of the rib superior to the intercostal space. In contrast, **to enter the pleural cavity** to aspirate fluid or to perform a biopsy, the needle is inserted near the superior border of the rib inferior to the intercostal space.

D. Intercostal Nerves and Blood Vessels
   1. **Intercostal nerves (see Figure 1-21)**
     a. Overview
      (1) **Anterior rami** of first 11 spinal nerves in intercostal spaces
      (2) Lie between internal and innermost intercostal muscles

Cardiac pain is often referred to the medial side of the left arm.

Cardiac pain is often **referred** to the medial side of the left arm because the T1 and T2 dermatomes continue there from the thoracic wall. Communication of the **intercostobrachial nerve** (T2) with the **medial brachial cutaneous nerve** (C8, T1) is one pathway for referred pain.

Shingles lesions follow a dermatomal pattern.

Herpes zoster (shingles) of an intercostal nerve produces **vesicular eruptions and burning pain** in the affected **dermatome.** Reactivation of the varicella-zoster virus follows a period of dormancy within the **posterior root ganglion** from years to decades after **chicken pox.** Elderly and immunocompromised individuals are particularly susceptible. Some patients experience severe residual pain for months or even years **(postherpetic neuralgia).** Contact with the shingles rash can cause chicken pox in a child who has never had it.

     b. **First intercostal nerve** is short because most of anterior ramus of T1 joins anterior ramus of C8 to form **lower trunk of brachial plexus**
     c. **Intercostobrachial nerve** is lateral cutaneous branch of second intercostal nerve (T2)

   d. **Subcostal nerve** is anterior ramus of T12 spinal nerve and lies immediately below rib 12

   e. **Thoracoabdominal nerves** are **seventh to eleventh intercostal nerves,** which leave intercostal space anteriorly to supply the anterolateral abdominal wall.

The T4 dermatome lies at the level of the nipple. The T10 dermatome lies at the level of the umbilicus.

Disease of the thoracic wall (e.g., in lower costal parietal pleura) may cause **abdominal pain and tenderness** and rigidity of abdominal muscles because the **thoracoabdominal nerves** continue into the anterior abdominal wall.

2. **Intercostal blood vessels**
   - Include 11 pairs of posterior intercostal arteries and veins and one pair of subcostal arteries and veins (see Section IX)

E. **The Breast**
   1. Overview
      a. **Mammary gland** embedded in superficial fascia with fat and secretory activity contributing to size and contour
      b. Overlies ribs 2-6 in young adult female; rudimentary in male and prepubertal female
      c. Pigmented, projecting **nipple** surrounded by circular, pigmented **areola.** In males and young females, nipple lies over **fourth intercostal space**
      d. Supported by **suspensory ligaments** that attach to overlying skin
      e. Separated from deep fascia over pectoralis major **(pectoral fascia)** by **retromammary space,** which allows movement on chest wall
   2. **Mammary gland**
      a. Has 15-20 **lobes,** each drained by a single corresponding **lactiferous duct** that opens on nipple
      b. **Lactiferous sinus,** expansion for each lactiferous duct deep to nipple, serves as **milk reservoir** during lactation
      c. May extend into axilla as **axillary tail**
   3. **Blood supply and innervation of breast**
      a. Supplied by mammary branches of **internal thoracic, intercostal,** and **lateral thoracic arteries**
      b. **Veins** are tributaries of internal thoracic, intercostal, and lateral thoracic veins.
      c. Innervation is by **intercostal nerves T2-T6.**
   4. **Lymphatic drainage of breast**
      a. Facilitates metastasis of breast cancer
      b. 75% of lymph passes to **axillary lymph nodes** but also may pass to lymph nodes near clavicle or lymph nodes draining upper abdominal wall.
      c. From medial quadrants is to **parasternal nodes** along internal thoracic artery or across midline to **opposite breast**

The mammary gland usually extends into the axilla as an axillary tail.

Seventy-five percent of the lymph from the breast drains to the axillary lymph nodes, particularly the pectoral group.

BRCA1 and BRCA2 gene mutations cause most hereditary breast cancer.

Radiographic examination of the breast by **mammographic screening** is used for early detection of small, nonpalpable **breast carcinomas** and is recommended annually for women over 40 or with a family history. BRCA1 and BRCA2 tumor suppressor gene mutations are responsible for most hereditary breast cancers, although these account for only about 7% of breast cancers.

Breast cancer may result in **dimpling of the skin** and **retraction of the nipple** caused by fibrosis and shortening of the **suspensory ligaments** or involvement of the ductal system. The skin may look like an orange peel **(peau d'orange)** because lymphatics are obstructed by the tumor. The breast may become fixed to the chest wall after the tumor invades the **retromammary space,** which is evident when the pectoralis major is contracted with the hand pressed against the hip.

The incidence of **breast cancer in males** is only 1% that of females, but often it is not diagnosed until extensive metastases have occurred. Males with **Klinefelter syndrome (47, XXY)** frequently exhibit **gynecomastia** and have an increased incidence of breast cancer.

Dimpling and an orange peel appearance of the skin and nipple retraction are signs of breast cancer.

Klinefelter syndrome males have an increased incidence of breast cancer.

Although less common than **metastasis** through lymphatics, cancer can spread from the breast through the **venous system** to the **vertebral column, spinal cord,** and **brain** through the **posterior intercostal veins** to the **vertebral venous plexuses,** and then superiorly to the **dural venous sinuses** of the cranial cavity.

Surgical removal of a breast carcinoma may involve only the tumor and adjacent tissue **(lumpectomy),** removal of the breast and axillary lymph nodes **(modified radical mastectomy),** or rarely the breast along with the axillary contents and pectoralis muscles **(radical mastectomy).** Surgery is often augmented by chemotherapy and/or radiation. During a **radical mastectomy,** the **long thoracic nerve,** which lies on the superficial surface of the serratus anterior muscle, is vulnerable. **Paralysis of the serratus anterior** prevents abduction of the arm above 90 degrees and causes a **winged scapula.** The **thoracodorsal nerve** also may be injured.

Breast cancer can metastasize through the venous system to the vertebral column, spinal cord, and brain.

II. Pleura (Figures 2-3 to 2-5)

A. Overview

1. Thin serous sac around each lung enclosing **pleural cavity,** which is potential space empty except for thin layer of serous fluid
2. Consists of **visceral pleura** adherent to lung surface and **parietal pleura** adherent to chest wall, diaphragm, and mediastinal structures (mainly fibrous pericardium)

B. Pleural Reflections (see Figure 2-5)

C. Cupula is cervical pleura extending above the first rib.

D. Pleural recesses contain no lung tissue during quiet respiration but fill with lung tissue during deep inspiration.

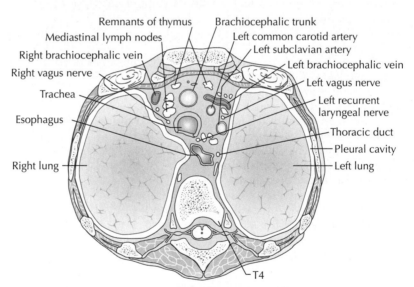

2-3: Transverse (axial) section through the superior mediastinum. Because structures within the mediastinum are closely packed, any space-occupying or invasive lesion may compromise their functions.

2-4: Axial CT near same level as Figure 2-3. Brachiocephalic trunk = 1; left common carotid artery = 2; left subclavian artery = 3; right brachiocephalic vein = 4; left brachioce-phalic vein = 5; trachea = 6; esophagus = 7; spinal cord = 8. *(From Weir, J, Abrahams, P: Imaging Atlas of Human Anatomy, 3rd ed. London, Mosby Ltd., 2003, p 92, b.)*

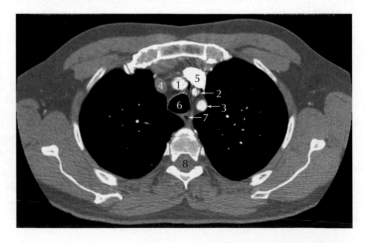

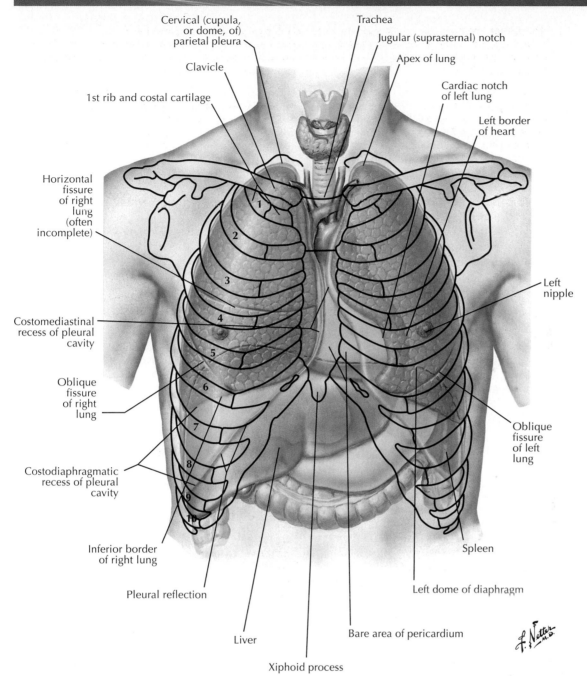

Cervical (cupula, or dome, of) parietal pleura

Trachea

Jugular (suprasternal) notch

Clavicle

Apex of lung

Cardiac notch of left lung

1st rib and costal cartilage

Left border of heart

Horizontal fissure of right lung (often incomplete)

Left nipple

Costomediastinal recess of pleural cavity

Oblique fissure of right lung

Oblique fissure of left lung

Costodiaphragmatic recess of pleural cavity

Inferior border of right lung

Spleen

Left dome of diaphragm

Pleural reflection

Liver

Bare area of pericardium

Xiphoid process

2-5: Surface projections of lungs and pleurae. *Numbers, ribs. (From Netter, F H: Atlas of Human Anatomy, 4th ed. Philadelphia, Saunders, 2006, Plate 196.)*

1. **Costodiaphragmatic recess** is the lowest part of the pleural cavity and may accumulate abnormal pleural fluid.
2. **Costomediastinal recess**

Pneumothorax is air in the pleural cavity that results in partial or total collapse of the lung. The **parietal pleura** may be **punctured** and the lung accidentally deflated **(open pneumothorax)** during a posterior approach to the kidney near rib 12, liver biopsy, nerve block of the stellate ganglion or brachial plexus at the root of the neck, or intravenous line insertion into the subclavian vein.

Pleural effusion is fluid in the pleural cavity from any of multiple causes, including infection, cancer, or **congestive heart failure. Thoracentesis** is surgical removal of fluid from the pleural cavity. A needle or incision over a lower intercostal space in the midaxillary line penetrates the skin, superficial fascia, serratus anterior, intercostal muscles, endothoracic fascia, and parietal pleura. The **long thoracic nerve** may be injured.

Pneumothorax is air in the pleural cavity, resulting in collapse of the lung.

To enter pleural cavity in midaxillary line the needle penetrates skin, fascia, serratus anterior, intercostal muscles, endothoracic fascia, and parietal pleura.

Parietal pleura injury is painful due to somatic afferent innervation, but visceral pleura is not painful due to visceral afferent innervation.

Pleuritis may cause chest pain and pleural friction rub.

Pleuritis (pleurisy) involving only **visceral pleura** may not be painful because innervation is from visceral afferent nerves. However, on inspiration a **sharp pain in the chest wall** is felt in pleuritis involving **parietal pleura** because innervation is from somatic nerves. Roughening of the pleura results in a **pleural friction rub** heard with a stethoscope, and **pleural adhesions** may develop between inflamed visceral and parietal pleurae.

Pain in the thorax, abdomen, or shoulder on deep inspiration suggests a pleural origin. **Shoulder pain** can be referred from **irritated diaphragmatic pleura.** Pleural pain related to **pneumonia** or **cancer of the lower lobe** may be **referred** to the anterior abdominal wall.

III. Trachea and Bronchi (Figure 2-6)

A. Trachea
1. Begins as continuation of **larynx** and ends by dividing into two **main (primary) bronchi** at level of sternal angle
2. Contains **carina,** posterior process of last tracheal cartilage that internally marks bifurcation of trachea as seen with **bronchoscope**
3. See **Figures 2-3 and 2-4** for relationships in **superior mediastinum.**

Distorted carina on bronchoscopy often indicates metastatic lung cancer.

During **bronchoscopy,** the **carina** is a critical landmark, and a deviation in its position may indicate **metastasis of lung cancer** to the **tracheobronchial lymph nodes** at the bifurcation of the trachea.

Insertion of an **endotracheal tube** during surgery or in emergency situations protects air flow to and from the lungs. **Insertion too deeply** may result in only one lung being ventilated, possibly causing **pneumothorax** and the other main bronchus being obstructed to cause **atelectasis** (see VI.A.3. following). Inadvertent insertion into the **esophagus** may result in aspiration of stomach contents and **aspiration pneumonia.**

The trachea may be **compressed** by an **enlarged thyroid gland** or by an **aortic arch aneurysm.**

An aspirated object or an endotracheal tube that is inserted too far is likely to enter the right main bronchus.

B. Right Main Bronchus
1. **Crossed superiorly by arch of azygos vein,** passing to superior vena cava
2. Aspirated objects will more likely enter **wider, more vertical** right main bronchus.

C. Left Main Bronchus
- Passes **inferior to arch of aorta** and **anterior to esophagus**

D. Eparterial Bronchus
- Another name for **right upper lobe bronchus** because it arises above level of pulmonary artery

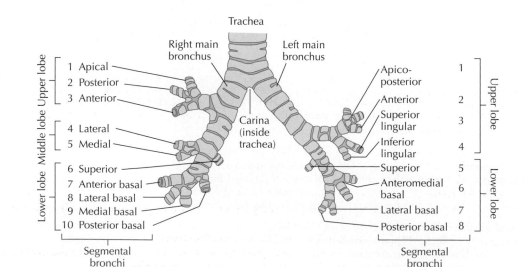

2-6: Trachea and bronchi, anterior view. The right lung has 10 segmental (tertiary) bronchi, and the left lung has 8-10.

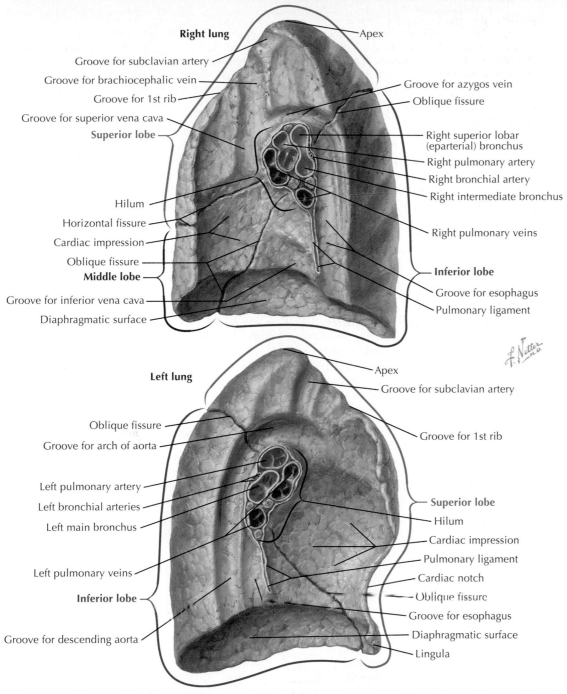

2-7: Medial views of right (*top*) and left (*bottom*) lungs. Oblique and horizontal fissures divide the right lung into three lobes while an oblique fissure divides the left lung into two lobes. The lingula of the left lung corresponds to the middle lobe of the right lung. The pulmonary ligament is a double layer of pleura inferior to the hilum. Adjacent structures produce contact impressions in embalmed lungs. *(From Netter, F H: Atlas of Human Anatomy, 4th ed. Philadelphia, Saunders, 2006, Plate 199.)*

IV. Lungs (Figure 2-7)

A. Overview

1. One **main bronchus**, one **pulmonary artery**, and two **pulmonary veins** divide within the substance of each lung.
2. **Surfaces** are **diaphragmatic, costal,** and **mediastinal.**
3. **Root of lung** consists of structures passing between the lung and mediastinum, and the **hilum** is the region where structures enter or leave the lung.

4. **Pulmonary ligament** is a double-layered vertical fold of pleura extending inferiorly from hilum to base.

An apical lung tumor (Pancoast tumor) may cause Horner syndrome.

> A **tumor of the apex of the lung (Pancoast tumor)** may involve the sympathetic chain and interrupt sympathetic innervation to the head, producing **Horner syndrome** (ipsilateral anhidrosis, miosis, ptosis, and vasodilation). The tumor also may involve the **inferior roots of the brachial plexus,** producing upper-extremity symptoms.

B. **Right Lung**
  1. Divided into **upper, middle, and lower lobes** by **oblique and horizontal fissures;** horizontal fissure is at level of **fourth rib and costal cartilage**
  2. Shorter than left because of higher **right dome of diaphragm**
  3. Contains **three lobar** (secondary) and **10 segmental** (tertiary) bronchi
  4. See **Figure 2-7** for relationships at hilum.
C. **Left Lung**
  1. Divided into **upper and lower lobes** at **oblique fissure**
  2. Includes **cardiac notch** that lies over **heart and pericardium** anteriorly **(see Figure 2-5); lingula** forms inferior margin of cardiac notch and corresponds to middle lobe of right lung
  3. **Two lobar** and **8-10 segmental** bronchi
  4. See **Figure 2-7** for relationships at hilum.
D. **Bronchopulmonary Segments (see Figure 2-6)**
  1. Pyramidal regions of lung supplied by one **segmental** (tertiary) **bronchus** and its accompanying **segmental branch of pulmonary artery**
  2. Drained in part by **intersegmental veins** used as **surgical landmarks**
  3. Usually number **10 in right lung** and **8-10 in left,** depending on fusion of segments

The cardiac notch allows a needle to enter the pericardium and heart through the left fifth intercostal space without damaging the lung and pleura.

Bronchopulmonary segments are independent functional and surgical units.

Patient position determines the location of inhaled foreign objects.

Intersegmental veins are surgical landmarks for segmentectomies.

> Gravity moves **foreign material** to different **bronchopulmonary segments of the right lung** depending on the patient's **position (Figure 2-8).** In a **standing or sitting** patient, the posterobasal segment is involved; in the **supine** patient, the superior segment of the lower lobe; in the **right-sided recumbent** position, the middle lobe or posterior segment of the right upper lobe. The arrangement of segments also means that a patient can be optimally positioned for **postural drainage** of an **infected bronchopulmonary segment** aided by percussion of the chest wall over the segment.
>
> Because bronchi and arteries of adjacent **bronchopulmonary segments** do not communicate, a segment can be resected without compromising the surrounding lung. **Intersegmental tributaries of pulmonary veins** are landmarks for **segmentectomies.**

E. **Blood Vessels of Lungs**
  1. **Pulmonary arteries** carry **deoxygenated blood** from right ventricle to lungs

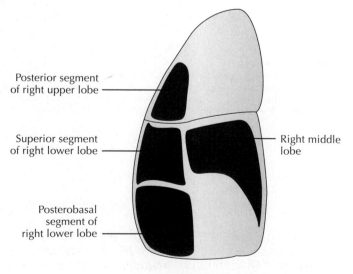

2-8: Bronchopulmonary segments of right lung where foreign material lodges depending on patient position. Standing or sitting: posterobasal segment. Supine position: superior segment of lower lobe. Right-sided recumbent: right middle lobe or posterior segment of right upper lobe. *(From Goljan, E F: Rapid Review Pathology, 3rd ed. Philadelphia, Mosby Elsevier, 2010, Box 16-1.)*

Posterior segment of right upper lobe

Superior segment of right lower lobe

Right middle lobe

Posterobasal segment of right lower lobe

Right lung

   a. **Left pulmonary artery** attached to aortic arch by **ligamentum arteriosum,** the remnant of the fetal **ductus arteriosus**
   b. **Right pulmonary artery** crosses under arch of aorta to reach hilum of right lung
2. **Pulmonary veins** carry **oxygenated blood** from lungs to the left atrium.

> Pulmonary arteries carry deoxygenated blood to the lungs; pulmonary veins return the oxygenated blood to the heart.

Lung cancer may **metastasize to the brain** through the **arterial system** when cancer cells enter the pulmonary veins and are returned to the left side of the heart. From the aorta, cancer cells pass through the common and internal carotid arteries or the subclavian and vertebral arteries.

3. **Bronchial arteries**
   a. Supply oxygenated blood to bronchial tree and visceral pleura
   b. Number **two on the left,** arising from descending thoracic aorta, but only **one on the right,** often branching from third right posterior intercostal artery
4. **Bronchial veins**

> Bronchial arteries supply oxygenated blood to lung tissues.

Lung cancer may **metastasize to the spinal cord and brain** through the **venous system** if cancer cells enter a **bronchial vein** and pass to the azygos system. Cancer cells may then pass to the **vertebral venous plexuses** and ascend to the **dural venous sinuses** in the cranial cavity.

F. **Lymphatic Drainage of Lungs**
   1. **Superficial lymphatic plexus** lies just beneath visceral pleura and drains toward hilum
   2. **Deep lymphatic plexus** follows bronchial tree to hilum and includes peribronchial **pulmonary nodes** lying within substance of lung
   3. **Bronchopulmonary nodes** at root of lung receive drainage from both superficial and deep plexuses.
   4. **Tracheobronchial nodes** at tracheal bifurcation receive lymph from bronchopulmonary nodes.
   5. Right and left **bronchomediastinal lymph trunks** drain tracheobronchial nodes and eventually reach a **venous angle,** either directly or through right lymphatic duct and thoracic duct, respectively

> Left and right venous angles formed at the union of internal jugular and subclavian veins.

The upper lobe of the left lung has lymphatic drainage to the left bronchiomediastinal trunk, but the **lower lobe of the left lung** has lymphatic drainage mainly to the **right bronchomediastinal lymph trunk.**

> Lung cancer cells can metastasize through arteries, veins, or lymphatic vessels.

G. **Nerve Supply of Lungs**
   1. **Pulmonary plexuses** contain **sympathetic, parasympathetic, and visceral afferent fibers** derived from the **deep cardiac plexus.**
   2. **Parasympathetic fibers** come from vagus nerves and produce **bronchial constriction and mucus secretion,**
   3. **Sympathetic fibers** are postganglionic fibers from upper five thoracic sympathetic ganglia; they **relax bronchial smooth muscle** and **constrict pulmonary vessels.**
   4. **Visceral afferent fibers** from vagus nerves
      a. Sensitive to stretch and participate in reflex control of respiration
      b. End in bronchial mucosa and participate in **cough reflex**

V. **Development of Respiratory System and Related Defects**
   A. **Development of Trachea and Bronchi**
      1. **Laryngotracheal (respiratory) diverticulum** forms during week 4 in floor of pharynx.
      2. **Tracheoesophageal septum** separates developing larynx and trachea from pharynx and esophagus
      3. **Lung buds** develop in week 5 at caudal end of laryngotracheal tube, growing into splanchnic mesoderm surrounding foregut to give rise to primary, secondary, and tertiary bronchi by week 6

> Esophageal atresia results in polyhydramnios.

A **congenital tracheoesophageal fistula** is an abnormal communication between the trachea and distal esophagus usually associated with **esophageal atresia** (blind-ending esophagus) **(Figure 2-9).** The resulting regurgitation and aspiration of swallowed milk (and possible reflux of gastric contents into lungs) cause **pneumonia.** Because esophageal atresia prevents the fetus from swallowing and absorbing amniotic fluid in the small intestine, the condition is often accompanied by excess amniotic fluid **(polyhydramnios).** An **acquired tracheoesophageal fistula** may result from malignancy, infection, or trauma.

> Tracheoesophageal fistula with esophageal atresia causes pneumonia.

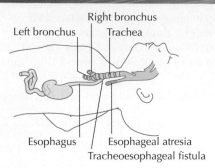

2-9: Tracheoesophageal fistula and esophageal atresia.

B. **Development of Lung**
1. **Pseudoglandular period**
   a. Comprises weeks 5-16 when conducting system is formed as far as terminal bronchiole
   b. Birth during this period is incompatible with life.
2. **Canalicular period**
   a. Comprises weeks 16-26 when terminal bronchioles give rise to respiratory bronchioles, each of which divides into alveolar ducts, and respiratory vasculature forms
   b. Some terminal sacs (primitive alveoli) develop toward end of period, so some infants born late in canalicular period may survive with intensive care
3. **Terminal sac period**
   • Comprises week 26-birth when more terminal sacs develop and pulmonary **surfactant** is produced by **type II alveolar cells** (pneumocytes)
4. **Alveolar period**
   • Comprises week 32 of gestation through age of 8 years when alveoli form and mature; boundary between terminal sac and alveolar period open to interpretation

Some infants born at 22-25 weeks survive with intensive care but often suffer lifelong disability.

Pulmonary surfactant produced by type II alveolar cells reduces surface tension to prevent alveolar collapse.

Maternal glucocorticoid treatment may prevent neonatal respiratory distress syndrome.

Surfactant reduces surface tension to allow inflation of alveoli. **Neonatal respiratory distress syndrome (hyaline membrane disease)** results from **deficient surfactant production** by type II alveolar cells in premature infants. **Glucocorticoid treatment** in at-risk pregnancies speeds up lung development and surfactant production. Treatment with **artificial surfactant** reduces neonatal mortality.

VI. **Respiration and Respiratory Diaphragm**
A. **Respiration**
   • Serous fluid adhesion between visceral and parietal pleura links volume of lungs with movements of diaphragm and thoracic wall and facilitates respiration
   1. **Inspiration** increases volume of thoracic cavity and lungs to create a **negative intrathoracic pressure** that draws air into lungs
      a. **Quiet inspiration**
         • Involves contraction of **diaphragm,** pulling it downward to increase **vertical dimension** of thorax
      b. **Forced inspiration**
         (1) **External intercostal muscles** contract, elevating ribs and carrying sternum upward and forward, and increase **anteroposterior and lateral diameters** of thorax
         (2) Recruits **accessory muscles of respiration** to assist elevating ribs, further increasing depth of inspiration
   2. **Expiration** decreases volume of thorax and lungs to create a **positive intrathoracic pressure** that forces air from lungs
      a. **Quiet expiration** is passive process largely caused by elastic recoil of lungs and relaxation of diaphragm

The diaphragm is the primary muscle of inspiration.

Patient with dyspnea may lean on upper extremities to allow accessory muscles to aid in respiration.

b. **Forced expiration** is active process involving contraction of anterior **abdominal wall muscles,** which depress ribs and sternum and increase intraabdominal pressure, and **internal intercostal muscles**

3. **Accessory muscles of respiration**
   - Include **head and neck muscles** and **upper limb muscles** attached to rib cage or sternum

---

In **spontaneous pneumothorax,** air enters the pleural cavity because of rupture of a bleb on a diseased lung. It occurs commonly in tall, slender males under 40 who smoke and **Marfan syndrome** patients.

> Spontaneous pneumothorax occurs in tall, slender male smokers under 40.

Tension pneumothorax is a life-threatening condition in which air enters the pleural cavity during inspiration due to a penetrating wound but cannot exit during expiration. Air pressure increases on the affected side, and the **mediastinum shifts away,** compressing the contralateral lung and compromising venous return to the heart **(Figure 2-10).** Bedside ultrasonography often replaces chest radiographs for diagnosis. The patient complains of **chest pain** and **dyspnea. Jugular venous distention** and a **tracheal shift** develop as the pressure increases.

> Tension pneumothorax may fatally compromise cardiopulmonary function.

Emphysema is destruction of the walls of airspaces distal to the terminal bronchioles. Because airspaces are consequently enlarged, surface area for gas exchange is reduced. Elastic tissue is destroyed, impairing expiration and requiring participation of accessory muscles of expiration.

Asthma is a variable obstruction of the airway caused by spasmodic contraction of smooth muscle in the bronchial tree, mucosal edema, and mucus plugging. Dyspnea, wheezing, coughing, and chest tightness are characteristic. Precipitating factors include ozone, inhalation of allergens, respiratory tract infections, emotions, exercise, and some drugs (e.g., aspirin).

Atelectasis is **collapse of lung tissue** from obstruction of airflow (e.g., by tumor, mucus, or aspirated body) and is a frequent **postoperative complication** because the patient cannot cough thick mucus loose from the bronchial lumen. The left main bronchus may be obstructed by an **endotracheal tube** inserted into the right main bronchus **(Figure 2-11).** Unlike tension pneumothorax, lung collapse in atelectasis results in **mediastinal shift toward the affected side.**

> Mediastinum shifts toward affected lung in atelectasis but away from affected lung in tension pneumothorax

---

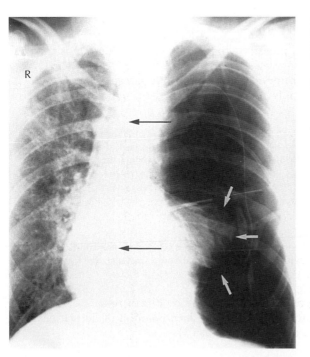

2-10: PA chest x-ray of tension pneumothorax showing collapsed left lung (*white arrows*), radiolucent air-filled pleural cavity, and flattened left hemidiaphragm. Mediastinal contents have been pushed to the right (*black arrows*). *(From Mettler, F A: Essentials of Radiology, 2nd ed. Philadelphia, Saunders, 2004, Figure 3-72.)*

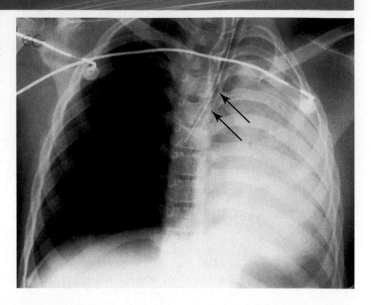

2-11: Atelectasis of left lung due to obstruction of left main bronchus by endotracheal tube (*arrows*) inserted too far and entering right main bronchus. Opacity increases as air is resorbed. Lung collapse results in mediastinal shift toward affected side. *(From Mettler, F A: Essentials of Radiology, 2nd ed. Philadelphia, Saunders, 2004, Figure 3-23.)*

Saddle embolus may fatally block pulmonary trunk bifurcation.

Fat embolism syndrome 1-3 days following long bone fracture or orthopedic surgery is acute respiratory failure, CNS dysfunction, and petechiae.

Thoracocentesis through lower intercostal space risks injury to diaphragm and liver on right and to diaphragm and spleen on left

Bronchiectasis is a pathologic condition involving chronic dilatation of portions of the bronchial tree that may be caused by prolonged atelectasis or respiratory infection. It is common in cystic fibrosis patients.

A **pulmonary embolus** usually originates in **deep veins of the lower extremity (usually the femoral vein).** It may pass through the right side of the heart and lodge in a pulmonary artery. The clot may cause **sudden death** if it lodges at the bifurcation of the pulmonary trunk **(saddle thrombus).**

Pulmonary emboli can arise from other sources, including the **fatty marrow of a long bone following fracture or orthopedic surgery.** These fat emboli are usually clinically silent but may cause **fat embolism syndrome** 1-3 days later with pulmonary insufficiency, neurologic symptoms, anemia, thrombocytopenia, and petechiae. **Amniotic fluid embolism** is an uncommon, but potentially fatal, complication of labor and the immediate postpartum period.

Phrenic nerves (C3,4,5) innervate the respiratory diaphragm.

Diaphragm openings: vena caval T8; esophageal T10; aortic T12

Diaphragm movements don't affect aortic blood flow because aortic hiatus is posterior to the diaphragm.

Paralyzed hemidiaphragm rises during inspiration on radiograph.

B. Respiratory Diaphragm (Figure 2-12)
1. Overview
   a. Includes **right dome** that arches superiorly to fifth rib and **left dome** that arches to fifth intercostal space
   b. Receives **motor and sensory innervation** from **phrenic nerves** except for peripheral part with sensory supply from **lower intercostal nerves**
2. Other features **(Table 2-2)**

Chronic, **intractable hiccups** sometimes are treated by **crushing one phrenic nerve.** A lesion of one phrenic nerve produces **hemiparalysis of the diaphragm** unless the lesion is proximal to union with an **accessory phrenic nerve.** On **radiographs,** paralysis is apparent by the diaphragm's **paradoxical movement** (i.e., diaphragm is elevated during inspiration by abdominal viscera).

Fracture of lower right ribs may injure liver, and fracture of lower left ribs may injure spleen

Because the diaphragm domes superiorly, **upper abdominal organs are enclosed by the thoracic rib cage.** Therefore, **fractures of the lower ribs** may damage not only the diaphragm but also the **liver,** right kidney, **spleen,** or left kidney.

3. **Development of respiratory diaphragm** occurs by incorporation of derivatives from the following four embryonic structures **(Figure 2-13).**
   a. **Septum transversum**

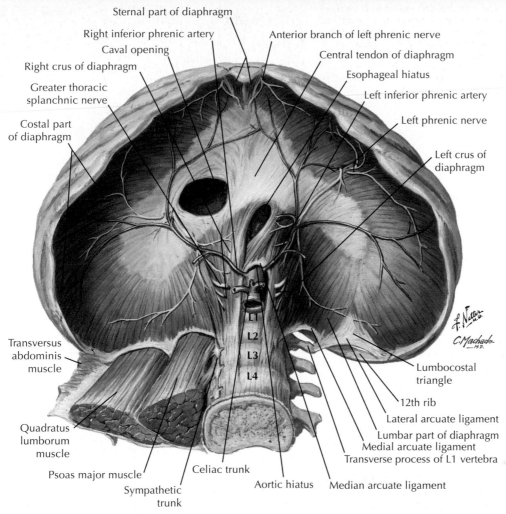

Sternal part of diaphragm
Right inferior phrenic artery
Caval opening
Right crus of diaphragm
Greater thoracic splanchnic nerve
Costal part of diaphragm
Anterior branch of left phrenic nerve
Central tendon of diaphragm
Esophageal hiatus
Left inferior phrenic artery
Left phrenic nerve
Left crus of diaphragm
Transversus abdominis muscle
Lumbocostal triangle
12th rib
Lateral arcuate ligament
Lumbar part of diaphragm
Medial arcuate ligament
Transverse process of L1 vertebra
Quadratus lumborum muscle
Psoas major muscle
Sympathetic trunk
Celiac trunk
Aortic hiatus
Median arcuate ligament

2-12: Respiratory diaphragm, inferior view. Openings allow the passage of the inferior vena cava (T8), esophagus (T10), and aorta (T12). Right crus splits to form esophageal hiatus. Phrenic nerves supply motor innervation and sensory innervation to all but peripheral part, which receives sensory supply from lower intercostal nerves. Inferior phrenic arteries contribute to blood supply. *(From Netter, F H: Atlas of Human Anatomy, 4th ed. Philadelphia, Saunders, 2006, Plate 195.)*

TABLE 2-2. FEATURES OF RESPIRATORY DIAPHRAGM

FEATURE	ATTACHMENTS OR LOCATION	COMMENTS
Central tendon	Receives insertions of sternal, costal, and lumbar parts	Cloverleaf-shaped central aponeurotic part
Median arcuate ligament	Unites crura across midline anterior to aorta	
Medial arcuate ligament	Body to transverse process of L1	Arches over psoas major
Lateral arcuate ligament	Transverse process of L1 to rib 12	Arches over quadratus lumborum
Right crus	Bodies of vertebrae L1-3	Larger and longer than left crus
Left crus	Bodies of vertebrae L1-2	
Opening		
Vena caval hiatus	Through central tendon at T8 vertebral level	Transmits inferior vena cava and right phrenic nerve
Esophageal hiatus	Through right crus at T10 level; left of midline	Transmits esophagus, vagal trunks, and esophageal branches of left gastric vessels
Aortic hiatus	Between crura behind median arcuate ligament at T12 level	Posterior to diaphragm so movements don't affect aortic flow; transmits aorta, thoracic duct, maybe azygos vein

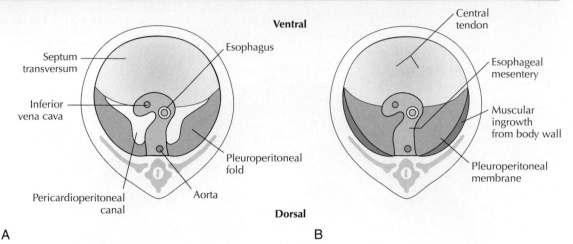

Ventral

Septum transversum

Esophagus

Inferior vena cava

Pericardioperitoneal canal

Pleuroperitoneal fold

Aorta

Central tendon

Esophageal mesentery

Muscular ingrowth from body wall

Pleuroperitoneal membrane

Dorsal

A   B

2-13: Progressive development (**A** and **B**) of the respiratory diaphragm, transverse section viewed from below. Septum transversum, pleuroperitoneal membranes and esophageal mesentery, and body wall mesoderm form the diaphragm.

Diaphragm origins: septum transversum, pleuroperitoneal membranes, esophageal mesentery, and body wall mesoderm

(1) **Lies in cervical region in week 4, adjacent to third, fourth, and fifth cervical somites,** which accounts for innervation of diaphragm by **phrenic nerves (C3,4,5)**
(2) Descends into thoracic region between developing heart and liver due to differential growth
(3) Gives rise to **central tendon** and to **myoblasts** that migrate into pleuroperitoneal membranes and esophageal mesentery

b. **Pleuroperitoneal membranes**
(1) Mesodermal tissue of **posterior body wall** that closes pericardioperitoneal canals by fusing with septum transversum and dorsal mesentery of esophagus
(2) Partition pleural cavity from peritoneal cavity

Intraembryonic body cavity divided into pericardial, pleural, and peritoneal cavities by pleuropericardial and pleuroperitoneal membranes

c. **Esophageal mesentery**
(1) Forms **middle** of diaphragm posteriorly
(2) Invaded by myoblasts that give rise to **crura** of diaphragm

d. **Body wall mesoderm**
• Forms **peripheral part** of diaphragm as a result of **excavation** by developing lungs and pleural cavities

Congenital diaphragmatic hernia: failure of pleuroperitoneal membrane to close pericardioperitoneal canal

A **congenital diaphragmatic hernia,** the most common congenital malformation of the diaphragm, results from **developmental failure of the pleuroperitoneal membrane** in week 6, usually posterolaterally on the left side (foramen of Bochdalek). Abdominal viscera then herniate into the thorax and compress the thoracic viscera; consequently, often fatal **pulmonary hypoplasia** occurs.

Congenital diaphragmatic hernia may cause fatal lung hypoplasia.

VII. Mediastinum (Figure 2-14)
A. **Overview**
1. Median partition of tissue lying between paired pleural sacs that contains all thoracic organs except lungs
2. Divided into **superior and inferior mediastinum** to assist clinical localizations; inferior mediastinum is subdivided into **anterior, middle, and posterior mediastinum**

Mediastinum is a median mass of tissue between pulmonary cavities.

B. **Subdivisions of mediastinum (Table 2-3)**

Fatal mediastinitis may result from the spread of a neck infection.

A **goiter** is prevented from expanding superiorly by the insertions of the sternothyroid muscles; therefore, it may extend inferiorly as a **retrosternal goiter,** possibly **compressing the trachea** and causing **dyspnea.** Less commonly the **esophagus** or **superior vena cava** is compressed.

In resecting a **parathyroid adenoma,** it is important to remember that the **inferior parathyroid glands** may be found in the superior mediastinum because they migrate with the **thymus** during development.

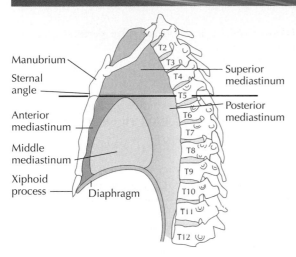

Manubrium
Sternal angle
Anterior mediastinum
Middle mediastinum
Xiphoid process
Diaphragm
T2 T3 T4 T5 T6 T7 T8 T9 T10 T11 T12
Superior mediastinum
Posterior mediastinum

2-14: Mediastinum, sagittal view. Horizontal plane at the sternal angle divides the superior and inferior mediastinum. The inferior mediastinum is subdivided by limits of the pericardium into middle, anterior, and posterior mediastinum.

TABLE 2-3. SUBDIVISIONS OF MEDIASTINUM

SUBDIVISION	BOUNDARIES	CONTENTS	COMMENTS
Superior mediastinum	Superior thoracic aperture to transverse plane connecting sternal angle and intervertebral disc T4/5	Remnants of thymus, right and left brachiocephalic veins uniting to form superior vena cava, arch of aorta and its branches, trachea, esophagus, thoracic duct, phrenic and vagus nerves	Trachea bifurcates at level of sternal angle; trachea and esophagus are mobile and may be shifted from midline position by tumors, etc.
Anterior mediastinum	Body of sternum to pericardium	Lymph nodes and loose connective tissue	May contain much of thymus in children
Middle mediastinum	Mostly enclosed within pericardial sac	Pericardium, heart, roots of great vessels, primary bronchi, phrenic nerves, arch of azygos vein	
Posterior mediastinum	Pericardium and sloping posterior surface of diaphragm to bodies of vertebrae T5-12	Descending thoracic aorta, esophagus and esophageal plexus, thoracic duct, azygos and hemiazygos veins	Some authors include thoracic sympathetic trunks

Infection that causes **mediastinitis** may travel a pathway of loose connective tissue (e.g., retropharyngeal space) from the neck to the mediastinum.

Because a **child's neck** is relatively short, the **left brachiocephalic vein** may be superior to the jugular notch, where it is at risk during a **tracheostomy**.

Child's left brachiocephalic vein may lie superior to the jugular notch in the root of the neck.

VIII. Pericardium and Heart
A. Pericardium
1. Overview
   a. Sac that encloses heart, proximal segments of great arteries, and terminal segments of great veins
   b. Consists of **outer fibrous layer** and **inner serous sac**
2. **Fibrous pericardium**
   a. Tough, indistensible, fibrous external layer
   b. Fused inferiorly with **central tendon of diaphragm**
3. **Serous pericardium**
   • Closed sac that covers heart as **visceral layer** and inner surface of fibrous pericardium as **parietal layer**
4. **Pericardial cavity**
   • **Potential space** normally empty except for a small amount of lubricating fluid that allows heart to move freely as it beats

5. **Pericardial sinuses**
   - Formed by reflection of visceral layer of serous pericardium onto parietal layer at roots of great vessels entering and leaving heart
   a. **Oblique pericardial sinus** is blind pocket dorsal to left atrium formed by pericardial reflections surrounding pulmonary veins and venae cavae.
   b. **Transverse pericardial sinus**
      (1) **Passageway** between right and left sides of pericardial cavity anterior to **superior vena cava,** posterior to **ascending aorta and pulmonary trunk,** and superior to **pulmonary veins and left atrium**
      (2) Critical to **cardiothoracic surgeon** who must identify and clamp great vessels

Transverse pericardial sinus allows clamping of great vessels for cardiopulmonary bypass during cardiac surgery.

Cardiac tamponade is life-threatening rapid fluid accumulation within the pericardial cavity.

Cardiac tamponade and tension pneumothorax both cause distended neck veins and hypotension.

Cardiac tamponade is a potentially fatal compression of the heart caused by rapid accumulation of fluids within the pericardial cavity, which compromises venous return. Tamponade may be caused by blood **(hemopericardium)** or serous **pericardial effusion.** Treatment is **pericardiocentesis** using a needle introduced in the left infrasternal angle or in the left fifth intercostal space near the sternum. The intercostal approach is possible because of the **cardiac notch** of the left lung and a corresponding pleural notch. Approaching through the infrasternal angle risks damage to the diaphragm and liver, whereas approaching through the fifth intercostal space risks the internal thoracic and coronary arteries and the parietal pleura.

Pericarditis can be misdiagnosed as myocardial infarction, but friction rub is present and pain is affected by positioning.

Pericarditis may be caused by **infection** or **myocardial infarction** or be **idiopathic.** When **acute,** the patient experiences severe **substernal chest pain** that is relieved by sitting leaning forward and is worsened by lying down. Roughening of the visceral and parietal layers of serous pericardium may create **pericardial friction rub** detectable on auscultation. In **constrictive pericarditis,** the thickened, fibrotic pericardium causes incomplete filling of the cardiac chambers and dyspnea. Causes include **tuberculosis** and post–myocardial infarction pericarditis.

B. **The Heart**
   1. General structure

The heart wall is mostly a thick myocardium of cardiac muscle fibers.

   a. Heart wall consists of outer **epicardium,** middle **myocardium,** and inner **endocardium**
   b. **Skeleton of heart**
      (1) Consists of **annuli fibrosi:** four firmly connected, fibrous connective tissue rings
      (2) Provides a relatively **rigid attachment** for myocardial fiber bundles and for **pulmonary, aortic, and atrioventricular valves**

Fibrous cardiac skeleton electrically insulates atria from ventricles

      (3) Separates and **electrically insulates** myocardial fibers of atria from those of ventricles
   2. **External features (Figure 2-15)**
      a. **Base** is **posterior** aspect of heart formed largely by **left atrium**
      b. **Apex**
         - Blunt inferolateral projection formed by **left ventricle**

2-15: Chest radiograph of a normal adult female, posteroanterior view. Variations in size, position, or density of thoracic shadows may reflect pathology.

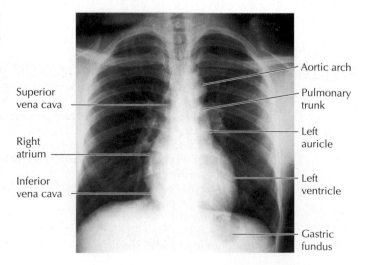

Aortic arch

Pulmonary trunk

Superior vena cava

Left auricle

Right atrium

Left ventricle

Inferior vena cava

Gastric fundus

c. **Diaphragmatic surface** is formed largely by the **left ventricle.**
d. **Sternocostal surface** is composed largely of **right ventricle** along with smaller parts of right atrium and left ventricle
e. **Right border** is formed by superior vena cava, right atrium, and inferior vena cava.
f. **Left border** is formed mainly by left ventricle with small contribution from left auricle

Although examination, palpation, percussion, and auscultation (the traditional techniques of physical diagnosis) provide key information about heart size and function, a **posteroanterior (PA) radiograph** can reveal **abnormal margins** that may indicate heart disease.

g. **Coronary sulcus** separates atria from ventricles.
3. **Internal features (Figure 2-16; Table 2-4)**
    a. **Atria (Table 2-5)**
    b. **Ventricles (Table 2-6)**
    c. **Valves**

The right ventricle is the heart chamber most likely to be injured by an anterior chest wound or blunt trauma.

Radiological left border of cardiovascular shadow is arch of aorta, pulmonary trunk, left auricle, and left ventricle **(see Figure 2-15)**

The apex beat lies to the left of the sternum in the fifth intercostal space.

Right heart failure (cor pulmonale) results from pulmonary hypertension and right ventricular hypertrophy.

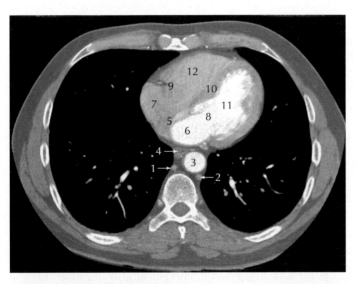

2-16: Axial CT of mediastinum. Azygos vein = 1; hemiazygos vein = 2; descending thoracic aorta = 3; esophagus = 4; interatrial septum = 5; left atrium = 6; right atrium = 7; mitral valve = 8; tricuspid valve = 9; interventricular septum = 10; left ventricle = 11; right ventricle = 12. *(From Weir, J, Abrahams, P: Imaging Atlas of Human Anatomy, 3rd ed. London, Mosby Ltd., 2003, p 95, r.)*

TABLE 2-4. HEART CHAMBERS

CHAMBER	BLOOD FROM	BLOOD TO
Right atrium	Superior and inferior venae cavae, coronary sinus	Right ventricle through tricuspid valve (right atrioventricular valve)
Right ventricle	Right atrium through tricuspid valve (right atrioventricular valve)	Pulmonary trunk through pulmonary semilunar valves
Left atrium	Pulmonary veins	Left ventricle through mitral valve (left atrioventricular valve)
Left ventricle	Left atrium through mitral valve (left atrioventricular valve)	Aorta through aortic semilunar valves

TABLE 2-5. INTERNAL FEATURES OF ATRIA

FEATURE	COMMENTS
Right atrium	Walls slightly thinner than left atrium
Sinus venarum	Smooth-walled part derived from incorporation of right horn of sinus venosus
Auricle	Corresponds to part of primitive atrium of embryonic heart; contains pectinate muscles
Crista terminalis	Separates sinus venarum from rough-walled part; superior end marks location of sinoatrial node
Fossa ovalis	Marks site of foramen ovale through which blood passes from right atrium to left atrium before birth
Valve of inferior vena cava	In embryonic heart, directs blood from inferior vena cava through foramen ovale into left atrium
Left atrium	
Smooth-walled part	Derived from incorporation of pulmonary veins
Rough-walled part (auricle)	Derived from embryonic atrium; contains pectinate muscles

TABLE 2-6. INTERNAL FEATURES OF VENTRICLES

FEATURE	COMMENTS
Common Features	
Papillary muscles	Anterior, posterior, and septal in right ventricle; anterior and posterior in left according to location of their bases
Trabeculae carneae	
Chordae tendineae	Fibrous strands connecting papillary muscles to cusps of atrioventricular valves
Right Ventricle	
Conus arteriosus (infundibulum)	Smooth-walled outflow tract to pulmonary trunk; separated from ventricle proper by supraventricular crest
Septomarginal trabecula (moderator band)	Trabecula carnea that carries fibers of right bundle branch to anterior papillary muscle
Left Ventricle	
Aortic vestibule	Smooth-walled outflow tract
Ventricle proper	Wall two to three times thicker than that of right ventricle
Chordae tendineae*	From papillary muscles connect to valve cusps

*False chordae tendineae are trabeculae carneae carrying fibers of the left bundle branch.

(1) **Tricuspid valve**
    (a) Contains **anterior, posterior,** and **septal cusps**
    (b) Allows blood flow from right atrium to right ventricle during diastole
    (c) Closes during systole and is prevented from being everted into right atrium by **papillary muscles** and **chordae tendineae** attached to its valve cusps

(2) **Mitral valve** has **anterior** and **posterior cusps.**

> Blood clots from left atrial fibrillation may cause stroke, renal failure, acute mesenteric ischemia, or myocardial infarction.

In **mitral valve prolapse,** the mitral valve everts into the left atrium when the left ventricle contracts, allowing regurgitation of blood into the left atrium. It can be inherited as an **autosomal dominant** disorder and often occurs with heritable connective tissue disorders, such as **Marfan syndrome.** Although relatively common and often benign, it may produce chest pain, shortness of breath, and cardiac arrhythmia. **Mitral stenosis** is the narrowing of the mitral orifice with left atrial enlargement due usually to recurrent **rheumatic fever** attacks **(Figure 2-17).** Frequent complications include pulmonary hypertension, atrial fibrillation, and thromboemboli. Right ventricular failure may occur.

(3) **Pulmonary valve**
    (a) Right, left, and anterior **semilunar cusps** and **pulmonary sinuses** named according to their fetal position
    (b) Forced closed by backflow of blood in pulmonary trunk during relaxation of right ventricle

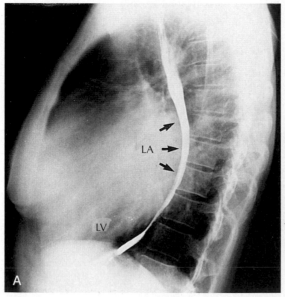
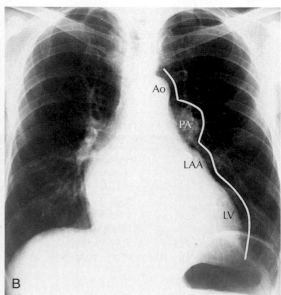

2-17: A, Mitral stenosis results in left atrial enlargement visible on lateral chest radiograph. Enlarged atrium displaces barium-filled esophagus posteriorly. **B,** Left auricle (LAA) bulges on PA chest x-ray. *(From Mettler, F A: Essentials of Radiology, 2nd ed. Philadelphia, Saunders, 2004, Figure 5-7.)*

(4) Aortic valve
  (a) Right, left, and posterior **semilunar cusps** and **aortic sinuses** named according to their fetal position
  (b) Related at **left and right aortic sinuses** to orifices of **left and right coronary arteries,** respectively
(5) **Heart sounds (Figure 2-18)**
  (a) First sound: coincides with **closure of atrioventricular valves** at start of systole
  (b) Second sound: produced by **closure of aortic and pulmonary valves** at end of systole

4. **Conducting system of heart (Figure 2-19)**
  a. Overview
    (1) Sequences atrial and ventricular contractions so atria contract together, followed by ventricles contracting together from apex toward base
    (2) Composed of **specialized cardiac muscle cells**
  b. **Sinoatrial node (SA node)**
    (1) Initiates heartbeat **(pacemaker of the heart)**
    (2) Lies in right atrial wall at **superior end of crista terminalis** near superior vena cava
    (3) Supplied by **SA nodal artery,** usually branching from **right coronary artery**
    (4) Possesses **inherent rhythmicity,** which is modified by autonomic nervous system
  c. **Atrioventricular node (AV node)**
    (1) Located in **interatrial septum** near opening of coronary sinus in right atrium
    (2) Receives impulse generated in sinoatrial node and passes it to atrioventricular bundle
    (3) Supplied by **atrioventricular nodal artery** usually branching from **right coronary artery**
  d. **Atrioventricular bundle (AV bundle)**
    (1) Begins at atrioventricular node and divides in muscular interventricular septum into **left and right bundle branches,** which comprise subendocardial **Purkinje fibers** in ventricular wall
    (2) Descends through fibrous cardiac skeleton to reach **membranous interventricular septum;** note this is the *only* connection between myocardium of atria and ventricles
    (3) Supplied mainly by **anterior interventricular branch of left coronary artery** (left anterior descending artery)

Pulmonary and aortic semilunar cusps are named for their original position in embryonic truncus arteriosus rather than the adult position.

Left and right coronary arteries originate in left and right aortic sinuses, respectively.

The sinoatrial node is the pacemaker of the heart.

AV bundle bridges fibrous skeleton of heart to electrically link atrial and ventricular myocardium

AV bundle and bundle branches are supplied by the left anterior descending artery.

Damage to the AV node or the AV bundle causes heart block with dissociation of atrial and ventricular contractions.

Septomarginal trabecula of right ventricle carries fibers of right bundle branch

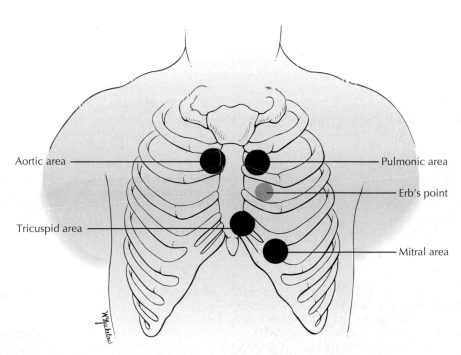

Aortic area

Tricuspid area

Pulmonic area

Erb's point

Mitral area

2-18: Surface projection of heart valve sounds. Position at which the sound of each valve is best heard *does not* correspond to the surface projection of the valve itself. *(From Swartz, M: Textbook of Physical Diagnosis: History and Examination, 5th ed. Philadelphia, Saunders, 2006, Figure 14-5.)*

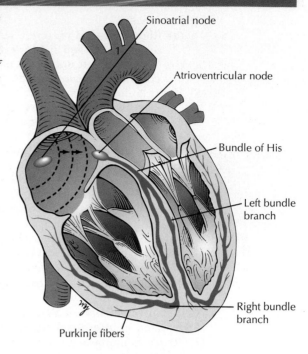

2-19: Conducting system of the heart. The sinoatrial node is the pacemaker. The atrioventricular node transmits impulses to the atrioventricular bundle (bundle of His), which divides into right and left bundle branches. A-V, atrioventricular; SA, sinoatrial. *(From Swartz, M: Textbook of Physical Diagnosis: History and Examination, 5th ed. Philadelphia, Saunders, 2006, Figure 14-2.)*

Sinoatrial node

Atrioventricular node

Bundle of His

Left bundle branch

Right bundle branch

Purkinje fibers

5. **Arterial supply to heart (Figure 2-20; Table 2-7)**
   - Blood flow through coronary arteries is greatest during diastole while myocardium is relaxed and aortic valve is closed.
   a. **Right coronary artery**
   b. **Left coronary artery (Figure 2-21)**
   c. **Variations in arterial supply**
       (1) **Right dominant** distribution is most common, with **posterior interventricular artery** arising from **right coronary artery**
       (2) **Left dominant** distribution is present when the **circumflex branch of left coronary** gives off **posterior interventricular artery**
       (3) **Balanced** distribution occurs when both right and left coronary arteries supply posterior interventricular arteries.

Myocardial infarction is the sudden occlusion of the coronary artery, producing myocardial necrosis.

Coronary artery occlusion in myocardial infarction: left anterior descending > right coronary > left circumflex artery

Sudden cardiac death in myocardial infarction is usually from ventricular fibrillation

Angina pectoris is exertion-induced chest pain relieved by rest or sublingual nitroglycerin.

Diabetic, elderly, and heart transplant patients may have silent myocardial ischemia.

Myocardial infarction is necrosis of an area of the myocardium caused by inadequate blood supply, usually due to **coronary artery thrombus formation** on top of an **atherosclerotic plaque.** Consequences depend on the location and extent of damage. **Sudden death** may result from **ventricular fibrillation** secondary to interruption of the conducting system. Most frequently, the **left anterior descending artery** is occluded. The **right coronary artery** and **circumflex branch of the left coronary artery** are the next most common sites for occlusion. **Thrombolytic enzymes** (e.g., streptokinase) are sometimes infused early to dissolve a coronary artery thrombus and limit damage.

Sites of **stenosis** can be identified by injection of a radiopaque contrast agent in **coronary angiography.** To circumvent the sites of stenosis, the patient may undergo **coronary artery bypass surgery.** The **internal thoracic artery** is freed from the thoracic wall and grafted to a blocked vessel, or the **radial artery** or **great saphenous vein** may be grafted to shunt blood from the aorta to the artery distal to the obstruction. Alternatively, the stenotic lesion may be dilated via percutaneous transluminal **coronary angioplasty.**

Angina pectoris is chest pain associated with **myocardial ischemia,** usually **during increased demand,** that occurs because coronary arteries are **functional end-arteries** without significant collateral circulation. Duration is limited, and the condition is relieved by rest or by **sublingual nitroglycerin.** In the variant known as **Prinzmetal angina,** chest pain occurs **at rest** due to **coronary artery vasospasm.** It has a characteristic **ST elevation** in an electrocardiogram during an attack.

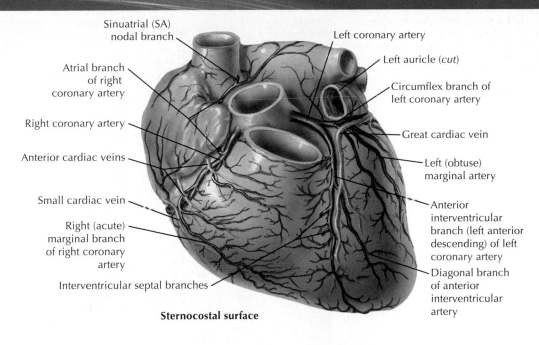

Sinuatrial (SA) nodal branch

Atrial branch of right coronary artery

Right coronary artery

Anterior cardiac veins

Small cardiac vein

Right (acute) marginal branch of right coronary artery

Interventricular septal branches

Left coronary artery

Left auricle (cut)

Circumflex branch of left coronary artery

Great cardiac vein

Left (obtuse) marginal artery

Anterior interventricular branch (left anterior descending) of left coronary artery

Diagonal branch of anterior interventricular artery

Sternocostal surface

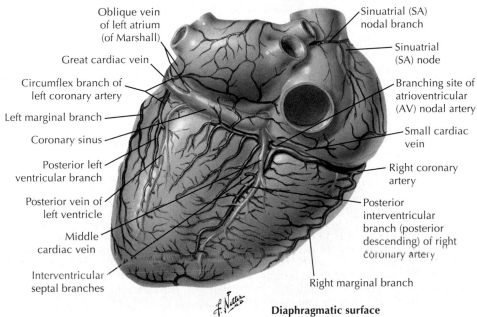

Oblique vein of left atrium (of Marshall)

Great cardiac vein

Circumflex branch of left coronary artery

Left marginal branch

Coronary sinus

Posterior left ventricular branch

Posterior vein of left ventricle

Middle cardiac vein

Interventricular septal branches

Sinuatrial (SA) nodal branch

Sinuatrial (SA) node

Branching site of atrioventricular (AV) nodal artery

Small cardiac vein

Right coronary artery

Posterior interventricular branch (posterior descending) of right coronary artery

Right marginal branch

Diaphragmatic surface

2-20: Coronary arteries and cardiac veins. Arteries to sinuatrial and atrioventricular nodes usually arise from right coronary artery. Anterior interventricular branch of left coronary artery supplies atrioventricular bundle. Most cardiac veins drain into coronary sinus, which empties into right atrium. *(From Netter, F H: Atlas of Human Anatomy, 4th ed. Philadelphia, Saunders, 2006, Plate 216.)*

TABLE 2-7. BRANCHES OF CORONARY ARTERIES

ARTERY	AREA OF HEART SUPPLIED
Right coronary	Right atrium, right ventricle, posterior part of interventricular septum
Artery to sinoatrial node	Right atrium and sinoatrial node
Artery to atrioventricular node	Atrioventricular node
Right marginal	Acute margin of right ventricle
Posterior interventricular (posterior descending)	Posterior $\frac{1}{3}$ of interventricular septum, right and left ventricles
Left coronary	Left atrium, left ventricle, most of interventricular septum
Anterior interventricular (left anterior descending)	Anterior $\frac{2}{3}$ of interventricular septum, left and right ventricles
Circumflex	Left atrium and left ventricle
Left marginal	Obtuse margin of left ventricle
Posterior ventricular	Posterior part of left ventricle

2-21: Left coronary arteriogram. Left coronary artery = 1; anterior interventricular artery = 2; diagonal arteries = 3; septal arteries = 4; circumflex artery = 5; left marginal artery = 6. *(From Weir, J, Abrahams, P: Imaging Atlas of Human Anatomy, 3rd ed. London, Mosby Ltd., 2003, p 111, a.)*

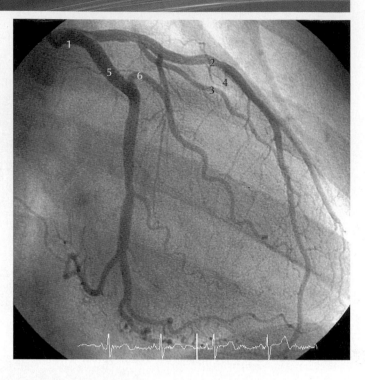

6. **Venous drainage of heart (Figure 2-22)**
    - Blood from coronary circulation mostly returns to the right atrium through the **cardiac veins;** largest cardiac vein is **coronary sinus**
    a. **Coronary sinus**
        (1) Direct continuation of **great cardiac vein**
        (2) Lies in posterior part of **coronary sulcus** and opens into **right atrium**
        (3) Receives all cardiac veins except anterior and smallest as tributaries

Coronary sinus drains cardiac veins into right atrium

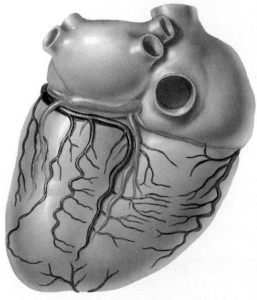

Posterior interventricular (posterior descending) branch is derived from circumflex branch of left coronary artery instead of from right coronary artery.

A

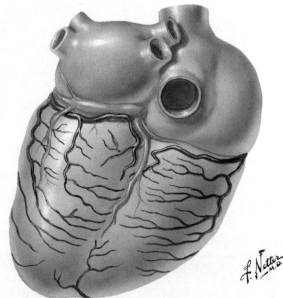

Posterior interventricular (posterior descending) branch is absent. Area supplied chiefly by small branches from circumflex branch of left coronary artery and from right coronary artery.

B

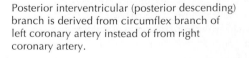

2-22: Variations in coronary arteries. **A,** Posterior interventricular artery arises from circumflex branch of left coronary artery in left dominant heart. **B,** Both right and left coronary arteries supply area of posterior interventricular sulcus in balanced (codominant) heart. *(From Netter, F H: Atlas of Human Anatomy, 4th ed. Philadelphia, Saunders, 2006, Plate 217.)*

b. **Great cardiac vein** ascends beside the **anterior interventricular artery.**

c. **Middle cardiac vein** ascends alongside the **posterior interventricular artery.**

d. **Small cardiac vein** runs along acute margin of right ventricle, paralleling **right marginal artery**

e. **Posterior vein of left ventricle** drains diaphragmatic surface of left ventricle

f. **Oblique vein of left atrium** represents remnant of embryonic **left sinus horn**

g. **Anterior cardiac veins** drain sternocostal surface of right ventricle **directly into right atrium**

h. **Smallest cardiac veins** arise in walls of heart and open directly into chambers

7. **Nerve supply of heart**
   - Originates largely in **cervical area,** attesting to original location of **cardiogenic area** at cranial end of embryonic germ disc

   a. **Sympathetic innervation**
      (1) Distributed to **conducting system** and **coronary arteries**
      (2) Derived mostly from **cardiac branches of cervical sympathetic ganglia** with some **thoracic cardiac nerves**

   b. **Parasympathetic innervation**
      (1) Decreases heart rate and force of contraction
      (2) Derived from cervical and thoracic cardiac branches of **vagus nerves**

   c. **Visceral afferent fibers traveling with sympathetic fibers**
      (1) Pass through cervical cardiac nerves and down cervical sympathetic trunk to cell bodies in **posterior root ganglia** of upper thoracic spinal nerves
      (2) Account for **referred pain from heart**

> **Pain from angina pectoris or myocardial infarction** is carried by **visceral afferent fibers that accompany sympathetic nerve fibers** to spinal cord segments **T1-5.** Cardiac pain is often **referred** to the **substernal and left pectoral regions, left shoulder,** and **medial side of the left arm** because cutaneous nerves supplying those dermatomes enter the same spinal cord segments. It also may be referred to neck, face, or right upper extremity because of the heart's early development in cardiogenic and neck regions.

   d. **Visceral afferent fibers traveling with parasympathetic fibers**
      - Provide sensory input for important **cardiac reflexes**

C. **Development of the Heart (Figure 2-23)**
   1. Overview
      a. Begins in splanchnic mesoderm of **cardiogenic area** at end of week 3

Sympathetic innervation increases heart rate and force of contraction.

Cardiac pain is referred when visceral afferent fibers from the heart enter the same spinal cord segments as somatic afferent fibers from involved dermatomes.

Parasympathetic innervation decreases heart rate and force of contraction.

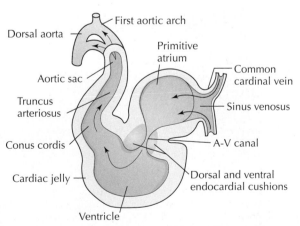

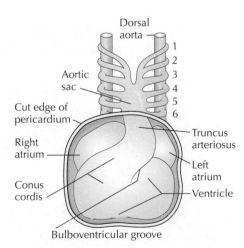

2-23: A, Blood flow through the primordial heart (week 4). **B,** Ventral view of the heart and aortic arches (week 5). Not all aortic arches are present at the same time. The heart tube forms the bulboventricular loop consisting of five dilatations: sinus venosus, primitive atrium, ventricle, conus cordis, and truncus arteriosus. All except sinus venosus are subsequently partitioned. *Arrows,* blood flow. *Numbers,* aortic arches.

b. Involves fusion of two endocardial tubes into single **heart tube** that bends on itself, forming U-shaped **bulboventricular loop** that includes one atrium and one ventricle

c. Includes partitioning of heart tube in weeks 4 and 5

2. **Partitioning of atrioventricular canal**

a. Accomplished by growth of **endocardial cushions** in dorsal and ventral walls of atrioventricular canal and their fusion

b. Divides common canal into **right** and **left atrioventricular canals**

3. **Partitioning of atrium and related defects (Figure 2-24)**

a. **Septum primum** is crescent-shaped membrane that grows into atrium from posterosuperior wall to fuse with endocardial cushions of atrioventricular canal

b. **Ostium primum** is opening between primitive atria that is gradually closed by growth of septum primum

c. **Ostium secundum** is opening created by programmed cell death in **septum primum,** providing new right-to-left shunt between atria

d. **Septum secundum**

(1) Second crescent-shaped membrane that grows from roof of atrium along right side of septum primum

(2) Stops growth and *does not* completely partition atrial cavity

e. **Foramen ovale**

(1) Opening at inferior margin of septum secundum resulting from its failure to fuse with endocardial cushions of atrioventricular canal (septum intermedium)

(2) Along with ostium secundum allows continued **right-to-left shunt**

f. **Atrial septal defect (Figure 2-25)**

(1) Occurs in area of **foramen ovale** and is relatively common

Fetal foramen ovale allows oxygenated blood returning from placenta to be shunted from right to left atrium

Fossa ovalis of right atrium marks the site of the fetal foramen ovale.

Probe patent foramen ovale occurs in 25% of the population but is clinically insignificant.

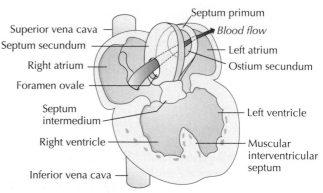

2-24: Partitioning of atria and interatrial shunting (week 7). Interatrial septum is formed by septum primum and septum secundum. A right-to-left shunt exists through foramen ovale until birth, when it is closed by fusion of valve of foramen ovale (remnant of septum primum) with septum secundum.

Superior vena cava —
Septum secundum —
Right atrium —
Foramen ovale —
Septum intermedium —
Right ventricle —
Inferior vena cava —

Septum primum
Blood flow
Left atrium
Ostium secundum
Left ventricle
Muscular interventricular septum

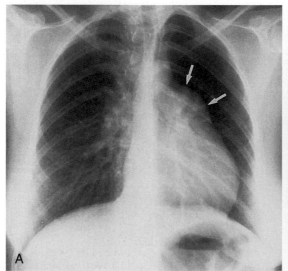
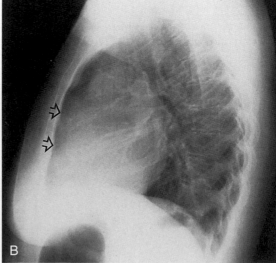

2-25: Atrial septal defect. **A,** The left-to-right shunt increases pulmonary blood flow with enlargement of the pulmonary trunk (*arrows*) in this PA radiograph. **B,** The extra blood flow causes right ventricular enlargement, which fills the anterior mediastinum (*open arrows*) in a lateral x-ray. (*From Mettler, F A: Essentials of Radiology, 2nd ed. Philadelphia, Saunders, 2004, Figure 5-16.*)

(2) May be **asymptomatic if small,** but right ventricle may **hypertrophy** with larger septal defects

(3) May result from **inadequate development of septum secundum** or **excessive resorption of septum primum**

4. **Partitioning of ventricle and related defects (Figure 2-26)**

   a. **Muscular interventricular septum** formation begins as muscular ridge in week 4 with increase in height due to expansion of ventricles on each side but stops in week 7, leaving septum incomplete

   b. **Membranous interventricular septum** formed by fusion of **truncoconal ridges** with **muscular interventricular septum** and extension from **endocardial cushion,** thus completing partitioning of ventricles by week 8

   c. **Ventricular septal defect**

      (1) Most common **congenital cardiac defect,** occurring most often in **membranous interventricular septum**

      (2) Results from failure of **truncoconal ridges** and **endocardial cushion** to fuse with **muscular interventricular septum**

Atrial septal defects and **ventricular septal defects** result in **left-to-right shunting** of blood after birth due to higher pressures on the left side of the heart. Over time, **pulmonary hypertension** results from large septal defects followed by **right ventricular hypertrophy** and potential failure **(see Figure 2-25).** Eventually pulmonary vascular resistance increases enough that the **shunt reverses to become right-to-left,** producing **late cyanosis** due to unoxygenated blood in the systemic circulation **(Eisenmenger syndrome).**

5. **Partitioning of conus cordis and truncus arteriosus and related defects**

   a. Overview

      (1) Accomplished by **fusion of paired truncoconal ridges** to form **aorticopulmonary septum (see Figure 2-26)**

      (2) Occurs in **spiral,** ensuring that **aorta** and **pulmonary trunk** twist around each other in a helix **(see Figure 2-28, B and D)**

   b. **Persistent truncus arteriosus**

      (1) Results from complete **failure in development of truncoconal ridges** and related membranous interventricular septum

      (2) Allows blood from both ventricles to leave heart through a **common vessel** with **partially oxygenated blood** passing both to lungs and systemic circulation

         • It is sometimes associated with the DiGeorge syndrome (absent parathyroid glands and thymus).

   c. **Transposition of great arteries**

      (1) Results from **failure of truncoconal ridges to spiral** as they partition outflow tract

      (2) Characterized by **aorta** arising from **right ventricle** and **pulmonary trunk** arising from **left ventricle**

Side notes (right margin):

Atrial septal defect results from excessive resorption of septum primum or underdeveloped septum secundum

Ventricular septal defects are the most common congenital heart defect and usually involve membranous interventricular septum.

Atrial septal defects and ventricular septal defects result in postnatal left-to-right shunts.

Eisenmenger syndrome is reversal of congenital left-to-right shunt when pulmonary hypertension develops

Right-to-left shunt of persistent truncus arteriosus, transposition of great arteries, and tetralogy of Fallot causes early cyanosis.

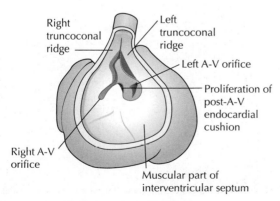
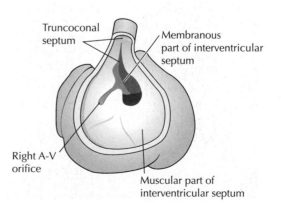

2-26: Formation (**A** and **B**) of membranous interventricular septum. A-V, atrioventricular.

(3) Must be accompanied by **ventricular or atrial septal defect** or a **patent ductus arteriosus** to be compatible with life

d. **Tetralogy of Fallot (Figure 2-27)**

(1) Caused primarily by **unequal partitioning** of outflow tract by **truncoconal ridges**

(2) Combines four defects: **pulmonary stenosis, ventricular septal defect, overriding aorta,** and **right ventricular hypertrophy**

(3) Associated with **early cyanosis** of lips and fingernails **(blue baby)** and assumption of a **squatting posture,** which increases peripheral vascular resistance and decreases the right-to-left shunt through the ventricular septal defect

D. **Aortic Arch Derivatives and Related Anomalies (Figure 2-28)**

- Six pairs of **aortic arches** usually develop, one for each pair of **pharyngeal arches,** but not all are present simultaneously, and the fifth pair may be absent.

1. **Derivatives of aortic arches (Table 2-8)**
2. **Patent ductus arteriosus (PDA)**

a. Results from **failure of ductus arteriosus to close after birth,** alone or in combination with other cardiac defects

b. Will cause **blood flow from aorta to pulmonary artery** because of considerable difference in pressure between the two vessels

c. May cause **obstructive pulmonary vascular disease** because of increased blood flow

Tetralogy of Fallot: pulmonary stenosis, right ventricular hypertrophy, overriding aorta, and ventricular septal defect

Tetralogy of Fallot causes boot-shaped heart on x-ray due to right ventricular hypertrophy.

Ductus arteriosus normally closes at birth to become ligamentum arteriosum.

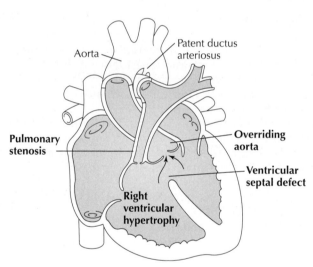

2-27: Tetralogy of Fallot. *Arrows,* blood flow.

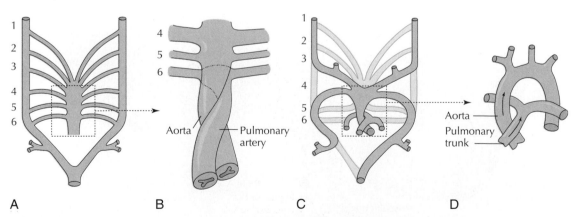

2-28: Development of great arteries of the thorax. The third pair of aortic arches contributes to the common and internal carotid arteries; the fourth right arch contributes to the right subclavian artery; and the fourth left arch contributes to the arch of the aorta. The sixth pair forms the proximal part of the pulmonary artery. **A** and **C,** Six pairs of arches develop, but not all are present simultaneously. **B,** Enlargement showing spiral partitioning. **C,** Parts of dorsal aortae and aortic arches normally disappear (*light red*). **D,** Enlargement showing final relationships. *Solid arrows,* blood flow. *Numbers,* aortic arches.

TABLE 2-8. THORACIC DERIVATIVES OF AORTIC ARCHES

AORTIC ARCH	DERIVATIVES
Third pair	Proximal part forms common carotid artery; distal part forms internal carotid artery
Fourth pair	Right arch forms proximal part of right subclavian artery; left arch forms part of arch of aorta
Fifth pair	No derivatives
Sixth pair	Right arch forms proximal part of right pulmonary artery; left arch forms proximal part of left pulmonary artery and ductus arteriosus

3. **Coarctation of aorta (Figure 2-29)**
   a. Relatively common malformation characterized by **constriction** of aorta proximal **(preductal)** or distal **(postductal)** to **ductus arteriosus**; preductal coarctation occurs with PDA
   b. Requires development of **extensive collateral circulation** in **postductal coarctation** to deliver blood into descending aorta; the preductal type requires early surgery for survival
   c. May cause characteristic **rib notching** on radiograph from enlarged **intercostal arteries**
   d. Results in **increased blood pressure in upper extremities, neck, and head,** with increased risk of cerebrovascular accident

E. **Fetal circulation and changes at birth (Figure 2-30; Table 2-9)**

IX. **Blood Vessels and the Nerves of the Thorax**
   A. **Blood Vessels of the Thorax**
      1. **Thoracic aorta and its branches (Figure 2-31)**
         • For descriptive purposes, the **aorta is divided into four parts:** three are in the thorax, and the fourth is the abdominal aorta.
         a. **Ascending aorta**
            (1) Begins within pericardial sac at aortic valve and ascends behind sternum to end in arch of aorta at level of **sternal angle**
            (2) Only right and left coronary arteries as branches
         b. **Arch of aorta**
            (1) Lies within **superior mediastinum** in front of **trachea,** arching over right pulmonary artery and left main bronchus
            (2) Gives rise to **brachiocephalic, left common carotid,** and **left subclavian arteries** that ascend in relation to **trachea (see Figures 2-3 and 2-4)**
            (3) May give rise to **thyroid ima artery** that ascends in midline of neck, where it may be damaged during **thyroid surgery** or **tracheotomy**
            (4) Prone to **aneurysms,** which may be revealed by **pulsatile swelling at jugular notch** or hoarseness

Preductal coarctation of aorta is common in Turner syndrome (45,X) patients.

Postductal coarctation of the aorta is compatible with survival into adulthood, but the preductal type requires early surgery.

Postductal coarctation of the aorta causes characteristic rib notching on x-rays, hypertension in upper extremities, and hypotension in lower extremities.

The umbilical vein may be catheterized in a neonate for transfusion.

Parts of aorta: ascending aorta, aortic arch, descending thoracic aorta, and abdominal aorta

A thoracic aortic aneurysm may cause superior vena cava syndrome, dyspnea, dysphagia, or hoarseness.

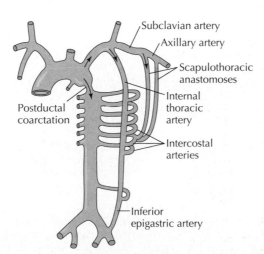

2-29: Postductal coarctation of aorta and resulting collateral circulation necessary to deliver blood into the descending aorta. *Arrows,* blood flow.

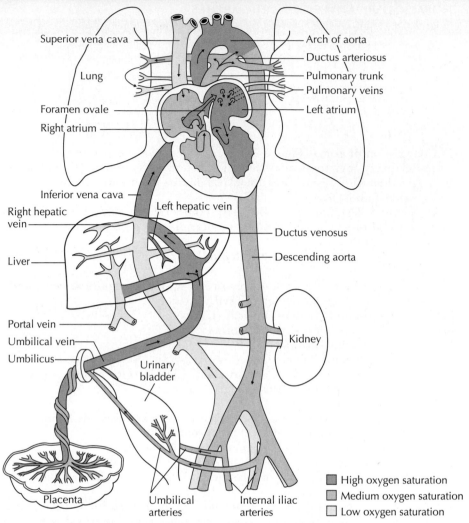

2-30: Fetal circulation. Ductus venosus shunts most blood past the liver, and the foramen ovale and the ductus arteriosus act as shunts to bypass pulmonary circulation. All of these shunts normally close at or shortly after birth, as do the umbilical vein and distal part of umbilical arteries. *Arrows,* blood flow.

TABLE 2-9. FEATURES OF FETAL CIRCULATION

STRUCTURE	LOCATION	FUNCTION	COMMENT
Umbilical vein	Connects placenta to fetal liver through umbilical cord	Carries oxygenated, nutrient-rich blood from placenta to fetus	Becomes round ligament of liver (ligamentum teres hepatis)
Ductus venosus	Venous shunt within liver connecting umbilical vein with inferior vena cava	Bypasses liver, carrying oxygenated blood directly to inferior vena cava	Becomes ligamentum venosum
Foramen ovale	Opening between right atrium and left atrium	Acts as shunt to bypass pulmonary circulation	Closes at birth to become fossa ovalis
Ductus arteriosus	Connects left pulmonary artery to arch of aorta	Acts as shunt to bypass pulmonary circulation	Closes shortly after birth to become ligamentum arteriosum
Umbilical artery	Connects fetal circulation (internal iliac artery) to placenta	Carries deoxygenated and nutrient-depleted blood from fetus to placenta	Atrophies to become medial umbilical ligament

Aortic aneurysms are localized **dilatations** of the aorta. They usually result from **atherosclerosis** or **cystic medial degeneration** (e.g., in Marfan syndrome), but **syphilis** was once a common cause. Many thoracic aneurysms are **asymptomatic** at diagnosis, but symptoms may result from **aortic regurgitation** into the left ventricle, **thromboemboli,** or a **mass effect.** The aneurysm may compress the superior vena

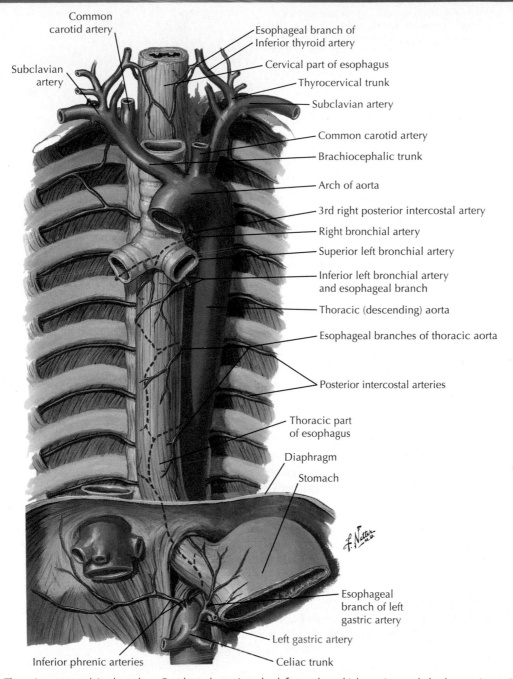

Common carotid artery

Subclavian artery

Esophageal branch of Inferior thyroid artery

Cervical part of esophagus

Thyrocervical trunk

Subclavian artery

Common carotid artery

Brachiocephalic trunk

Arch of aorta

3rd right posterior intercostal artery

Right bronchial artery

Superior left bronchial artery

Inferior left bronchial artery and esophageal branch

Thoracic (descending) aorta

Esophageal branches of thoracic aorta

Posterior intercostal arteries

Thoracic part of esophagus

Diaphragm

Stomach

Esophageal branch of left gastric artery

Left gastric artery

Celiac trunk

Inferior phrenic arteries

2-31: Thoracic aorta and its branches. Esophageal arteries, the left two bronchial arteries, and the lower nine pairs of posterior intercostal arteries branch from the thoracic aorta. The right bronchial artery often arises from the third right posterior intercostal artery. The first two posterior intercostal arteries on each side arise from the supreme intercostal branch of the costocervical trunk, not the aorta. *(From Netter, F H: Atlas of Human Anatomy, 4th ed. Philadelphia, Saunders, 2006, Plate 237.)*

cava to cause **superior vena cava syndrome,** trachea or main stem bronchus to cause **dyspnea,** the esophagus to cause **dysphagia,** or the left recurrent laryngeal nerve to cause **hoarseness. Pulsatile swelling** may occur at the suprasternal notch. **Chest pain** and interscapular **back pain** may be present. **Rupture** results in usually fatal **hemorrhage.**

Blood may enter a tear in the intima in **aortic dissection** and erode between layers of the vessel wall with or without aneurysmal enlargement. Death often occurs from **hemorrhage.**

Thoracic aortic aneurysms are less common than abdominal aortic aneurysms.

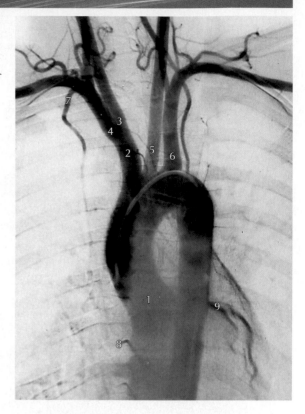

2-32: Subtraction aortogram, left anterior oblique image. Ascending aorta = 1; brachiocephalic trunk = 2; right common carotid artery = 3; right subclavian artery = 4; left common carotid artery = 5; left subclavian artery = 6; internal thoracic artery = 7; intercostal artery = 8; left coronary artery = 9. *(From Weir, J, Abrahams, P: Imaging Atlas of Human Anatomy, 3rd ed. London, Mosby Ltd., 2003, p 115, b.)*

c. **Descending thoracic aorta (Figures 2-16 and 2-32)**
  • Descends in **posterior mediastinum** to become abdominal aorta at aortic hiatus. Important **branches** include:
    (1) Lower nine pairs of **posterior intercostal arteries** and **subcostal arteries**
    (2) Two or more **bronchial arteries**
    (3) Two to five **esophageal arteries**

2. **Other arteries of thorax**
  a. **Supreme (superior) intercostal artery** arises from **costocervical trunk** of subclavian artery to supply first two **posterior intercostal arteries**
  b. **Internal thoracic artery** arises in root of neck and descends vertically just lateral to sternum. **Branches** include:
    (1) **Anterior intercostal arteries** to first five or six intercostal spaces
    (2) **Musculophrenic artery,** a terminal branch to the diaphragm and seventh to ninth intercostal spaces
    (3) **Superior epigastric artery,** a terminal branch descending in the rectus sheath to supply abdominal wall and anastomose with inferior epigastric artery

3. **Great systemic veins**
  a. **Right brachiocephalic vein**
    (1) Begins in union of **right internal jugular** and **subclavian veins**
    (2) Receives **right internal thoracic vein** and **right supreme intercostal vein** as tributaries
  b. **Left brachiocephalic vein**
    (1) Begins in union of **left internal jugular** and **subclavian veins** (left venous angle)
    (2) Descends obliquely to right behind manubrium
    (3) Receives **left internal thoracic vein, left supreme and superior intercostal veins,** and **inferior thyroid veins** as tributaries
  c. **Superior vena cava**
    (1) Formed by union of **right and left brachiocephalic veins**
    (2) Enters **right atrium** behind right third costal cartilage
    (3) Receives arch of **azygos vein** before it enters pericardial sac

The left and right brachiocephalic veins unite to form the superior vena cava.

Compression by bronchogenic carcinoma or thrombosis from a central venous catheter may cause superior vena cava syndrome.

In **superior vena cava syndrome,** an obstructed superior vena cava may lead to **edema and venous distension** in the head, neck, and upper extremities. **Laryngeal** and **cerebral edema** may cause dyspnea, hoarseness, and mental status changes. The syndrome most often results from compression of the superior vena cava by a tumor, usually **bronchogenic carcinoma,** but may be secondary to **thrombosis from a central venous catheter.**

> Superior vena cava syndrome results in head, neck, and upper extremity edema and jugular venous distention.

A **left superior vena cava** results from **persistence of the left anterior and common cardinal veins** and degeneration of the right anterior and common cardinal veins. The left superior vena cava drains into the right atrium via the coronary sinus.

> Left superior vena cava results from persistent left anterior and common cardinal veins.

  d. **Inferior vena cava**
      (1) Formed in abdomen by union of **common iliac veins**
      (2) Passes through diaphragm at level of T8 and pierces pericardial sac to end in right atrium
  e. **Development of great systemic veins (Figure 2-33)**
      (1) **Left brachiocephalic vein** forms from **anastomosis** between **anterior cardinal veins.**
      (2) **Proximal part of inferior vena cava** is derived from proximal part of **right vitelline vein.**
      (3) **Superior vena cava** forms from **right anterior and common cardinal veins.**
  4. **Azygos system of veins (Figures 2-16 and 2-34)**
      a. Drains most blood from **posterior thoracic wall**
      b. Consists of **variable longitudinal veins** lying along thoracic vertebral bodies
      c. Forms **caval-caval anastomosis** between inferior vena cava and superior vena cava if either is obstructed
      d. Communicates with **vertebral venous plexus**

> The azygos system provides venous return to the heart in vena caval obstruction.

B. **Nerves of the Thorax**
  1. **Phrenic nerves**
      a. Arise in neck from anterior rami of spinal nerves **C3,4,5**
      b. Supply **sole motor innervation** to respiratory diaphragm
      c. Transmit **referred pain** from pericardium, mediastinal pleura, and pleural and peritoneal coverings of central diaphragm to base of neck and **shoulder**
      d. Descend through **middle mediastinum** between fibrous pericardium and mediastinal pleura

> The phrenic nerve transmits referred pain to the shoulder from the pericardium or from the pleura or peritoneum covering the diaphragm.

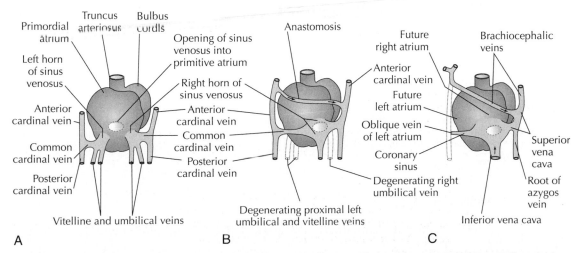

2-33: Remodeling of venous return to the heart. The anterior cardinal veins and anastomosis between them **(B)** form the brachiocephalic veins and the superior vena cava **(C).** The left sinus horn **(A and B)** forms the oblique vein of the left atrium and coronary sinus **(C).** Vitelline veins form the hepatic veins and portal vein. The proximal part of the inferior vena cava develops from the proximal part of the right vitelline vein. *Arrows,* blood flow.

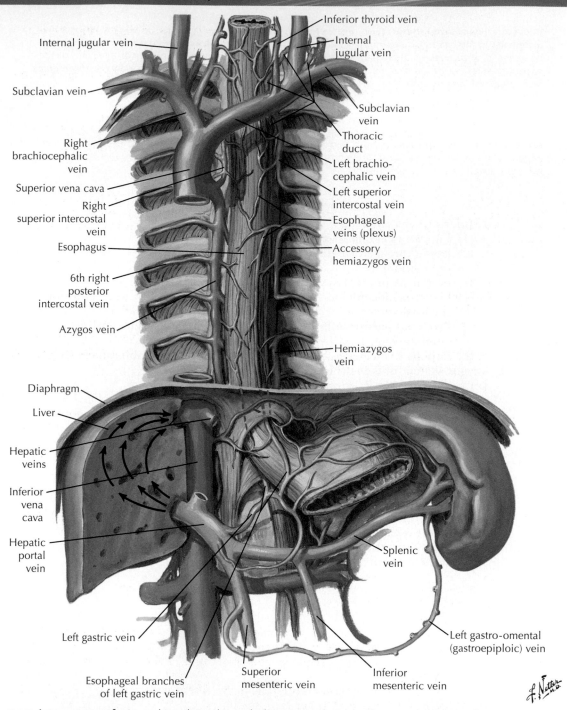

2-34: Azygos system of veins and its relationship to the hepatic portal system. The azygos vein drains the posterior walls of the thorax and abdomen and some mediastinal viscera. Tributaries include hemiazygos, accessory hemiazygos, and right posterior intercostal veins. Anastomoses between esophageal tributaries of the azygos and portal systems of veins become important in portal hypertension (discussed in Chapter 3). *(From Netter, F H: Atlas of Human Anatomy, 4th ed. Philadelphia, Saunders, 2006, Plate 238.)*

2. **Vagus nerves**
   a. Overview
      (1) Supply **parasympathetic** and **general visceral afferent** innervation to thoracic viscera
      (2) **Parasympathetic preganglionic** cell bodies located in **brainstem** and **postganglionic** cell bodies in **terminal ganglia** in autonomic plexuses or in wall of organ supplied
      (3) Include **visceral afferent fibers** from cell bodies in **vagal ganglia**

b. **Right vagus nerve**
   - Descends on right side of trachea, **posterior to root of right lung,** and onto posterior esophagus, contributing to **esophageal plexus**

c. **Left vagus nerve**
   - Descends across left side of aortic arch, **posterior to root of left lung,** and onto anterior esophagus, contributing to **esophageal plexus**

d. **Branches of vagus in thorax**
   (1) **Branches to cardiac, pulmonary, and esophageal plexuses**
   (2) **Left recurrent laryngeal nerve** curves below arch of aorta to left of **ligamentum arteriosum** and ascends between trachea and esophagus

A **hoarse voice** may be the first sign of injury to the **left recurrent laryngeal nerve,** which can be damaged by an **aortic arch aneurysm,** bronchogenic or esophageal **carcinoma,** surgery on a patent ductus arteriosus, a **Pancoast tumor,** or an **enlarged left atrium** (e.g., in advanced mitral stenosis) that pushes the left pulmonary artery against the aortic arch.

Persistent hoarseness may indicate an intrathoracic left recurrent laryngeal nerve lesion.

3. **Autonomic plexuses of thorax (Table 2-10)**
   a. Contain **sympathetic and parasympathetic fibers** that are motor to **cardiac muscle, smooth muscle,** and **glands of thoracic viscera**
   b. Also contain accompanying **general visceral afferent fibers** that serve as sensory limb of autonomic reflex arcs; GVA fibers accompanying **sympathetic fibers** carry **pain from thoracic viscera**

4. **Sympathetic nerves of thorax**
   a. Overview
      (1) Contain **postganglionic sympathetic fibers** from cell bodies located in thoracic **sympathetic chain ganglia;** preganglionic cell bodies are in spinal cord intermediolateral cell column
      (2) Contain **visceral afferent fibers** with cell bodies located in **posterior root ganglia** of thoracic spinal nerves
   b. **Thoracic sympathetic trunk**
      (1) Descends along sides of vertebral bodies
      (2) Has 11 or 12 **sympathetic ganglia (paravertebral ganglia)** corresponding to spinal nerves, with first thoracic ganglion often fused with inferior cervical ganglion to form **cervicothoracic (stellate) ganglion**
   c. **Rami communicantes** (see Chapter 1)
   d. **Visceral branches from upper five thoracic ganglia**
      - Distribute through aortic, pulmonary, and esophageal plexuses
   e. **Thoracic splanchnic nerves**
      (1) Overview
         (a) Visceral branches of T5-T12 sympathetic ganglia to **abdominal organs**
         (b) Contain **preganglionic sympathetic fibers,** which pass through their respective paravertebral ganglia to synapse in abdominal **prevertebral ganglia**
         (c) Carry general **visceral afferent nerve fibers** with cell bodies in **T5-T12 posterior root ganglia**

Pain from thoracic viscera is carried only in visceral afferent nerve fibers accompanying sympathetic fibers.

Paravertebral ganglia: sympathetic chain ganglia. Prevertebral ganglia: ganglia at major branches of abdominal aorta

TABLE 2-10. AUTONOMIC PLEXUSES OF THORAX

PLEXUS	LOCATION	COMMENTS
Superficial cardiac	Below arch of aorta	Communicates with deep cardiac plexus and left coronary plexus
Deep cardiac	Between arch of aorta and bifurcation of trachea	Contributes to coronary, pulmonary, and aortic plexuses
Coronary	Along coronary arteries	Provides innervation to heart
Pulmonary	Divided into anterior and posterior plexuses at roots of lungs	Constitutes innervation of lungs
Esophageal	Anterior and posterior surfaces of esophagus	At lower end of esophagus forms anterior and posterior vagal trunks

TABLE 2-11. LYMPHATIC DRAINAGE OF THORAX

STRUCTURE	LOCATION	AFFERENTS	EFFERENTS
Bronchomediastinal lymph trunk	Formed in superior mediastinum	Parasternal, brachiocephalic, and tracheobronchial nodes	Thoracic duct or subclavian vein on left side and right lymphatic duct or subclavian vein on right side
Thoracic duct	Begins at cisterna chyli, ascends through aortic hiatus and posterior and superior mediastina to end in root of neck	Body below respiratory diaphragm; lower right and all left posterior intercostal nodes; left jugular, subclavian, and bronchomediastinal lymph trunks	Union of left internal jugular and subclavian veins (left venous angle)

(2) Greater splanchnic nerves arise from **T5-T9** ganglia.
(3) **Lesser splanchnic nerves** arise from **T10-T11** ganglia.
(4) **Least splanchnic nerves** arise from **T12** ganglia.

Greater, lesser, and least splanchnic nerves carry preganglionic sympathetic fibers to the abdominal prevertebral ganglia.

C. Lymphatic Drainage of Thorax (Table 2-11)

Chylothorax may result from a thoracic duct injury in the thorax.

Thoracic duct drains the body below the diaphragm, the left half of the body above the diaphragm, and the lower right intercostal region.

Surgery, trauma, or **malignancy** may injure the **thoracic duct** as it ascends through the posterior or superior mediastinum, which can cause lymphatic fluid to enter the pleural cavity **(chylothorax). Blockage** of the thoracic duct by a tumor often causes no signs and symptoms because of alternative routes for lymphatic drainage to the venous system.

X. Esophagus and Thymus
  A. Esophagus
    1. Overview
      a. Muscular tube that begins in neck as **continuation of pharynx** and ends in abdomen, where it **joins stomach**
      b. Voluntary skeletal muscle superiorly and involuntary smooth muscle inferiorly
      c. Follows a **curved path in thorax**: starts left of midline, is pushed right by aortic arch, then inclines back toward left near diaphragm
    2. **Barium swallow** demonstrates the following **thoracic esophageal constrictions:**
      a. Origin at **cricopharyngeus** part of inferior pharyngeal constrictor
      b. Point where esophagus is crossed by arch of aorta and left main bronchus
      c. Point behind left atrium **when left atrium is enlarged (see Figure 2-17)**
      d. Point where esophagus passes through diaphragm (esophageal hiatus at T10)

Esophageal constrictions are likely sites for swallowed **foreign bodies** to lodge and for **strictures** to develop after swallowing corrosive fluids. In **left-sided heart failure, barium swallow** may help to assess the size of the left atrium.

An esophageal perforation from iatrogenic or other injury may produce fatal mediastinitis.

    3. **Relationships in superior mediastinum (see Figures 2-3 and 2-4)**
      • **To right:** only terminal part of azygos vein, easing surgical approach to midesophagus from right
    4. **Relationships in posterior mediastinum (see Figure 2-16)**
      a. **Anterior:** left main bronchus, pericardium, and left atrium
      b. **Left above** and **posterior below:** descending thoracic aorta
    5. **Blood vessels of esophagus**
      a. Arterial supply is from **inferior thyroid** artery to its upper third, **esophageal** branches of **aorta** to its middle third, and **left gastric** and **inferior phrenic** arteries to its lower third
      b. Venous drainage is to **inferior thyroid veins** in upper third, **azygos vein** in middle third, and **left gastric vein** in lower third

In **portal hypertension, esophageal varices** develop at **portocaval anastomosis** in the lower esophagus between tributaries of the **left gastric vein** of the hepatic portal system and the **azygos vein** of the superior vena caval system. They may be the source of a fatal **hemorrhage.**

Esophageal varices resulting from portal hypertension may cause a fatal hemorrhage.

6. **Nerve supply of esophagus**
   a. To voluntary muscle of **upper esophagus** is from **recurrent laryngeal nerves**
   b. To middle and lower esophagus is via **esophageal plexus**
      (1) **Sympathetic fibers** are primarily **vasomotor.**
      (2) Vagal **parasympathetic fibers** primarily stimulate **peristalsis** and **visceral afferent fibers** are concerned with **reflex activity.**

Achalasia of the esophagus is the **failure of the lower esophageal sphincter to relax** due to **degeneration of the postganglionic parasympathetic neurons** in the wall of the esophagus (Auerbach plexus). The passage of food is **obstructed,** resulting in **dysphagia** and **distention of the esophagus.** On the radiograph of a barium swallow, there is a characteristic **"bird beak" appearance** at the lower esophageal sphincter. **Aspiration pneumonia** may result from regurgitation of food, and there is an increased risk of **esophageal carcinoma.**

Achalasia shows a bird's beak deformity at the lower esophageal sphincter on a radiograph of barium swallow.

Lymphatic drainage from the upper esophagus is to **deep cervical nodes** of the neck. The middle esophagus drains to the **posterior mediastinal nodes.** From the lower third of the esophagus, lymphatic drainage is through the esophageal hiatus to the **left gastric nodes** of the abdomen. Therefore, **esophageal cancer** may metastasize in multiple directions.

B. **Thymus**
   1. Bilobed lymphoid organ lying behind sternum in superior mediastinum (**see Figure 2-3)**
   2. Source of **T-lymphocytes** and crucial to establish **immune competence** after birth
   3. **Largest at birth** relative to body size and continues to grow until **puberty,** when it begins **involution** and is mostly replaced by fat
   4. Supplied by branches of **internal thoracic** and **inferior thyroid arteries**
   5. Venous drainage largely to **left brachiocephalic vein**

The thymus undergoes involution after puberty.

The thymus may develop **thymic hyperplasia** or a **thymoma,** which is a tumor often associated with immune disorders such as **myasthenia gravis.** The phrenic nerves are in danger during a thymectomy.

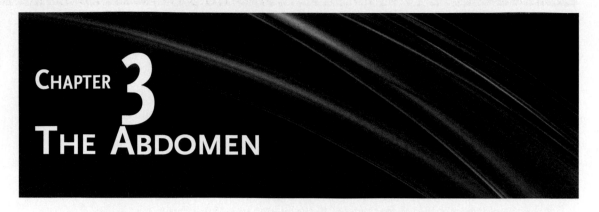

I. Anterior Abdominal Wall
   A. **Surface Projections of Abdominal Organs (Figures 3-1 and 3-2; Table 3-1)**
   B. **Fasciae of Anterior Abdominal Wall**
      1. **Superficial layer of superficial fascia** (Camper fascia)
         • **Fatty layer** continuous with superficial fascia of thorax and thigh
      2. **Deep layer of superficial fascia** (Scarpa fascia)
         a. **Membranous layer** continuous with superficial fascia of penis, dartos layer of scrotum, and superficial perineal fascia (Colles fascia)
         b. Laterally fuses with **fascia lata** of thigh
         c. Forms **fundiform ligament of penis** in lower midline

Membranous layer of superficial abdominal fascia is continuous with corresponding layer of penis, scrotum, and perineum.

Extravasated urine from a ruptured penile urethra may accumulate deep to Scarpa's fascia.

Anterolateral abdominal incisions penetrate the skin, superficial and deep fasciae, muscle layers, transversalis fascia, extraperitoneal connective tissue, and parietal peritoneum.

> When incising the anterior abdominal wall lateral to the rectus abdominis, the blade penetrates successively the skin, the superficial fascia, the deep fascia, the external and internal oblique and transversus abdominis muscle layers, the transversalis fascia, the extraperitoneal connective tissue, and the parietal peritoneum.

> When suturing lower abdominal wall incisions, surgeons may include the **membranous layer of superficial fascia** for added strength.

The inguinal canal is an oblique passage through the abdominal wall connecting the deep and superficial inguinal rings.

   C. **Muscles of Anterior Abdominal Wall (Figure 3-3, A)**
      1. Connect rib cage to hip bone as three large flat sheets: external and internal abdominal oblique and transversus abdominis
      2. Innervated by thoracoabdominal (intercostal T7-T11), subcostal (T12), and iliohypogastric and ilioinguinal (L1) nerves
   D. **Formation of Rectus Sheath (Figure 3-3, B)**
   E. **Inguinal Region (Figure 3-4; Table 3-2)**
      1. **Inguinal canal**
         a. Joins **deep and superficial inguinal rings** above medial half of **inguinal ligament**, transmitting spermatic cord in male and round ligament of uterus in female

Persistent processus vaginalis predisposes to indirect inguinal hernia and hydrocele development.

The canal of Nuck may contain a herniated ovary and a uterine tube.

The inguinal ligament is the rolled-under inferior border of the external oblique aponeurosis between the ASIS and the pubic tubercle.

         b. May contain **persistent processus vaginalis** in male that will predispose to **indirect inguinal hernia** and will frequently form a **hydrocele of the testis**
         c. May contain persistent **processus vaginalis in female,** termed the **canal of Nuck,** predisposing to development of **indirect inguinal hernia**
         d. **Boundaries**
            (1) **Roof:** arching fibers of transversus abdominis and internal abdominal oblique muscles
            (2) **Floor:** medial half of inguinal ligament and lacunar ligament
            (3) **Anterior wall:** external oblique aponeurosis medially and internal oblique muscle fibers arising from inguinal ligament laterally
            (4) **Posterior wall:** conjoint tendon medially and transversalis fascia laterally

The inguinal canal transmits the spermatic cord in males and the round ligament of the uterus in females.

      2. **Inguinal triangle (Hesselbach triangle) (Figure 3-5)**
         a. Lies posterior to **superficial inguinal ring**
         b. Posterior wall formed by transversalis fascia and **conjoint tendon**
         c. Site where **direct inguinal hernia** exits abdominal cavity

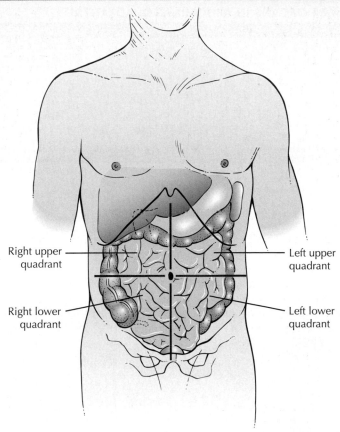

3-1: Localization of abdominal organs by four quadrants defined by horizontal transumbilical plane and vertical median plane. *(From Swartz, M: Textbook of Physical Diagnosis: History and Examination, 5th ed. Philadelphia, Saunders, 2006, Figure 17-1.)*

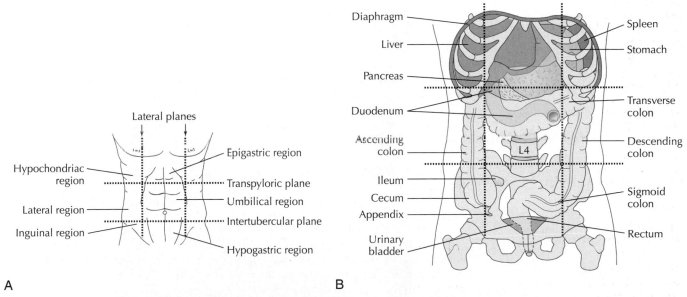

3-2: A, Division of the abdomen into nine regions for localization of abdominal organs. The transpyloric plane is a hypothetical plane that passes through the L1 vertebra posteriorly and lies midway between the jugular notch and pubic symphysis anteriorly. Computed tomography and magnetic resonance imaging scans are interpreted with reference to this plane. **B,** Surface projections of abdominal viscera, anterior view.

3. Indirect and direct inguinal hernias (Figure 3-6; Table 3-3)

A hernia is the protrusion of a structure from the space it normally occupies through a weakness in the surrounding walls. Abdominal hernias occur most frequently in the **inguinal region** (groin) and usually involve a loop of **small intestine,** which may have its lumen obstructed **(bowel obstruction)** and/or its blood supply compromised (strangulation). Both are surgical emergencies. In females, an **ovary** or **uterine tube** may be the herniating structure.

A hernia is protrusion of an organ from the space it usually occupies.

Indirect inguinal hernias are the most common type of hernia in both sexes but are much more frequent in males.

TABLE 3-1. LOCATION OF ORGANS IN ABDOMINAL QUADRANTS

RIGHT UPPER QUADRANT	LEFT UPPER QUADRANT
Liver, right lobe	Liver, left lobe
Gallbladder	Spleen
Pylorus	Stomach
Duodenum, parts 1-3	Jejunum and proximal ileum
Pancreas, head	Pancreas, body and tail
Right kidney and suprarenal gland	Left kidney and suprarenal gland
Right colic (hepatic) flexure	Left colic (splenic) flexure
Ascending colon, superior part	Transverse colon, left half
Transverse colon, right half	Descending colon, superior part

RIGHT LOWER QUADRANT	LEFT LOWER QUADRANT
Cecum	Sigmoid colon
Appendix	Descending colon, inferior part
Ascending colon, inferior part	Left ovary and uterine tube
Right ovary and uterine tube	Left ureter
Right ureter	Left spermatic cord
Right spermatic cord	Uterus (if enlarged)
Uterus (if enlarged)	Urinary bladder (if very full)
Urinary bladder (if very full)	

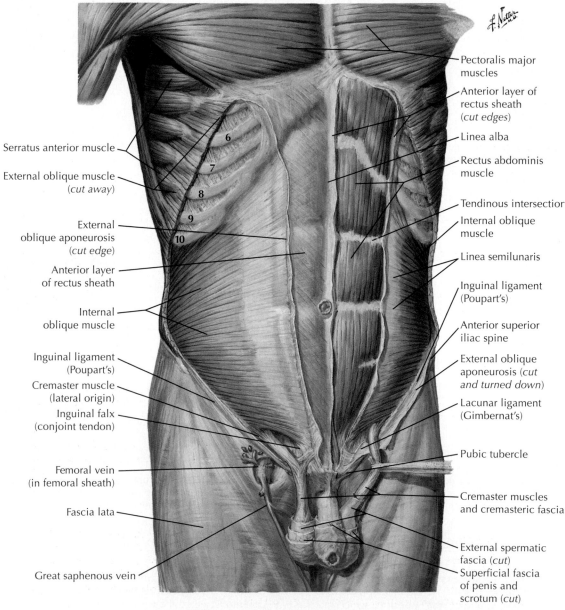

Labels (left side, top to bottom): Serratus anterior muscle; External oblique muscle (*cut away*); External oblique aponeurosis (*cut edge*); Anterior layer of rectus sheath; Internal oblique muscle; Inguinal ligament (Poupart's); Cremaster muscle (lateral origin); Inguinal falx (conjoint tendon); Femoral vein (in femoral sheath); Fascia lata; Great saphenous vein

Labels (right side, top to bottom): Pectoralis major muscles; Anterior layer of rectus sheath (*cut edges*); Linea alba; Rectus abdominis muscle; Tendinous intersection; Internal oblique muscle; Linea semilunaris; Inguinal ligament (Poupart's); Anterior superior iliac spine; External oblique aponeurosis (*cut and turned down*); Lacunar ligament (Gimbernat's); Pubic tubercle; Cremaster muscles and cremasteric fascia; External spermatic fascia (*cut*); Superficial fascia of penis and scrotum (*cut*)

3-3: Muscles of the anterior abdominal wall. The external oblique muscle has been removed on both sides to expose the internal oblique muscle. The anterior layer of the rectus sheath has been removed on the cadaver's left side. (*From Netter, F H: Atlas of Human Anatomy, 4th ed. Philadelphia, Saunders, 2006, Plate 250.*)

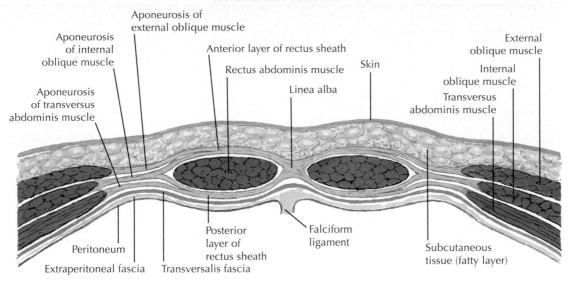

Section above arcuate line

Aponeurosis of external oblique muscle

Aponeurosis of internal oblique muscle

Aponeurosis of transversus abdominis muscle

Anterior layer of rectus sheath

Rectus abdominis muscle

Linea alba

Skin

External oblique muscle

Internal oblique muscle

Transversus abdominis muscle

Peritoneum

Extraperitoneal fascia

Transversalis fascia

Posterior layer of rectus sheath

Falciform ligament

Subcutaneous tissue (fatty layer)

Aponeurosis of internal oblique muscle splits to form anterior and posterior layers of rectus sheath. Aponeurosis of external oblique muscle joins anterior layer of sheath; aponeurosis of transversus abdominis muscle joins posterior layer. Anterior and posterior layers of rectus sheath unite medially to form linea alba.

Section below arcuate line

Aponeurosis of external oblique muscle

Aponeurosis of internal oblique muscle

Aponeurosis of transversus abdominis muscle

Anterior layer of rectus sheath

Rectus abdominis muscle

Skin

External oblique muscle

Internal oblique muscle

Transversus abdominis muscle

Transversalis fascia

Peritoneum

Extraperitoneal fascia

Median umbilic alligament (obliterated urachus) in median umbilical fold

Medial umbilical ligament and fold

Subcutaneous tissue (fatty and membranous layers)

Aponeurosis of internal oblique muscle does not split at this level but passes completely anterior to rectus abdominis muscle and is fused there with both aponeurosis of external oblique muscle and that of transversus abdominis muscle. Thus, posterior wall of rectus sheath is absent below arcuate line, and rectus abdominis muscle lies on transversalis fascia.

3-4: Formation of rectus sheath above (*upper figure*) and below (*lower figure*) arcuate line. The arcuate line (see Figure 3-7) is located midway between the umbilicus and pubic crest and marks the level below which all three aponeurotic layers pass anterior to the rectus abdominis muscle, which lies against transversalis fascia posteriorly. The arcuate line is also the point at which the inferior epigastric vessels enter the rectus sheath. (*From Netter, F H: Atlas of Human Anatomy, 4th ed. Philadelphia, Saunders, 2006, Plate 252.*)

Indirect inguinal hernias exit the abdominal cavity lateral to the inferior epigastric vessels, and direct inguinal hernias medial to them.

Inguinal hernia bulges are superior to the pubic tubercle, but femoral hernia bulges are inferior and lateral to the pubic tubercle.

Indirect inguinal hernias are by far the **most frequent abdominal hernias in both sexes** but are **6-7 times more common in males.** The herniating structure exits the abdominal cavity at the deep inguinal ring **lateral to the inferior epigastric vessels,** traverses the inguinal canal, and exits the superficial inguinal ring to descend into the scrotum or labium majus. It follows the **path of descent of the embryonic testis** and is due to persistence of a saclike evagination of the peritoneal cavity, the **processus vaginalis,** that normally is obliterated shortly after birth.

TABLE 3-2. INGUINAL REGION

STRUCTURE	DERIVED FROM	COMMENTS
Superficial inguinal ring	Aponeurosis of external abdominal oblique	Lies above and lateral to pubic tubercle; transmits spermatic cord or round ligament
Deep inguinal ring	Oval defect in transversalis fascia	Lies lateral to inferior epigastric vessels and just above inguinal ligament
Inguinal ligament	Lower border of external oblique aponeurosis	Extends from anterior superior iliac spine to pubic tubercle. Curves inward, forming shallow trough that contains structures in inguinal canal
Lacunar ligament	Medial portion of inguinal ligament	Passes posteroinferiorly, forming medial border of femoral ring
Conjoint tendon	Aponeuroses of transversus abdominis and internal abdominal oblique muscles	Reinforces posterior wall of superficial inguinal ring
Pectineal ligament	Lacunar ligament	In inguinal hernia repair will hold sutures anchoring conjoint tendon
Iliopubic tract	Thickened inferior margin of transversalis fascia	Landmark on internal aspect of inguinal ligament on laparoscopic view

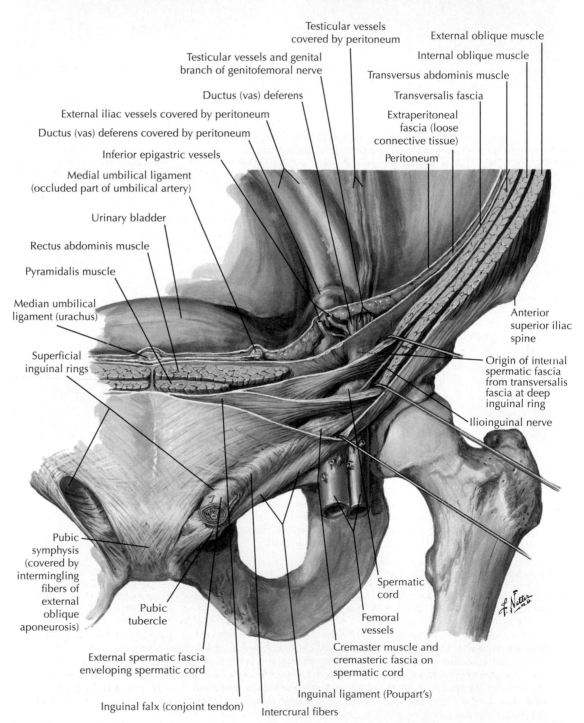

3-5: Relationship of spermatic cord and inguinal canal to layers of anterior abdominal wall. The left spermatic cord was cut shortly after emerging from the superficial inguinal ring. *(From Netter, F H: Atlas of Human Anatomy, 4th ed. Philadelphia, Saunders, 2006, Plate 260.)*

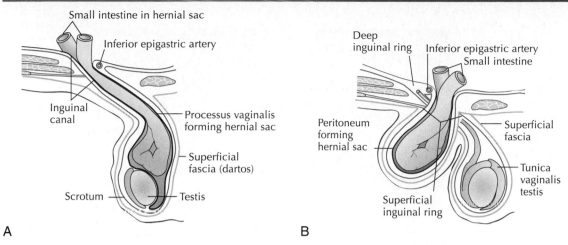

3-6: A, Indirect inguinal hernia exits abdominal cavity at deep inguinal ring lateral to inferior epigastric artery. **B,** Direct inguinal hernia exits through inguinal triangle medial to inferior epigastric artery.

TABLE 3-3. DIRECT AND INDIRECT INGUINAL HERNIAS

CHARACTERISTIC	INDIRECT INGUINAL HERNIA	DIRECT INGUINAL HERNIA
Incidence	Most common type of hernia in both sexes but much more common in males, especially male children	50% or less frequency of indirect inguinal hernias; more common in males over 40
Predisposing Factors	Persistent processus vaginalis	Weak or narrow conjoint tendon, large superficial inguinal ring
Course through Abdominal Wall	Passes lateral to inferior epigastric vessels and through deep inguinal ring, inguinal canal, and superficial inguinal ring; often descends into scrotum or labium majus	Passes medial to inferior epigastric vessels through inguinal triangle and superficial inguinal ring; rarely descends into scrotum
Covering(s) of Herniating Structure	Same three covering layers as spermatic cord—external spermatic fascia, cremasteric layer, and internal spermatic fascia	External spermatic fascia after pushing through superficial inguinal ring
Complications	Prone to obstruction and strangulation of herniating intestine; surgical repair on diagnosis	More easily reduced than indirect hernias and less likely obstruction and strangulation

Direct inguinal hernias are less common than indirect inguinal hernias. The herniating structure exits the abdominal cavity through the **inguinal triangle,** which is **medial to the inferior epigastric vessels,** and pushes through the superficial inguinal ring but seldom descends into the scrotum or labium majus. These hernias are more common in **older males** and are usually due to a **weak or narrow conjoint tendon.**

F. Posterior Aspect of Lower Anterior Abdominal Wall (Figure 3-7)

Features of the internal surface of the anterior abdominal wall are important in **laparoscopic repair** of abdominal hernias. Five **peritoneal folds** are raised over blood vessels or the fibrous remnants of fetal structures. The **median umbilical fold** is parietal peritoneum raised over the **median umbilical ligament,** a remnant of the fetal **urachus.** The paired **medial umbilical folds** overlie the obliterated distal portions of the **umbilical arteries.** The **lateral umbilical folds** are raised over the **inferior epigastric arteries and veins.** Depressions, or **peritoneal fossae,** bounded by these folds on each side of the midline are potential sites of hernias. The **supravesical fossa** lies between the median and medial umbilical folds. The **medial inguinal fossa** between medial and lateral umbilical folds corresponds to the **inguinal triangle,** where a **direct inguinal hernia** exits the abdominal cavity. The **lateral inguinal fossa** is the location of the **deep inguinal ring,** where an **indirect inguinal hernia** leaves the abdominal cavity.

On laparoscopic view, the medial inguinal fossa is the site of a direct inguinal hernia, while the lateral inguinal fossa is the site of an indirect inguinal hernia.

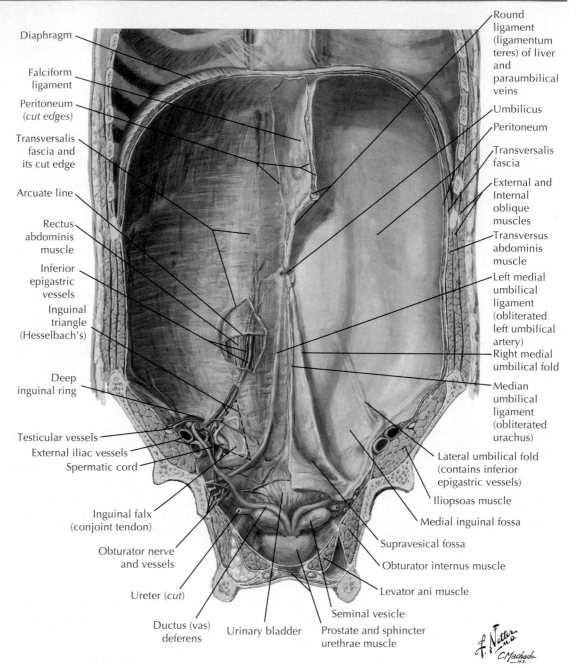

Diaphragm

Falciform ligament

Peritoneum (*cut edges*)

Transversalis fascia and its cut edge

Arcuate line

Rectus abdominis muscle

Inferior epigastric vessels

Inguinal triangle (Hesselbach's)

Deep inguinal ring

Testicular vessels

External iliac vessels

Spermatic cord

Inguinal falx (conjoint tendon)

Obturator nerve and vessels

Ureter (*cut*)

Ductus (vas) deferens

Urinary bladder

Round ligament (ligamentum teres) of liver and paraumbilical veins

Umbilicus

Peritoneum

Transversalis fascia

External and Internal oblique muscles

Transversus abdominis muscle

Left medial umbilical ligament (obliterated left umbilical artery)

Right medial umbilical fold

Median umbilical ligament (obliterated urachus)

Lateral umbilical fold (contains inferior epigastric vessels)

Iliopsoas muscle

Medial inguinal fossa

Supravesical fossa

Obturator internus muscle

Levator ani muscle

Seminal vesicle

Prostate and sphincter urethrae muscle

3-7: Posterior aspect of anterior abdominal wall with peritoneum removed from left side. The arcuate line marks the inferior border of the posterior layer of the rectus sheath. The inguinal triangle (*dashed lines*), which is bounded laterally by the inferior epigastric vessels, medially by the rectus abdominis, and inferiorly by the inguinal ligament, is the site of a direct inguinal hernia. Note the conjoint tendon (inguinal falx) in the posterior wall of the inguinal triangle. (*From Netter, F H: Atlas of Human Anatomy, 4th ed. Philadelphia, Saunders, 2006, Plate 253.*)

G. Spermatic Cord, Scrotum, Testis, and Epididymis (Figure 3-8)

1. **Spermatic cord** is collection of structures that traverse inguinal canal passing to or from testis (**see Figure 3-5**)
   a. **Ductus deferens**
   b. **Artery of ductus deferens**
   c. **Testicular artery**
   d. **Pampiniform plexus coalescing to become single testicular vein**
   e. **Cremasteric artery**
   f. **Genital branch of genitofemoral nerve**
   g. **Periarterial sympathetic plexus**
   h. **Testicular lymph vessels**

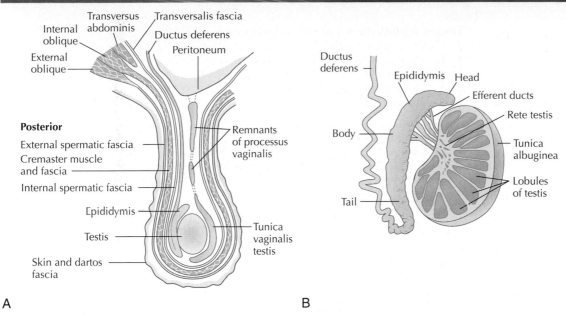

3-8: A, Scrotum and coverings of the spermatic cord and testis, lateral view. Note that the transversus abdominis muscle does *not* contribute a layer to the spermatic cord. **B,** Epididymis and testis, lateral view.

2. **Processus vaginalis**
   a. Saclike evagination of peritoneal cavity into inguinal canal and scrotum in fetus
   b. Normally disappears except for **tunica vaginalis testis** in male
3. **Gubernaculum testis**
   a. Fibrous cord connecting developing testis to floor of scrotum
   b. Guides descent of testis, then remains as **scrotal ligament** (often still labeled as gubernaculum)
   c. Homologous to female **round ligament of uterus** and **ovarian ligament proper**

> The gubernaculum is a fibrous cord that guides the descent of the fetal testis or ovary.

Cryptorchidism is the failure of one or both testes to descend into the scrotum. The **undescended testis** may lie anywhere along the path of the usual descent but usually is in the **inguinal canal.** Cryptorchidism results in increased risk of **testicular cancer** and **decreased fertility.** The normally descended testicle is also at risk.

> Cryptorchidism is an undescended testis with the risk of testicular cancer and decreased fertility.

Torsion of the spermatic cord produces acute pain and swelling and can result in **testicular necrosis and atrophy** if not reduced promptly. The condition usually occurs just above the superior pole of the testis. Repair requires a high scrotal incision to untwist the cord, and the testis is sutured to the scrotal septum to prevent recurrence. Torsion frequently **follows vigorous exercise in 10- to 20-year-olds** and may be associated with **congenital anomalies** (e.g., a mobile, horizontally oriented testis [bell-clapper deformity] or cryptorchidism). In children, **acute scrotal pain and swelling** are assumed to be testicular torsion until proven otherwise.

> Untreated testicular torsion results in testicular necrosis and atrophy.

The **genital branch of the genitofemoral nerve** innervates the **cremaster muscle** and is the efferent limb of the **cremasteric reflex (L1),** which is tested in males by stroking the upper medial thigh. Absence of the cremasteric reflex in children with acute scrotal pain and swelling supports a diagnosis of torsion.

> Acute scrotal pain and swelling in children are assumed to be torsion of the testis until proven otherwise.

4. **Scrotum**
   a. **Dartos layer** is membranous superficial fascia **containing smooth muscle** that elevates scrotum to conserve heat
   b. Divided into right and left halves by **scrotal septum,** an inward extension of dartos layer
   c. Receives **cutaneous innervation** from branches of ilioinguinal, genitofemoral, pudendal, and posterior femoral cutaneous nerves

5. **Testis**
   a. **Tunica albuginea** is a dense connective tissue capsule.
   b. **Tunica vaginalis testis**
      • Serous sac derived from fetal **processus vaginalis**
   c. **Testicular artery** from abdominal aorta supplies blood
   d. **Pampiniform plexus** via **testicular vein** drains to inferior vena cava on right and **left renal vein on left**

The right gonadal vein drains to the inferior vena cava, and the left gonadal vein drains to the left renal vein.

Testicular cancer metastasizes to aortic nodes, but scrotal cancer metastasizes to superficial inguinal nodes.

Transillumination of a scrotal mass detects hydrocele.

Varicocele is **engorgement of the pampiniform plexus** that produces a **scrotal mass** palpable as a **"bag of worms."** Formation is usually on the left side due to incompetent venous valves and is benign, but varicocele on either side may indicate a **retroperitoneal malignancy or fibrosis** obstructing the testicular vein. A rapidly developing **left-sided varicocele** may be due to a **renal tumor** (renal cell carcinoma) that has spread along the renal vein.

Testicular cancer is the most common malignancy in young adult males. It spreads to the **aortic (lumbar) nodes** through the lymphatics accompanying the testicular artery. Blood supply and lymphatic drainage reflect the developmental origin of the testis from the posterior abdominal wall.

The **tunica vaginalis testis** or other **remnants of the processus vaginalis** may accumulate serous fluid **(hydrocele)** or blood **(hematocele)**. With **transillumination,** a hydrocele produces a reddish glow, whereas light usually will not penetrate other scrotal masses such as a hematocele, solid tumor, or herniated bowel.

---

6. **Epididymis** is a **convoluted tube** that stores spermatozoa until transport into the **ductus deferens (Figure 3-8, *B*).**

Epididymitis is a common cause of acute scrotal pain and swelling in young, sexually active males.

A **spermatocele** is a **sperm-filled cyst** that occurs near the head of the epididymis. It is usually asymptomatic and discovered on routine physical examination. **Epididymitis** is inflammation of the epididymis causing **acute scrotal pain and swelling.** It is common in young males with sexually transmitted infections or older males with urinary tract infections secondary to benign prostatic hyperplasia or other genitourinary problems.

H. **Important Blood Vessels of Anterior Abdominal Wall**
   1. **Arteries**
      a. **Superior epigastric artery**
         • Terminal branch of **internal thoracic artery** that descends in rectus sheath to anastomose with inferior epigastric artery

Umbilical vessels can be catheterized in newborns to administer fluids or collect samples.

Superior-inferior epigastric artery anastomoses provide collateral circulation in postductal coarctation of the aorta.

In **postductal coarctation of the aorta,** anastomoses between the superior and inferior **epigastric arteries** provide **collateral circulation** between the subclavian and external iliac arteries.

---

      b. **Inferior epigastric artery**
         (1) Arises from **external iliac artery** and ascends medial to deep inguinal ring to enter rectus sheath
         (2) May be source of **aberrant obturator artery** in danger during **femoral hernia repair**
      c. Posterior intercostal (7-11), subcostal (12), and lumbar segmental (1 and 2) arteries
         • Anastomose with superior and inferior epigastric arteries
   2. **Collateral venous drainage**
      • Provides **collateral connections** between superior and inferior vena caval systems when inferior vena cava is blocked by **thrombus** or by **retroperitoneal tumor**
      a. **Superior and inferior epigastric veins**
         • Connect brachiocephalic vein (superior vena cava) to external iliac vein (inferior vena cava)
      b. **Posterior intercostal veins (7-11), subcostal vein,** and **lumbar segmental veins** (1 and 2)
         • Connect azygos system of veins (superior vena cava) to inferior epigastric vein (inferior vena cava)

Thoracoepigastric and superior-inferior epigastric veins provide caval-caval anastomoses to bypass vena caval obstruction.

c. **Thoracoepigastric vein**
   (1) Connects **lateral thoracic vein** (superior vena cava) to **superficial epigastric vein** (inferior vena cava)
   (2) May enlarge as part of collateral drainage accompanying **portocaval anastomoses** and **caput medusae**

II. Nerves of Anterior Abdominal Wall (Figure 3-9)
   a. Continue from anterior rami of spinal nerves T7-L1
   b. Provide **motor innervation to muscles** and **cutaneous innervation** of anterior abdominal wall

III. Peritoneum and Peritoneal Cavity (Figure 3-10)
   ### A. Peritoneum
   • Serous sac lining abdominopelvic cavity and forming covering layer for viscera invaginating it from behind
   1. **Parietal peritoneum**
      a. Lines walls of abdominopelvic cavity and inferior surface of respiratory diaphragm
      b. Innervated by **somatic nerves**

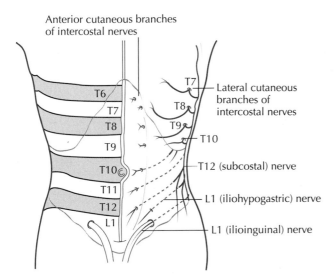

Anterior cutaneous branches of intercostal nerves

T6
T7
T8
T9
T10
T11
T12
L1

T7
T8
T9
T10

Lateral cutaneous branches of intercostal nerves

T12 (subcostal) nerve

L1 (iliohypogastric) nerve

L1 (ilioinguinal) nerve

3-9: Thoracoabdominal nerves and corresponding dermatomes. T10 dermatome is at the level of the umbilicus, so pain from an organ innervated by T10 may be referred to the umbilicus; pain carried by L1 may be referred to the groin region. Disease of the lower thoracic wall may refer pain to the abdominal distribution of the thoracoabdominal nerves, mimicking abdominal disease. *Broken lines,* Paths of nerves.

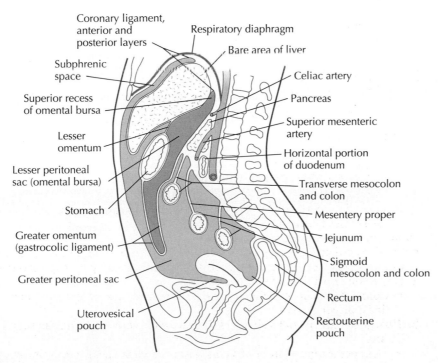

Coronary ligament, anterior and posterior layers

Respiratory diaphragm

Bare area of liver

Subphrenic space

Celiac artery

Superior recess of omental bursa

Pancreas

Lesser omentum

Superior mesenteric artery

Lesser peritoneal sac (omental bursa)

Horizontal portion of duodenum

Transverse mesocolon and colon

Stomach

Mesentery proper

Greater omentum (gastrocolic ligament)

Jejunum

Greater peritoneal sac

Sigmoid mesocolon and colon

Rectum

Uterovesical pouch

Rectouterine pouch

3-10: Abdominal cavity, sagittal view.

TABLE 3-4. PERITONEAL LIGAMENTS AND MESENTERIES

STRUCTURE	EMBRYOLOGIC ORIGIN	COMMENTS
Greater omentum	Dorsal mesogastrium	Can prevent spread of infection by adhering to and localizing areas of inflammation
Gastrosplenic ligament		Contains short gastric arteries and veins
Gastrocolic ligament		Contains gastro-omental (gastroepiploic) vessels
Splenorenal ligament		Contains tail of pancreas and splenic vessels
Lesser omentum	Septum transversum	Ventral mesentery of stomach and anterior wall of lesser peritoneal sac
Hepatogastric ligament		Contains right and left gastric vessels along lesser curvature
Hepatoduodenal ligament		Contains common bile duct, proper hepatic artery, and portal vein
Falciform ligament	Septum transversum	In its free edge contains ligamentum teres hepatis, remnant of left umbilical vein of fetus
Mesentery proper	Embryonic common dorsal mesentery	Contains vessels, nerves, and lymphatics supplying jejunum and ileum
Transverse mesocolon	Embryonic common dorsal mesentery	Contains middle colic vessels
Sigmoid mesocolon	Embryonic common dorsal mesentery	Contains sigmoidal arteries and veins
Mesoappendix	Embryonic common dorsal mesentery	Transmits appendicular artery and vein

Somatic pain from the parietal peritoneum is sharp and localized; visceral pain from the visceral peritoneum is diffuse and aching or cramping.

Mesenteries carry vessels and nerves between the body wall and the organs.

Intraperitoneal organs invaginate the peritoneal sac, while retroperitoneal organs remain posterior to the sac.

2. **Visceral peritoneum**
   a. Covers abdominal organs that have invaginated peritoneal sac
   b. Innervated by GVA fibers in abdominal **autonomic plexuses**
3. **Peritoneal mesenteries and ligaments (Table 3-4)**
   • Suspend organs within abdominal cavity and transmit vessels and nerves between body wall and organs
4. **Intraperitoneal, retroperitoneal, and secondarily retroperitoneal organs (Table 3-5)**
   a. **Intraperitoneal organs** invaginate peritoneal sac and receive coat of visceral peritoneum.
   b. **Retroperitoneal organs** lie within abdominal cavity behind posterior parietal peritoneum and were never intraperitoneal during development
   c. **Secondarily retroperitoneal organs** developed "intraperitoneally" but fused secondarily with posterior body wall, so they are covered only anteriorly by peritoneum
B. **Peritoneal Cavity**
   • Potential space containing thin film of fluid to lubricate visceral movements and resist infection

Peritonitis results from the introduction of sterile material or bacteria into the peritoneal cavity.

Common clinical disorders of the peritoneum are peritonitis and ascites. **Peritonitis** is **inflammation of the peritoneum** due to entrance into the peritoneal cavity of sterile materials such as bile **(aseptic peritonitis)** or bacterial contamination **(septic peritonitis)**. Septic peritonitis commonly is due to a perforated viscus, such as the appendix or a peptic ulcer, and also typically develops over time in aseptic peritonitis. Septic peritonitis *without* bowel perforation **(spontaneous bacterial peritonitis)** may occur when ascites is present in cirrhosis of the liver or the nephrotic syndrome (massive protein loss in the urine with decreased serum albumin).

TABLE 3-5. CLASSIFICATION OF PERITONEAL ORGANS

INTRAPERITONEAL	RETROPERITONEAL	SECONDARILY RETROPERITONEAL
Duodenum, first part	Kidneys	Duodenum, second, third, and fourth parts
Liver and gallbladder	Ureters	Colon, ascending and descending
Pancreas, tail	Suprarenal glands	Rectum
Stomach	Abdominal aorta	Pancreas, head, neck, and body
Spleen	Inferior vena cava	
Jejunum		
Ileum		
Cecum		
Appendix		
Transverse colon		
Sigmoid colon		

Ascites is **excess fluid in the peritoneal cavity.** It most commonly results from **cirrhosis** of the liver but may follow **peritoneal malignancy, right-sided heart failure,** or **peritoneal tuberculosis.** A needle is inserted into the peritoneal cavity to collect a sample for analysis or to drain fluid to relieve respiratory distress or abdominal pain **(paracentesis).**

> The peritoneal cavity is subdivided into greater and lesser peritoneal sacs connected by the omental foramen.
>
> Ascites is excess fluid in the peritoneal cavity due most often to cirrhosis.

1. **Greater peritoneal sac**
   a. **Subphrenic recess**
      • Potential peritoneal space between liver and inferior surface of diaphragm

A **liver abscess** in the subphrenic recess may erode through the diaphragm into the thorax. **Cancer** can spread quickly to adjacent organs.

   b. **Hepatorenal recess** (Morison pouch)
      (1) Potential space between right lobe of liver and right kidney
      (2) Lowest point of peritoneal cavity when patient is supine
   c. **Paracolic gutters**
      • Lie lateral to ascending and descending colons and extend over pelvic brim into pelvis

> The hepatorenal recess is the lowest point of the peritoneal cavity in a supine patient and may be infected from subphrenic recess or omental bursa.
>
> Paracolic gutters are pathways for the spread of infection and cancer cells.

Fluid draining from the **subphrenic recess** or **omental bursa** collects in the **hepatorenal recess** in supine patients. In upright patients, the **paracolic gutters** provide a **path for infection and cancer cells** to spread into the lower abdomen or pelvis. Patients with **peritonitis due to bacterial infections** are treated with antibiotics and may be positioned sitting up to facilitate drainage into the pelvis, where absorption of toxins is slower.

2. **Lesser peritoneal sac (omental bursa)**
   a. Lies posterior to stomach, liver, and lesser omentum
   b. Communicates with greater peritoneal sac through **omental foramen**

In **acute pancreatitis** fluid may accumulate within or around the pancreas as a **pancreatic pseudocyst,** and most often enters the **omental bursa (Figure 3-11).** Pseudocysts may become infected and **may compress or erode adjacent structures.** The majority of cases of acute pancreatitis are due to **alcohol abuse** or a **gallstone obstructing the distal bile duct.** Patients show constant severe **epigastric pain radiating to the back** with **fever, nausea, and vomiting.** Seventy percent of acute pancreatitis patients have elevated serum amylase **(hyperamylasemia)** for about 3 days. In **necrotizing pancreatitis** blood may dissect along fascial planes to produce **ecchymoses** in the flank **(Grey-Turner sign)** or periumbilical region **(Cullen sign).**

> Pancreatic pseudocyst is a fluid collection in pancreatitis, most frequently in the omental bursa.
>
> Flank or periumbilical ecchymoses may signal necrotizing pancreatitis.

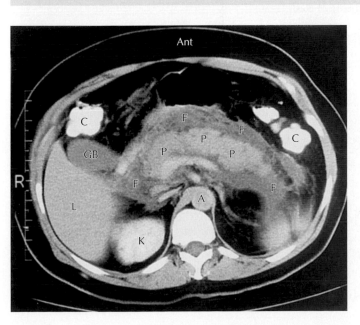

3-11: Axial CT scan showing acute pancreatitis with fluid collection around the pancreas in a patient with hyperlipidemia. A pancreatic pseudocyst often causes fluid within the omental bursa. Pancreas = P; peripancreatic fluid = F; liver = L; gallbladder = GB; colon = C; right kidney = K; aorta = A. *(From Mettler, F A: Essentials of Radiology, 2nd ed. Philadelphia, Saunders, 2004, Figure 6-58.)*

3. **Omental (epiploic) foramen**
   a. Only communication between greater and lesser peritoneal sacs
   b. Bounded anteriorly by **hepatoduodenal ligament,** posteriorly by **inferior vena cava,** superiorly by **caudate lobe of liver,** and inferiorly by **first part of duodenum**
   c. May be site of **internal hernia**

The omental foramen is bounded by the first part of the duodenum, hepatoduodenal ligament, caudate lobe, and inferior vena cava.

Inflammation caused by **acute pancreatitis** or a **perforated posterior gastric ulcer** may obstruct the **omental foramen.** Accumulated fluid in the lesser peritoneal sac (e.g., pancreatic pseudocyst) is evident on a CT scan. Rarely, a loop of **small intestine** may become entrapped in the omental foramen as an **internal hernia** and is in danger of **bowel obstruction** and **strangulation.** Since none of the boundaries of the foramen can be incised, the swollen intestine may have to be decompressed to allow extraction.

Differential diagnosis of small bowel obstruction includes an internal hernia in the absence of surgery or trauma history.

IV. Gastrointestinal Viscera
A. Distal Esophagus

A Mallory-Weiss tear is a mucosal tear of the gastroesophageal junction from retching.

Longitudinal mucosal tears through the **gastroesophageal junction,** or gastric cardia **(Mallory-Weiss tears)** may cause severe **upper gastrointestinal bleeding** and vomiting of blood **(hematemesis).** They usually result from severe retching or vomiting in those with alcoholism or bulimia. A rupture of the distal esophagus in similar patients is **Boerhaave syndrome.** Severe epigastric pain and dyspnea are present, and the condition is **fatal without treatment.**

The most common causes of upper-GI bleeding are peptic ulcers, esophageal varices, and Mallory-Weiss tears.

B. Stomach (Figures 3-12 and 3-13)

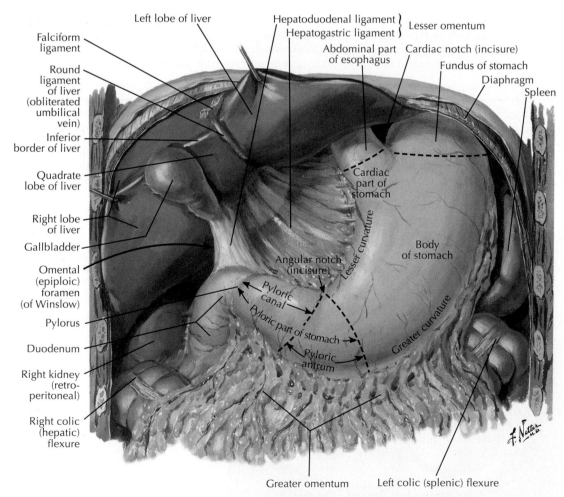

3-12: Stomach in situ with its parts labeled. *(From Netter, F H: Atlas of Human Anatomy, 4th ed. Philadelphia, Saunders, 2006, Plate 275.)*

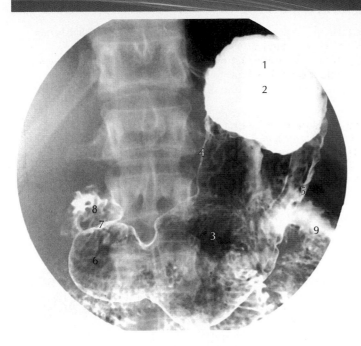

3-13: Radiograph of supine patient following double-contrast barium meal showing features of normal stomach. Fundus of stomach = 1; barium pooling in fundus = 2; body of stomach = 3; lesser curvature = 4; greater curvature = 5; antrum of stomach = 6; pyloric sphincter = 7; duodenal cap = 8; small intestine = 9. *(From Weir, J, Abrahams, P: Imaging Atlas of Human Anatomy, 3rd ed. London, Mosby Ltd., 2003, p 133, a.)*

1. **Cardia** lies adjacent to junction with esophagus and is related to physiological **lower esophageal (cardiac) sphincter** that prevents regurgitation into esophagus **(gastroesophageal reflux)**.
2. **Pylorus** is divided into proximal **pyloric antrum** and distal **pyloric canal** and has smooth muscle **pyloric sphincter** that controls gastric emptying under vagal parasympathetic control

In a **sliding hiatal hernia,** the **gastroesophageal junction** herniates through the **esophageal hiatus** of the diaphragm with part of the stomach **(Figure 3-14)**, predisposing to **gastroesophageal reflux.** Heartburn from hiatal hernia can mimic the substernal pain of **myocardial infarction** but differs in that the pain is usually lessened when the patient sits upright or takes antacids. In the less common **paraesophageal hiatal hernia** the gastroesophageal junction remains in place, but the adjacent **fundus** herniates into the thorax. A paraesophageal hernia usually does *not* cause reflux.

> Heartburn from gastroesophageal reflux can mimic myocardial infarction but is relieved by position change or antacids.

Gastric ulcers, which occur less frequently than duodenal ulcers, usually form along the lesser curvature near the pyloric antrum and have been linked to **chronic use of aspirin** and other **NSAIDs,** to **cigarette smoking,** and to *Helicobacter pylori* **infection (the most common cause).** Gastric ulcers have a **higher mortality rate** than duodenal ulcers because they may cause **posterior erosion** with **fatal hemorrhage** from the **splenic artery.** Alternatively, erosion into the pancreas causes **pancreatitis.**

> Posterior gastric ulcer perforation may fatally erode the splenic artery.

3. **Relationships of stomach (see Figures 3-2, 3-10, 3-29, and 3-31)**
4. **Blood supply to stomach (Figure 3-15; Table 3-6)**
5. **Venous drainage of stomach**
   - Accompanies arterial supply to ultimately end in **portal vein**

Increased pressure in the portal vein and its tributaries due to obstructed blood flow through the liver is **portal hypertension.** In portal hypertension blood is shunted via the **left gastric vein** to **anastomoses with tributaries of the azygos vein** in the lower esophagus **(portocaval anastomoses).** These anastomoses may become grossly enlarged as **esophageal varices** and **rupture,** causing life-threatening **hemorrhage.**

> Anastomoses between the left gastric and the azygos veins form esophageal varices in portal hypertension.

6. **Lymphatic drainage of stomach**
   - Accompanies arterial supply to ultimately end in **celiac nodes**

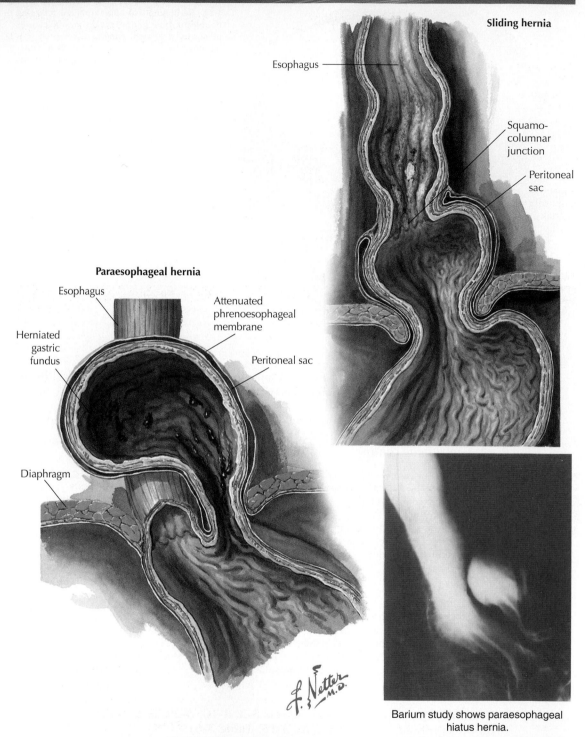

Sliding hernia

Esophagus

Squamo-
columnar
junction

Peritoneal
sac

Paraesophageal hernia

Esophagus

Attenuated
phrenoesophageal
membrane

Herniated
gastric
fundus

Peritoneal sac

Diaphragm

Barium study shows paraesophageal
hiatus hernia.

3-14: Hiatal hernias. A sliding hiatal hernia (*upper right figure*) involves the cardia of the stomach and may cause gastroesophageal reflux disease. A less common paraesophageal hiatal hernia (*left and lower right figures*) usually doesn't cause regurgitation of gastric contents. (*From Hansen, J T, Lambert, D R: Netter's Clinical Anatomy, Icon Learning Systems, 2005, p 404.*)

C. Small Intestine
   1. **Duodenum (Figure 3-16)**
      • Extends from pylorus to jejunum as C-shaped tube surrounding head of pancreas
     a. **First part** (superior part)
       (1) First 2 cm is called **duodenal bulb (duodenal cap)** because walls look smooth on radiograph using barium contrast; bulb is only intraperitoneal part of duodenum
       (2) Joined to liver by **hepatoduodenal ligament**
       (3) Crossed posteriorly by portal vein, bile duct, and **gastroduodenal artery**

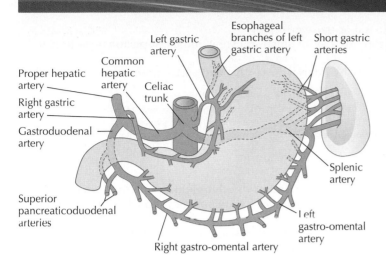

3-15: Arteries of the stomach, anterior view. All three branches of the celiac trunk supply blood to the stomach.

TABLE 3-6. DERIVATIVES OF DEVELOPING GUT

REGION	BLOOD SUPPLY	ADULT DERIVATIVE
Caudal foregut	Celiac artery*	Liver parenchyma, pancreas, stomach, first part of duodenum, half of second part of duodenum
Midgut	Superior mesenteric artery	Second part of duodenum, third and fourth parts of duodenum, jejunum, ileum, cecum, appendix, ascending colon, transverse colon
Hindgut	Inferior mesenteric artery	Descending colon, sigmoid colon, rectum, upper anal canal

*The celiac artery also supplies the spleen, but this structure derives from the mesoderm of the dorsal mesentery rather than the foregut.

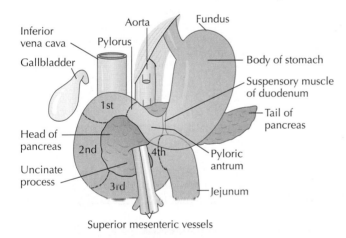

3-16: Stomach, duodenum, and pancreas.

Gnawing or burning epigastric pain 1-3 hours after a meal or at night can indicate a **duodenal ulcer,** which usually develops in the **duodenal bulb.** Epigastric tenderness is the most common physical sign. An ulcer on the posterior wall may perforate and erode the **gastroduodenal artery,** causing severe **hemorrhage,** or permit contents to enter the peritoneal cavity, causing **peritonitis.** Erosion into the pancreas causes **pancreatitis.**

Duodenal ulcer perforation may result in hemorrhage, peritonitis, or pancreatitis.

b. **Second part** (descending part)
(1) Receives termination of **bile duct** and **main pancreatic duct** at **hepatopancreatic ampulla** that opens at **major duodenal papilla**
(2) Receives termination of **accessory pancreatic duct** at **minor duodenal papilla**

Bile duct and main pancreatic duct drain into hepatopancreatic ampulla that opens into second part of duodenum

---

A **gallstone** or **tumor** can **block** the common opening of the **bile duct** and **main pancreatic duct** at the **hepatopancreatic ampulla** and cause bile to reflux into the pancreas, producing **acute pancreatitis.** The patient may have **obstructive jaundice. Spasm of the hepatopancreatic sphincter** (of Oddi) can have the same results.

c. **Third part** (horizontal or transverse part)
   (1) Crossed anteriorly by root of small intestine and by **superior mesenteric vessels**
   (2) Crossed posteriorly by inferior vena cava and aorta anterior to vertebra L3

Superior mesenteric artery syndrome is a life-threatening small bowel obstruction by SMA compression.

> The **superior mesenteric artery** can compress the **third part of the duodenum** against the aorta, causing life-threatening **small bowel obstruction (superior mesenteric artery syndrome).** This rare condition may occur following **rapid weight loss** or **scoliosis surgery.**

d. **Fourth part** (ascending part)
   (1) Ascends to left side of L2 to end at **duodenojejunal flexure,** which is attached to right crus of diaphragm by **suspensory muscle of duodenum (ligament of Treitz)**
   (2) May have associated **peritoneal recesses,** the **superior and/or inferior duodenal recesses,** which can trap section of small intestine as an **internal hernia**

The suspensory muscle of the duodenum is a surgical landmark and indicates the boundary between upper- and lower-GI bleeding.

> The **duodenojejunal flexure** marks the transition between **upper** and **lower gastrointestinal bleeding.** Black, tarry stools **(melena)** distinguish most upper-GI bleeding, whereas stools from lower-GI bleeding contain red blood **(hematochezia).**

2. **Jejunum and ileum (Table 3-7)**
   • Intraperitoneal, suspended from posterior abdominal wall by **mesentery proper**

Ileus differs from mechanical bowel obstruction by the absence of crampy abdominal pain and bowel sounds.

> **Ileus** is the temporary loss of peristalsis, most commonly following abdominal surgery. **Postoperative ileus** results in vague abominal pain and bloating and may cause nausea and vomiting. Bowel sounds are hypoactive or absent **(silent abdomen).** It usually resolves within 2-3 days. **Other causes of ileus** include peritonitis, compromised intestinal blood supply, drugs (e.g., anticholinergics), intraabdominal hematomas (ruptured aortic aneurysm), lower lobe pneumonia, and head injury.

3. **Blood supply to small intestine (Figures 3-17 to 3-19; see Table 3-6)**
4. **Venous drainage of small intestine (see Figure 3-26)**
   a. **Duodenum** is drained by veins ending in portal vein or its tributaries.
   b. **Jejunum** and ileum are drained by **superior mesenteric vein,** which helps form the portal vein
D. **Large Intestine (see Figures 3-2, 3-20, and 3-21)**
   • Characterized by **teniae coli, haustra,** and **omental (epiploic) appendices**
   1. **Cecum** is blind pouch that receives **ileocecal orifice** and **opening of appendix**
   2. **Ileocecal valve** is rudimentary and does not prevent reflux into ileum
   3. **Appendix** is intraperitoneal and suspended by **mesoappendix**

An unapparent appendix may be found by tracing the convergence of the teniae coli at its base.

> The **appendix** has a complete layer of longitudinal smooth muscle, while the colon as far distally as the rectosigmoid junction has only three longitudinal bands: the **teniae coli.** Therefore, an appendix that is difficult to locate during surgery can be found by tracing the convergence of the teniae coli at its base.

Acute appendicitis pain changes from diffuse periumbilical to sharp, localized right lower quadrant pain.

> The appendix is usually located in a **retrocecal** position, but its position is quite variable. **Pain of acute appendicitis** usually projects first to the **periumbilical region** and then migrates to the **right lower quadrant** as the parietal peritoneum becomes irritated. Maximum tenderness is often near the **McBurney point.** Extension of the right hip may elicit pain **(psoas sign).**

TABLE 3-7. COMPARISON OF JEJUNUM AND ILEUM

FEATURE	JEJUNUM	ILEUM
Diameter	Slightly larger	Slightly smaller
Wall	Thicker	Thinner
Vessels	Fewer arcades, longer vasa recta, fewer anastomoses	More arcades, shorter vasa recta, more anastomoses
Amount of fat	Less	More
Plicae circulares	Numerous	Rudimentary
Peyer patches	Few	Many

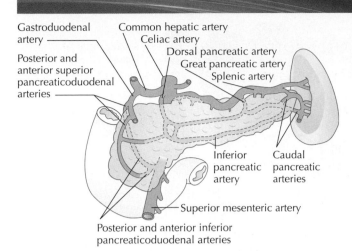

Gastroduodenal artery

Posterior and anterior superior pancreaticoduodenal arteries

Common hepatic artery
Celiac artery
Dorsal pancreatic artery
Great pancreatic artery
Splenic artery

Inferior pancreatic artery

Caudal pancreatic arteries

Superior mesenteric artery

Posterior and anterior inferior pancreaticoduodenal arteries

3-17: Arteries of the pancreas and duodenum, anterior view. Branches of the celiac and superior mesenteric arteries nourish the pancreas and duodenum. The spleen is supplied by the splenic branch of the celiac trunk.

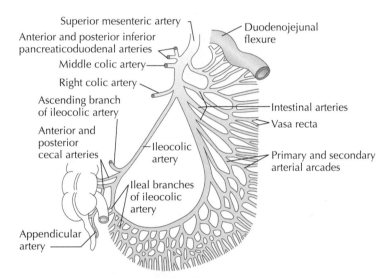

Superior mesenteric artery
Anterior and posterior inferior pancreaticoduodenal arteries
Middle colic artery
Right colic artery
Ascending branch of ileocolic artery
Anterior and posterior cecal arteries
Ileocolic artery
Ileal branches of ileocolic artery
Appendicular artery

Duodenojejunal flexure

Intestinal arteries
Vasa recta
Primary and secondary arterial arcades

3-18: Arteries of the jejunum and ileum. The number of arterial arcades increases and the vasa recta become shorter from proximal to distal.

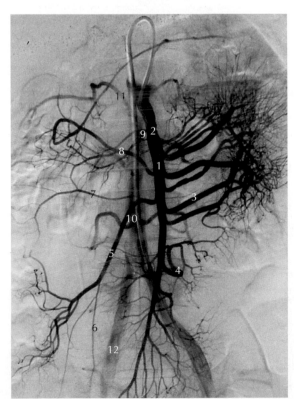

3-19: Subtracted superior mesenteric arteriogram. Superior mesenteric artery (1) with catheter tip (2); jejunal branches = 3; ileal branches = 4; ileocolic artery = 5; appendicular artery = 6; right colic artery = 7; middle colic artery = 8; inferior pancreaticoduodenal artery = 9. Note also posterior abdominal arteries: aorta = 10; lumbar arteries = 11; and right common iliac artery = 12. *(From Weir, J, Abrahams, P: Imaging Atlas of Human Anatomy, 3rd ed. London, Mosby Ltd., 2003, p 142, a.)*

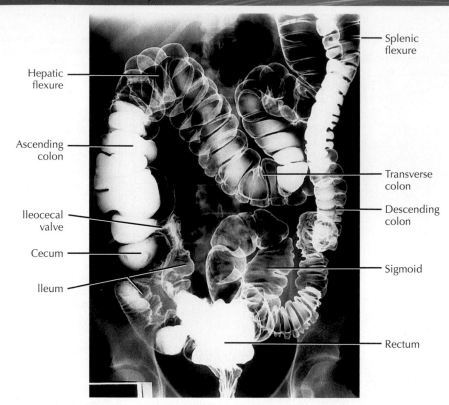

3-20: Supine radiograph of normal colon following double-contrast barium enema. Transverse colon loops down a variable distance in front of the small intestine. A long sigmoid colon and sigmoid mesocolon are more susceptible to volvulus. *(From Mettler, F A: Essentials of Radiology, 2nd ed. Philadelphia, Saunders, 2004, Figure 6-66.)*

3-21: Arteries of the large intestine. The marginal artery formed by anastomoses between branches of the superior and inferior mesenteric arteries may provide collateral circulation in vessel occlusion.

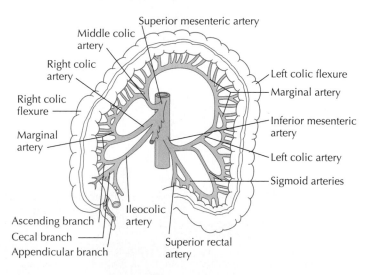

4. **Ascending colon**
   a. Secondarily retroperitoneal
   b. Covered by peritoneum except on its posterior side, which is fused to posterior abdominal wall

A mobile ascending colon predisposes to volvulus.

> Failure of fusion of the **proximal part of the ascending colon** to the posterior abdominal wall means that it retains a **mesentery.** The abnormal mobility makes it vulnerable to twisting around its mesentery **(volvulus)** with **bowel obstruction** and **strangulation.**

The celiac artery supplies the foregut. The superior mesenteric artery supplies the midgut. The inferior mesenteric artery supplies the hindgut.

5. **Transverse colon**
   a. Intraperitoneal, suspended from posterior body wall by **transverse mesocolon**
   b. Related to liver at **hepatic (right colic) flexure** and to spleen at **splenic (left colic) flexure**

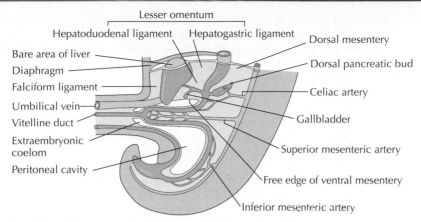

3-22: Blood supply of the embryonic gut. Caudal foregut (celiac artery), midgut (superior mesenteric artery), and hindgut (inferior mesenteric artery) at the end of week 5.

6. **Descending colon**
   a. Secondarily retroperitoneal
   b. Covered by peritoneum except on posterior side, which is fused to posterior abdominal wall

The **ascending and descending colon** become **secondarily retroperitoneal** by fusion of their peritoneal covering with the posterior abdominal wall, and their vessels and nerves reach them from near the midline. Thus, they can be **safely mobilized via a lateral approach** during surgery.

Both the ascending and descending colon are surgically mobilized via a lateral approach.

7. **Sigmoid colon**
   • Intraperitoneal, suspended from posterior body wall by sigmoid mesocolon

Volvulus is most frequently seen in the **sigmoid colon;** it may occur when the sigmoid colon and **sigmoid mesocolon** are abnormally long. Development of outpouchings of the mucosa and submucosa in middle-aged and older patients **(diverticulosis)** also occurs most commonly in the sigmoid colon, particularly in patients with long-standing constipation. Diverticulosis is a common cause of massive **lower-GI bleeding,** and diverticula may become infected **(diverticulitis)** and rupture, resulting in a **pericolic abscess** or **peritonitis.**

The sigmoid colon is the most common location of volvulus and diverticulosis.

A **marginal artery** often is formed along the inner margin of the large intestine from the ileocolic to the rectosigmoid junction by anastomosing branches of the superior and inferior mesenteric arteries. If the marginal artery provides sufficient collateral circulation, surgeons may be able to ligate or even remove the **inferior mesenteric artery** (e.g., during resection of the sigmoid colon). However, the **left colic flexure** is a "watershed area," and systemic hypotension or inferior mesenteric artery insufficiency may result in **ischemia** and **ulceration (called ischemic colitis).**

A marginal artery may allow the safe ligation of the inferior mesenteric artery.

8. **Blood supply to large intestine (Figures 3-19 and 3-21; see Table 3-6)**
   a. **Superior mesenteric artery** supplies colon to near left colic flexure

Superior mesenteric ischemia is decreased intestinal blood flow due to **occlusion** of the superior mesenteric artery or its branches by **atherosclerosis, emboli** (e.g., from left atrial fibrillation), or **external compression** (e.g., adhesions, tumors). Collateral circulation may compensate for partial or slow-onset occlusions. **Nonocclusive ischemia** results from **hypotension** due to heart failure or **shock.** Severe, poorly localized **abdominal pain** is often the main symptom of acute mesenteric ischemia, but abdominal distention, nausea, vomiting, and bloody diarrhea also occur. Chronic, intermittent ischemia may result in abdominal pain only after meals. **Venous thrombosis** also is a cause of mesenteric ischemia.

Superior mesenteric artery ischemia may cause intestinal necrosis from decreased blood flow.

Foregut derivatives refer pain to the epigastric region, midgut derivatives to the umbilical region, and hindgut derivatives to the hypogastric region.

      b. **Inferior mesenteric artery** supplies descending and sigmoid colons, proximal rectum, and upper half of anal canal

      c. **Marginal artery** provides **collateral circulation** between adjacent branches of superior and inferior mesenteric arteries

9. **Venous drainage of large intestine**
   a. **Cecum, appendix, ascending and transverse colons**
      - Drainage is to the **superior mesenteric vein**
   b. **Descending and sigmoid colons**
      - Drainage is to **inferior mesenteric vein** and then to splenic vein or superior mesenteric vein, which join to form portal vein

10. **Lymphatic drainage of large intestine**
    a. **Cecum, appendix, ascending and transverse colons**
       - Drainage is via regional nodes to superior mesenteric nodes and through intestinal lymph trunk to cisterna chyli
    b. **Descending and sigmoid colons**
       - Drainage is via regional nodes to inferior mesenteric nodes and through intestinal lymph trunk to cisterna chyli

V. Development of Midgut (Figure 3-22)

A. **Midgut Loop** (Primary Intestinal Loop)
   1. Formed by rapid lengthening of gut tube
   2. Communicates with **yolk sac** by way of **vitelline duct** (yolk stalk)
   3. **Cranial** and **caudal limbs** demarcated by attachment of vitelline duct

B. **Physiological Herniation of Midgut**
   1. Occurs into **extraembryonic coelom** of umbilical cord as elongating intestine becomes too large for abdominal cavity
   2. Lasts from week 6 to week 10

C. **Rotation of Midgut**
   1. Occurs about axis formed by **superior mesenteric artery**
   2. Totals 270° counterclockwise

D. **Retraction of Midgut**
   1. Begins in week 10, with **jejunum** coming to lie in **upper left quadrant**
   2. Completed with **caudal limb** (cecal bud) coming to lie in upper right quadrant before later descending into **lower right quadrant**

E. **Anomalies of Midgut Development**
   1. **Omphalocele**
      a. **Herniation of abdominal viscera into umbilical cord** due to **failure of midgut to return to abdominal cavity**
      b. Herniated gut is covered by **amnion.**
      c. Occurs with other severe malformations (e.g., cardiac) and has high mortality rate
   2. **Gastroschisis**
      a. **Herniation of abdominal viscera** through body wall **lateral to umbilicus**
      b. Not associated with extraintestinal anomalies
      c. Herniated gut is *not* covered by the peritoneum or amnion and may be damaged by amniotic fluid.
   3. **Ileal diverticulum** (Meckel diverticulum)
      - Represents **persistence of vitelline duct**

Omphalocele is the failure of the embryonic midgut to return to the abdominal cavity, and gastroschisis is a herniation through an abdominal wall defect.

High amniotic alpha-fetoprotein levels occur with anterior abdominal wall defects such as gastroschisis.

Ileal diverticulum rule of 2s: ~2% of population, 2x as common in males, ~2 feet from ileocecal junction, ~2 inches long

The connection of an **ileal diverticulum** to the **umbilicus** of a newborn may be retained (**vitelline fistula**), which allows feces to leak from the umbilicus.

Although usually asymptomatic, an ileal diverticulum may ulcerate, bleed, or perforate if **heterotopic pancreatic tissue** or **gastric mucosa** is contained. It may become infected (**Meckel diverticulitis**) with symptoms similar to appendicitis. Telescoping of the proximal portion of bowel into the distal portion (**intussusception**) or **volvulus** may occur at a Meckel diverticulum and result in bowel obstruction.

    4. **Rotational anomalies**
      a. Result from nonrotation, incomplete rotation, or reversed rotation of midgut
      b. Result in abnormal positioning of adult intestines
      c. May cause **volvulus** with a compromised blood supply

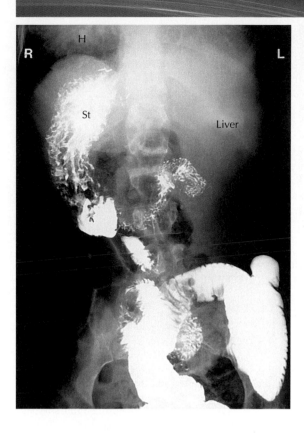

3-23: Radiograph of complete situs inversus showing heart and stomach on the right side and liver on the left. *(From Mettler, F A: Essentials of Radiology, 2nd ed. Philadelphia, Saunders, 2004, Figure 6-38.)*

5. **Situs inversus (Figure 3-23)**
   - Mirror-image reversal of thoracic and abdominal viscera due to anomalous determination of right and left sidedness during gastrulation

Individuals with **situs inversus** have **transposition of organs** in the thorax and the abdomen. The heart lies on the right side of the thorax **(dextrocardia),** the stomach and spleen are located on the right side of the abdomen, and the liver is on the left side. The heart loops and the gut rotates opposite their usual directions. The left lung has three lobes and the right lung has two. Situs inversus usually is asymptomatic but may cause diagnostic confusion if a physician is unaware of it (e.g., **appendicitis produces lower left quadrant pain**). It can be inherited as an **autosomal recessive** condition. Numerous partial reversals of organ positions can occur as variations.

> Situs inversus is the complete mirror-image reversal of thoracic and abdominal organs, causing potentially confusing signs and symptoms.

6. **Duodenal atresia**
   a. Results from **incomplete recanalization** distal to bile duct opening
   b. Common in **Down syndrome** infants
   c. Results in **double-bubble sign** on radiographs or ultrasound scans due to gas-filled stomach and proximal duodenum **(Figure 3-24)**
   d. Causes **polyhydramnios** due to absence of normal amniotic fluid absorption in intestines

> Double-bubble sign on newborn radiograph or ultrasound scan indicates duodenal atresia or anular pancreas.

7. **Congenital megacolon (Hirschsprung disease)**
   a. Most common cause of **neonatal bowel obstruction,** usually involving **sigmoid colon and rectum**
   b. Occurs more frequently in infants with **Down syndrome**
   c. Causes **dilation of normal colon proximal to aganglionic segment** from lack of peristalsis in aganglionic segment; bowel is obstructed because intestinal contents cannot be moved

> Congenital megacolon results from the absence of parasympathetic neurons in the wall of the large intestine.

VI. **Liver, Biliary System, Pancreas, and Spleen**
   A. **Liver (Figure 3-25; see Figures 3-2 and 3-10)**
      1. Overview
         a. Intraperitoneal organ covered by **visceral peritoneum** except where it directly contacts diaphragm
         b. Relatively larger in newborn and child than in adult

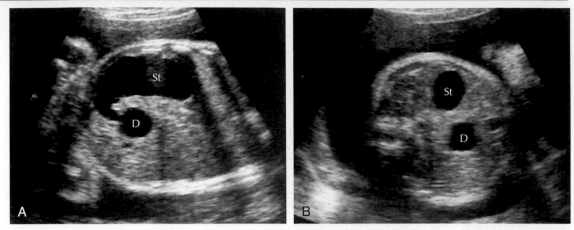

3-24: Ultrasound scans of fetus at 33 weeks of gestation showing duodenal atresia. **A,** Oblique scan shows dilated stomach (St) and proximal duodenum (D). **B,** Transverse scan shows characteristic "double-bubble" appearance of stomach and duodenum in duodenal atresia. *(From Moore, K L, Persaud, T V N: The Developing Human: Clinically Oriented Embryology, 8th ed. Philadelphia, Saunders, 2008, Figure 11-7.)*

Lower thoracic wall trauma on the right may injure the liver and on the left may injure the spleen.

To **biopsy the liver,** a needle is inserted under ultrasound guidance through the thoracic wall at a lower intercostal space (7-10) in the right midaxillary line. To reach liver parenchyma, the instrument must pass through the skin, superficial fascia, intercostal muscles, endothoracic fascia, costal pleura, costodiaphragmatic recess, diaphragmatic pleura, diaphragm, diaphragmatic peritoneum, subphrenic recess, and visceral peritoneum on the liver. Potential complications include hemorrhage, bile peritonitis, and pneumothorax/hemothorax. A **transjugular liver biopsy** may be performed in patients with a severe coagulopathy. The catheter is inserted into the right internal jugular vein and advanced through the superior vena cava, right atrium, and inferior vena cava into a hepatic vein.

Because the diaphragm domes, the **liver may be injured** by **trauma or clinical procedures** involving the right lower thoracic wall.

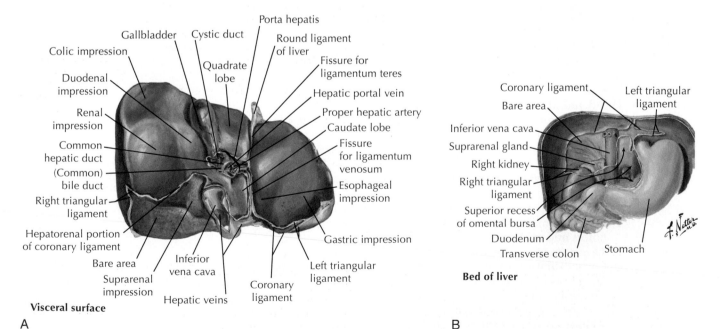

3-25: Visceral surface and bed of liver. **A,** Visceral surface of liver seen by tilting inferior border upward. Fissures for the ligamentum teres hepatis and ligamentum venosum separate the functional left lobe into medial and lateral parts with the medial part formed by the caudate and quadrate lobes. **B,** Bed of liver showing organs that produce contact impressions on its visceral surface. *(From Netter, F H: Atlas of Human Anatomy, 4th ed. Philadelphia, Saunders, 2006, Plate 287.)*

2. **Surfaces and borders of liver**
   a. **Diaphragmatic surface** has **bare area** that directly contacts diaphragm with no intervening peritoneum
   b. **Visceral surface** contacts other abdominal organs.

The smooth inferior edge of the **right lobe** of a normal liver can occasionally be palpated below the right costal margin, and it descends in **hepatomegaly**. Causes of an enlarged liver include cirrhosis, space-occupying masses (e.g., tumors, abscesses), biliary tract obstruction, and right-sided heart failure.

3. **Lobes of liver**
   • **Caudate and quadrate lobes** are functionally part of left lobe (Note: some experts consider the caudate an independent lobe.)
4. **Visceral surface of liver**
   a. **Porta hepatis** transmits hepatic ducts, hepatic arteries, branches of portal vein, autonomic nerves, and lymphatics.
   b. **Groove for inferior vena cava** lies within the bare area and contains terminations of hepatic veins.
   c. **Fissure for ligamentum venosum**, remnant of fetal **ductus venosus**
   d. **Fissure for ligamentum teres hepatis** (round ligament of the liver), remnant of **umbilical vein**
5. **Peritoneal ligaments of liver (see Table 3-4)**

Paraumbilical veins paralleling the **ligamentum teres** in the **falciform ligament** connect the portal vein and superficial (systemic) veins around the umbilicus. In **portal hypertension**, dilation of the superficial veins radiating from the umbilicus may produce **caput medusae (see Figure 3-40).**

Portal hypertension results in caput medusae.

6. **Blood vessels of liver**
   • Blood supplied by **proper hepatic artery** from **celiac trunk** (20%) and **portal vein** (80%); drainage from liver is by **hepatic veins**
   a. **Right hepatic artery**
      (1) Supplies right lobe of liver
      (2) May arise as aberrant branch of **superior mesenteric artery**
   b. **Left hepatic artery**
      (1) Supplies left, quadrate, and caudate lobes
      (2) May arise as aberrant branch of **left gastric artery**
   c. **Portal vein (Figure 3-26)**
      (1) Formed by **union of superior mesenteric and splenic veins** posterior to neck of pancreas
      (2) Reaches liver through **hepatoduodenal ligament**

Aberrant right hepatic artery may branch from SMA, and aberrant left hepatic artery may branch from the left gastric artery.

Portal vein thrombosis, usually in association with cirrhosis or acute appendicitis, results in **prehepatic portal hypertension.**

   d. **Hepatic veins**
      • Empty directly into **inferior vena cava**

Budd-Chiari syndrome is the obstruction of venous outflow from the liver. It often is due to **hepatic vein thrombosis** related to diverse factors such as hypercoagulable states (oral contraceptives; polycythemia), metastasis, infection, and pregnancy. Occlusion of the **hepatic veins** usually occurs subacutely over weeks with abdominal pain, hepatomegaly, ascites, and jaundice. Untreated acute hepatic vein obstruction results in fatal liver failure. Hepatic venous flow may be restored by **interventional radiologic procedures** (e.g., angioplasty or transjugular intrahepatic portosystemic shunts), or the liver may be decompressed by **surgically shunting blood** from the portal system into the inferior vena cava.

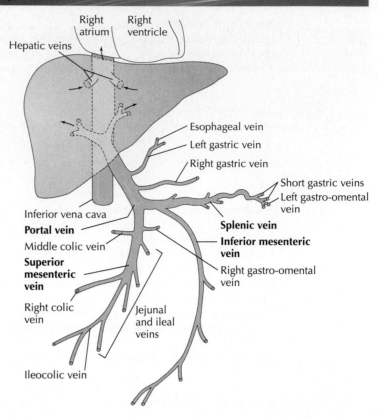

3-26: Hepatic portal venous system. *Arrows,* blood flow.

B. **Biliary System (Figure 3-27)**
   1. **Gallbladder**
      a. Pear-shaped sac on visceral surface of liver that **stores and concentrates bile**
      b. Consists of blunt-ended **fundus, body,** and narrow S-shaped **neck**

Situs inversus: left lower quadrant pain in appendicitis, left upper quadrant pain in cholecystitis

The **gallbladder fundus** may be palpable as it projects below the liver at the right costal margin **(9th costal cartilage) near the lateral border of the rectus abdominis.** An abnormal sacculation **(Hartman pouch)** may develop at the junction of the neck of the gallbladder and cystic duct and harbor **gallstones.**

   2. **Bile ducts**
      a. **Common hepatic duct**
         (1) Formed near **porta hepatis** by union of **right and left hepatic ducts**
         (2) Accompanied by **portal vein** and **proper hepatic artery**

3-27: Ducts of the liver, gallbladder, and pancreas, anterior view. Bile duct and main pancreatic duct join to form hepatopancreatic ampulla opening into second part of duodenum.

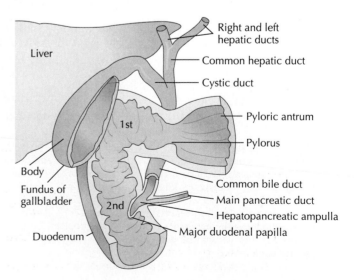

TABLE 3-8. REFERRED PAIN PATHWAYS FROM ABDOMINAL VISCERA*

VISCERA	VISCERAL AFFERENT PATHWAY	SPINAL CORD LEVEL(S) OF TERMINATION	AREAS OF REFERRAL
Foregut derivatives supplied by celiac trunk	Greater splanchnic nerves	T5-9	Epigastric region and T5-9 dermatomes of back**
Midgut derivatives supplied by superior mesenteric artery	Greater and lesser splanchnic nerves	T8-11	Umbilical region
Hindgut derivatives	Least and lumbar splanchnic nerves	T12-L2	Hypogastric region, inguinal region, and flanks

*Note that there is overlapping innervation by splanchnic nerves, depending on the synapses of the preganglionic fibers in the prevertebral ganglia.
**Inflamed foregut derivatives also may irritate diaphragmatic peritoneum, with pain referred to the ipsilateral shoulder via the phrenic nerve (C3,4).

    b. **Cystic duct**
       • Lined by mucous membrane organized into spirally arranged folds **(spiral valve)** that keep lumen open

> Cystic duct obstruction causes acute cholecystitis with Murphy sign.

Cystic duct obstruction, usually by **gallstones,** results in **acute inflammation of the gallbladder (cholecystitis)** that initially presents as epigastric pain, but pain may be **referred to T5-T9 dermatomes** of the back below the right scapula. Pain is referred to these dermatomes because **visceral afferent fibers from foregut derivatives** accompany sympathetic fibers of the **greater splanchnic nerve (Table 3-8).** Pain may also be referred to the **right shoulder** if the **diaphragmatic peritoneum** is irritated. Inflammation that involves the **parietal peritoneum** of the body wall produces pain localized in the **right upper quadrant.** The patient shows a sudden catch in breath on deep inspiration as the examiner's fingers contact the area over the fundus of the inflamed gallbladder **(Murphy sign). Gallstone obstruction** of the cystic duct causes **jaundice. Perforation of the gallbladder** results in formation of an abscess or **bile peritonitis.**

During surgical removal of the gallbladder **(cholecystectomy)** the **cystohepatic triangle**—bounded by the cystic duct, common hepatic duct, and liver—is an important surgical landmark. The **cystic artery** usually arises from the **right hepatic artery** in the cystohepatic triangle.

> Pain impulses from viscera supplied by the celiac trunk ascend the greater splanchnic nerve and are referred to dermatomes T5-T9.
>
> Cystohepatic triangle: cystic duct, common hepatic duct, and liver

An inflamed gallbladder may adhere to the first part of the duodenum or transverse colon, resulting in a **cholecystenteric fistula.** A gallstone entering the duodenum this way can obstruct the **ileocecal valve,** producing **gallstone ileus.** This usually occurs in elderly women.

> The cystic artery often arises from the right hepatic artery in the hepatocystic triangle, a key landmark for cholecystectomy.

    c. **Bile duct** (common bile duct)
      (1) Formed by **union of common hepatic and cystic ducts**
      (2) Descends in **hepatoduodenal ligament** to right of proper hepatic artery and anterior to portal vein
      (3) Passes behind first part of duodenum
      (4) Pierces **head of pancreas** and joins **main pancreatic duct** to form **hepatopancreatic ampulla,** which opens into **second part of duodenum** at **major duodenal papilla**

A **gallstone** or **adenocarcinoma** may obstruct the **hepatopancreatic ampulla,** causing **obstructive jaundice.** When the hepatopancreatic ampulla is obstructed, patients often develop **pancreatitis.**

Biliary stricture most commonly results from iatrogenic injury. The **bile duct** and **main pancreatic duct** can be examined for stricture by a radiograph following injection of contrast media at the **hepatopancreatic ampulla** in **endoscopic retrograde cholangiopancreatography (ERCP) (Figure 3-28).**

> Gallbladder pain may be referred to the right shoulder.

    C. **Pancreas (Figures 3-29 and 3-30; see Figures 3-2 and 3-10)**
      • Lies in bed of stomach behind parietal peritoneum except for tail
      1. **Head**
        a. Lies in curvature of duodenum and shares blood supply with it
        b. Traversed by bile duct
        c. Hooklike **uncinate process** lies **posterior to superior mesenteric vessels**

> Pancreatic cancer is the fourth leading cause of cancer deaths in the United States.

3-28: Normal endoscopic retrograde cholangiopancreatography (ERCP). Contrast medium is injected at hepatopancreatic ampulla, allowing radiographic examination of bile duct (CBD), intrahepatic ducts (HD), and main pancreatic duct (PD). Duodenum = D. *(From Mettler, F A: Essentials of Radiology, 2nd ed. Philadelphia, Saunders, 2004, Figure 6-52.)*

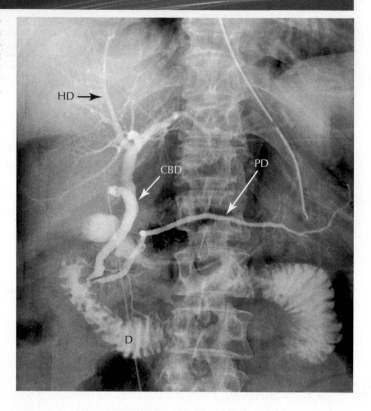

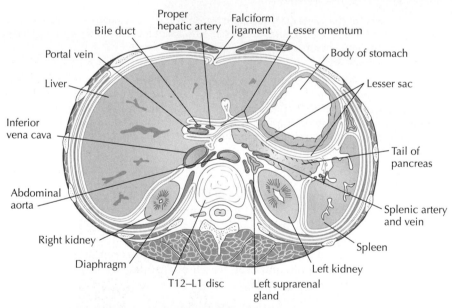

3-29: Horizontal section of the abdomen at the level of the disc between vertebrae T12 and L1, inferior view. Note that the left lobe of the liver lies to the left of midline and that the more superior left kidney is cut closer to the renal sinus than the right kidney.

Cancer of the pancreatic head obstructs the bile duct to produce jaundice.

Superior mesenteric artery involvement is a contraindication for pancreatic cancer surgery.

Pancreatic cancer is the fourth leading cause of cancer death in the United States, with a five-year survival rate of less than 5%. It occurs more commonly after age 50 and has **smoking** and **chronic pancreatitis** as other risk factors. Approximately 70% of pancreatic cancers develop in the head and neck of the pancreas, almost always from the **exocrine portion. Carcinoma of the head of the pancreas** typically obstructs the **bile duct,** causing **obstructive jaundice,** and also causes epigastric pain and weight loss. The gallbladder is frequently palpable from increased back-pressure (Courvoisier sign). New-onset **diabetes mellitus** after age 50 in the absence of a family history may be a sign of pancreatic cancer. Since **carcinomas of the body and tail** do not impinge on the bile duct, they usually continue growing and metastasize long before discovery.

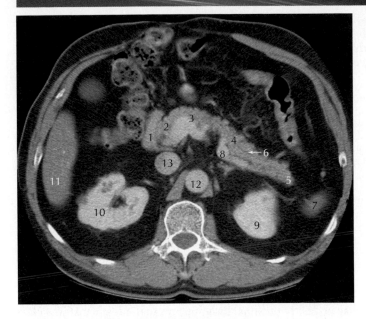

3-30: Axial CT during venous phase of contrast injection. Descending part of duodenum = 1; head of pancreas = 2; neck of pancreas = 3; body of pancreas = 4; tail of pancreas = 5; main pancreatic duct = 6; spleen = 7; splenic vein = 8; left kidney = 9; right kidney = 10; right lobe of liver = 11; aorta = 12; inferior vena cava = 13. (*From Weir, J, Abrahams, P: Imaging Atlas of Human Anatomy, 3rd ed. London, Mosby Ltd., 2003, p 125, m.*)

2. **Neck** is constricted where it is **crossed posteriorly by superior mesenteric vessels** and origin of the **portal vein.**
3. **Body** extends across midline, overlying aorta, left renal vein, splenic vein, and termination of inferior mesenteric vein
4. **Tail** enters **splenorenal ligament** and ends at hilum of spleen
5. **Main pancreatic duct (see Figures 3-27 and 3-28)**
    a. Traverses length of pancreas
    b. Joins bile duct to form **hepatopancreatic ampulla**

Acute pancreatitis may be caused by pancreatic enzymes escaping from the ductal system, perhaps after **obstruction or edema of the hepatopancreatic ampulla.** In middle-aged individuals, the condition frequently follows **excessive alcohol intake** or a **heavy meal.** The collection of fluid in the omental bursa from an injured or inflamed pancreas produces a **pancreatic pseudocyst.**

6. **Accessory pancreatic duct**
    a. Drains **uncinate process** and lower part of head
    b. Opens independently into second part of duodenum at **minor duodenal papilla**
D. **Spleen (Figures 3-29, 3-30, and 3-31; see also Figure 3-2)**

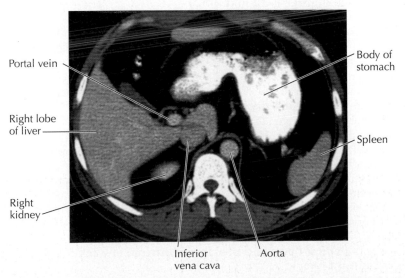

3-31: Computed tomography image at the level of about T12. The right kidney is uncharacteristically higher than the left kidney. The liver and spleen both lie deep to the lower ribs, where they are vulnerable to injury in thoracic wall trauma.

Pain from spleen may be referred to the left shoulder via the phrenic nerve.

Accessory spleens may be present near splenic hilum.

The spleen is the most frequently injured abdominal organ with potentially fatal hemorrhage.

Splenic artery aneurysm rupture is fatal in 70% of pregnant patients.

1. Lies posterior to midaxillary line in left hypochondriac region **deep to ribs 9-11** with long axis along rib 10 but is **separated from ribs by diaphragm and pleura**
2. Related on visceral surface to **left colic flexure,** stomach, and left kidney
3. **Peritoneal ligaments related to spleen (see Table 3-4)**

The **spleen** is the most frequently injured abdominal organ, often by **blunt trauma** that fractures the lower left ribs. Rupture results in intraperitoneal **hemorrhage** and requires spleen removal. The spleen enlarges **(splenomegaly)** and may have to be removed also in some hemolytic anemias, in which it destroys blood cells at abnormally high rates. **Splenectomy** usually has minimal consequences, but young children may develop **overwhelming postsplenectomy sepsis,** most frequently due to *Streptococcus pneumoniae.* The **tail of the pancreas** may be damaged during splenectomy because it extends in the **splenorenal ligament** to the hilum of the spleen.

Splenic artery aneurysms are the third most common intraabdominal aneurysm (after aortic and iliac artery aneurysms). They occur more commonly in women and are usually discovered during **pregnancy.** They may be an incidental finding or present with left-sided abdominal pain, nausea, and vomiting. **Aneurysmal rupture** results in hypotension and sudden collapse and is fatal in up to 25% of nonpregnant patients and 70% of pregnant patients.

Liver parenchyma develops from foregut endoderm; supporting cells arise from septum transversum mesoderm.

Septum transversum forms the central tendon of diaphragm, lesser omentum, and falciform ligament.

An anular pancreas may cause duodenal obstruction.

E. **Lymphatic Drainage of Liver, Biliary System, Pancreas, and Spleen**
   • From regional nodes to celiac nodes to intestinal lymph trunk that ends in cisterna chyli
VII. **Development of Liver, Pancreas, and Spleen**
   A. **Liver (Figure 3-32; see Figure 3-22)**
      1. Overview
         a. Engages in **hematopoiesis** from week 6 until late in fetal development
         b. Begins **bile formation** in week 12
      2. **Hepatic diverticulum (liver bud)**
         a. Ventral outgrowth of **caudal foregut endoderm** in week 4
         b. Invades **septum transversum** and proliferates to form **liver parenchyma**
      3. **Cystic diverticulum**
         • Outgrowth of **bile duct** giving rise to **cystic duct** and **gallbladder**
      4. **Septum transversum**
         a. Mesodermal mass lying between developing pericardial and peritoneal cavities
         b. Gives rise to Kupffer cells and connective tissue cells of liver
         c. Becomes attenuated by growth of liver, forming **lesser omentum, falciform ligament,** and **central tendon of diaphragm**
      5. **Extrahepatic biliary atresia**
         a. Produces **obstruction of bile ducts,** usually near porta hepatis, requiring surgery or liver transplant for survival
         b. Results from **failure of developing bile ducts to recanalize** from solid phase of development
   B. **Pancreas (see Figures 3-22 and 3-32)**
      1. Overview
         a. Arises from **ventral and dorsal pancreatic buds** of endoderm from caudal foregut
         b. Formed by migration of ventral bud (head of pancreas) to fuse with dorsal bud (rest of pancreas)
      2. **Main pancreatic duct**
         • Formed from fusion of duct of ventral bud with distal part of duct of dorsal bud
      3. **Accessory pancreatic duct**
         • Formed from proximal part of duct of dorsal bud
      4. **Anular pancreas**
         a. Results when tissue of a bifid ventral bud migrates in opposite directions to surround duodenum
         b. May result in partial or complete **obstruction of duodenum**
      5. **Pancreas divisum**
         a. Occurs when ventral and dorsal pancreatic buds fail to fuse
         b. May result in **stenosis** of minor duodenal papilla and **pancreatitis**
   C. **Spleen**
      1. Arises from **mesoderm of dorsal mesogastrium** in week 5 and is *not* an embryologic derivative of foregut
      2. Functions as a **hematopoietic organ** until late in fetal life
      3. Characterized by **lobules** in fetus that largely disappear by birth

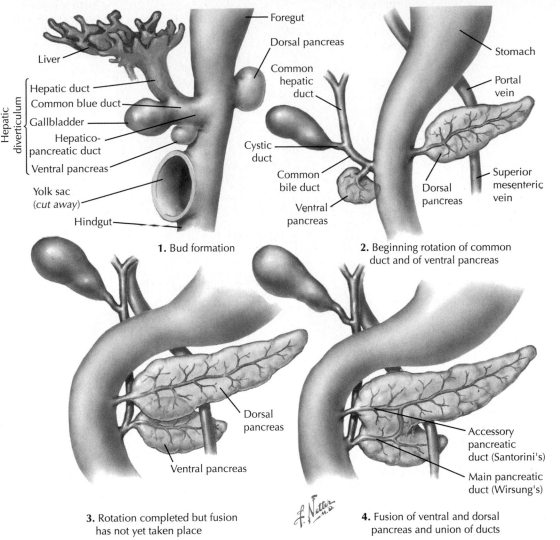

Liver

Hepatic diverticulum
- Hepatic duct
- Common blue duct
- Gallbladder
- Hepatico-pancreatic duct
- Ventral pancreas

Yolk sac (*cut away*)

Hindgut

Foregut

Dorsal pancreas

Common hepatic duct

Ventral pancreas

1. Bud formation

Stomach

Portal vein

Superior mesenteric vein

Dorsal pancreas

Cystic duct

Common bile duct

Ventral pancreas

2. Beginning rotation of common duct and of ventral pancreas

Dorsal pancreas

Ventral pancreas

3. Rotation completed but fusion has not yet taken place

Accessory pancreatic duct (Santorini's)

Main pancreatic duct (Wirsung's)

4. Fusion of ventral and dorsal pancreas and union of ducts

3-32: Progressive development (1-4) of the pancreas and biliary system in weeks 5 and 6. The pancreas is formed by dorsal and ventral pancreatic buds, with the ventral bud migrating around the caudal foregut to fuse with the dorsal bud. Ducts of the ventral bud and distal part of dorsal bud fuse to form the main pancreatic duct. (*From Cochard, L: Netter's Atlas of Human Embryology, Icon Learning Systems. Philadelphia, Saunders, 2002, Figure 6.11.*)

VIII. Posterior Abdominal Wall
A. Lumbar Plexus (Figure 3-33)
1. Supplies **extensor** and **adductor** compartments of thigh
2. Formed within psoas major muscle by **anterior rami** of **spinal nerves L1-4**
3. Upper part of larger **lumbosacral plexus**

B. Kidney (Figures 3-34 and 3-35)
1. Overview
   a. Retroperitoneal organ lying at vertebral levels T12-L3
   b. Usually lies lower on right side than left to accommodate large right lobe of liver
2. **Hilum**
   • Transmits renal vessels, renal pelvis, and autonomic nerves
3. **Renal pelvis**
   a. Funnel-shaped expansion of upper end of ureter
   b. Drains **major calyces,** each of which drains two to three **minor calyces;** each minor calyx drains one **renal papilla.**
4. **Ureter**
   a. Descends **retroperitoneally** on anterior surface of **psoas major**
   b. Receives **blood supply** primarily from renal, gonadal, common iliac, and vesical arteries

Superior pole of kidney extends to rib 12 on the right and to rib 11 on the left.

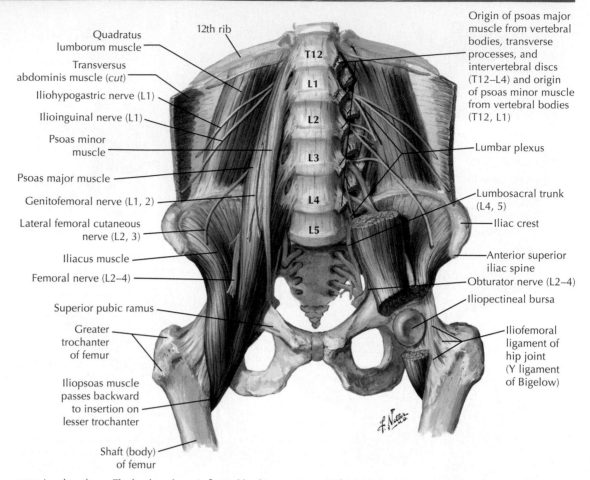

Quadratus lumborum muscle

12th rib

Origin of psoas major muscle from vertebral bodies, transverse processes, and intervertebral discs (T12–L4) and origin of psoas minor muscle from vertebral bodies (T12, L1)

T12

L1

Transversus abdominis muscle (cut)

Iliohypogastric nerve (L1)

L2

Ilioinguinal nerve (L1)

Psoas minor muscle

L3

Lumbar plexus

Psoas major muscle

Genitofemoral nerve (L1, 2)

L4

Lumbosacral trunk (L4, 5)

L5

Iliac crest

Lateral femoral cutaneous nerve (L2, 3)

Anterior superior iliac spine

Iliacus muscle

Obturator nerve (L2–4)

Femoral nerve (L2–4)

Iliopectineal bursa

Superior pubic ramus

Greater trochanter of femur

Iliofemoral ligament of hip joint (Y ligament of Bigelow)

Iliopsoas muscle passes backward to insertion on lesser trochanter

Shaft (body) of femur

3-33: Lumbar plexus. The lumbar plexus is formed by the anterior rami of spinal nerves L1-4 within the substance of the psoas major muscle, which has been partially removed on the cadaver's left side. The spinal cord levels that contribute to each branch of the lumbar plexus are indicated in parentheses. (From Netter, F H: Atlas of Human Anatomy, 4th ed. Philadelphia, Saunders, 2006, Plate 496.)

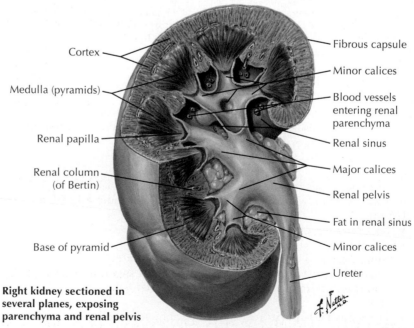

Cortex

Fibrous capsule

Minor calices

Medulla (pyramids)

Blood vessels entering renal parenchyma

Renal papilla

Renal sinus

Renal column (of Bertin)

Major calices

Renal pelvis

Fat in renal sinus

Base of pyramid

Minor calices

Ureter

Right kidney sectioned in several planes, exposing parenchyma and renal pelvis

3-34: Kidney sectioned in several planes. (From Netter, F H: Atlas of Human Anatomy, 4th ed. Philadelphia, Saunders, 2006, Plate 334.)

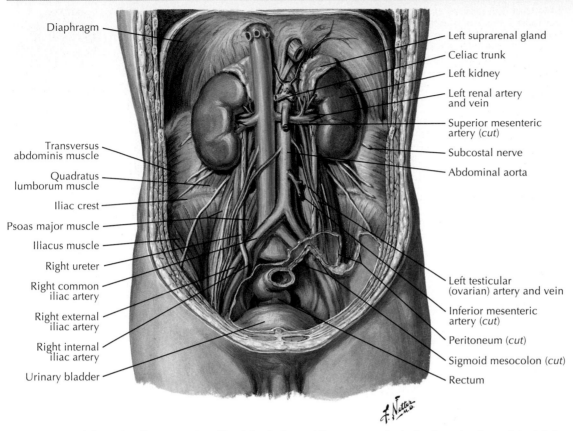

Diaphragm

Transversus abdominis muscle

Quadratus lumborum muscle

Iliac crest

Psoas major muscle

Iliacus muscle

Right ureter

Right common iliac artery

Right external iliac artery

Right internal iliac artery

Urinary bladder

Left suprarenal gland

Celiac trunk

Left kidney

Left renal artery and vein

Superior mesenteric artery (*cut*)

Subcostal nerve

Abdominal aorta

Left testicular (ovarian) artery and vein

Inferior mesenteric artery (*cut*)

Peritoneum (*cut*)

Sigmoid mesocolon (*cut*)

Rectum

3-35: Posterior abdominal wall, anterior view. The abdominal aorta bifurcates over the body of vertebra L4, and the inferior vena cava is formed to its right at the level of L5. The ureter descends retroperitoneally on the psoas major muscle and crosses the pelvic brim at the bifurcation of the common iliac artery. (*From Netter, F H: Atlas of Human Anatomy, 4th ed. Philadelphia, Saunders, 2006, Plate 329.*)

    c. Receives **innervation** from autonomic and afferent fibers derived from renal, aortic, and superior hypogastric plexuses

Ureter obstruction usually occurs where the ureter joins the **renal pelvis,** crosses the **pelvic brim,** or enters the **bladder wall. Renal calculi** (kidney stones) entering the ureter typically lodge at these narrow points, resulting in backup of urine with dilation of the ureter **(hydroureter)** and the renal pelvis and calyces **(hydronephrosis) (Figure 3-36).** Hydronephrosis causes progressive **renal atrophy;** unfortunately, if unilateral it may be asymptomatic until permanent kidney damage has occurred. A calculus in the ureter causes its smooth muscle to undergo intense peristaltic contractions in an attempt to dislodge the stone, causing severe intermittent pain referred to the lumbar region, inguinal region, external genitalia, and medial upper thigh. T11-L2 dermatomes are involved in a pattern called **"loin-to-groin" pain.**

The passage of ureteric stone causes loin-to-groin pain.

A ureter also may be obstructed by **external compression,** such as a tumor or idiopathic retroperitoneal fibrosis.

Obstruction of a ureter by calculi usually occurs at the ureteropelvic junction, pelvic brim, or bladder wall.

    5. **Renal fat and fascia**
      • Support and cushion kidney
      a. **Renal fascia**
        • Membranous condensation of connective tissue that surrounds **kidney** and **suprarenal gland** and divides fat into two regions

Urinary tract obstruction causes hydroureter and hydronephrosis with kidney atrophy.

Because the **renal fascia** is open inferiorly along the ureter, it provides a **path for infection** between the kidney and the pelvis.

Renal fascia directs the spread of perinephric infection inferiorly into the pelvis.

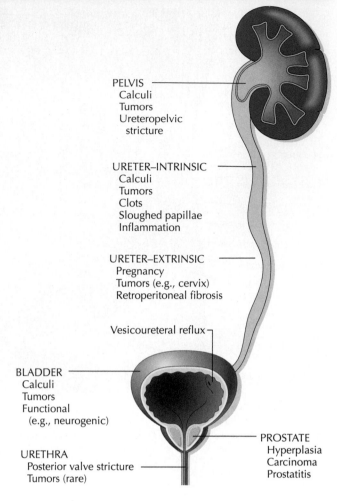

3-36: Obstructive lesions of the urinary tract that may cause hydroureter and hydronephrosis. *(From Kumar, V, Abbas, A, Fausto, N, Aster, J: Robbins and Cotran's Pathologic Basis of Disease, 8th ed. Philadelphia, Saunders, 2010, Figure 20-49.)*

PELVIS
Calculi
Tumors
Ureteropelvic
   stricture

URETER–INTRINSIC
Calculi
Tumors
Clots
Sloughed papillae
Inflammation

URETER–EXTRINSIC
Pregnancy
Tumors (e.g., cervix)
Retroperitoneal fibrosis

Vesicoureteral reflux

BLADDER
Calculi
Tumors
Functional
   (e.g., neurogenic)

PROSTATE
Hyperplasia
Carcinoma
Prostatitis

URETHRA
Posterior valve stricture
Tumors (rare)

b. **Renal fat**
   (1) **Perirenal (perinephric) fat** surrounds kidney inside renal fascia
   (2) **Pararenal (paranephric) fat** lies outside the renal fascia.
6. **Blood vessels of kidney (see Figure 3-35)**
   a. **Renal arteries** divide at the hilum into anterior and posterior branches that give rise to **segmental arteries,** one to each of **five kidney segments.**
   b. **Segmental renal arteries**
      (1) Essentially **end arteries** without functional anastomoses
      (2) If **occluded,** will result in **infarction** of that kidney segment

> Segmental renal arteries are **end arteries** with no effective collateral circulation. If a segmental artery is occluded, usually by a **thromboembolus** from the left atrium or **thrombosis of an atheromatous lesion,** the affected segment undergoes **infarction.** A renal infarct may be clinically silent or cause pain with costovertebral angle tenderness and hematuria. The lack of collateral circulation also means that a renal segment can be **surgically resected,** leaving the adjacent segments functioning.

   c. **Accessory renal arteries**
      • **Segmental arteries** that do not pass through renal hilum to enter kidney
   d. **Renal veins**
      (1) Paired tributaries of **inferior vena cava,** one from each kidney
      (2) **Intersegmental** in their distribution (in contrast to renal arteries)
      (3) Each passes **anterior** to **renal artery** and **renal pelvis** at hilum
   e. **Left renal vein**
      (1) Passes **anterior to aorta** just below origin of superior mesenteric artery
      (2) Receives **left suprarenal** and **left gonadal veins** and communicates with ascending lumbar vein, providing **collateral drainage if ligated**

Unilateral renal artery stenosis may cause surgically correctable hypertension.

A segmental renal artery is an end artery, and occlusion results in the infarction of the involved segment.

Accessory renal arteries are at risk during renal surgery and may compress the ureteropelvic junction to obstruct urine outflow.

Left renal vein in some patients can be safely ligated between inferior vena cava and termination of left suprarenal and left gonadal veins.

The **left renal vein** crosses toward the inferior vena cava through the **angle between the superior mesenteric artery and aorta (see Figure 3-35)**. The vein may be compressed in **renal vein entrapment syndrome (nutcracker syndrome)**, causing left flank pain and hematuria. Male patients may develop **varicocele** and left testicular pain. Note that renal vein entrapment syndrome differs from the **superior mesenteric artery syndrome**, in which the third part of the duodenum is compressed in the same angle.

Renal cell carcinomas often grow within the renal vein toward the inferior vena cava **(Figure 3-37)**. They may invade the vena cava and reach the right atrium. Hepatocellular carcinomas are another cancer with a tendency to invade veins.

The left renal vein may be compressed between the superior mesenteric artery and the aorta.

Renal cell carcinoma often spreads along the renal vein.

   f. **Right renal vein** passes posterior to second part of duodenum and head of pancreas
 7. **Lymphatic drainage of kidney**
   - To **aortic nodes**
C. **Suprarenal (adrenal) gland (see Figure 3-35)**
 1. Overview
   a. Paired **retroperitoneal** organ lying on upper pole of each kidney
   b. Enclosed by **perirenal fat** but easily separated surgically from kidney because of intervening renal fascial septum
   c. Consists of outer **cortex** and inner **medulla**
 2. **Suprarenal medulla**
   a. Consists of modified **postganglionic sympathetic neurons** known as **chromaffin cells** that secrete **epinephrine** and **norepinephrine**
   b. Receives innervation directly from **preganglionic sympathetic fibers**
 3. **Suprarenal cortex**
   - Secretes **steroid hormones** under influence of ACTH secreted by anterior lobe of pituitary
 4. **Blood vessels of suprarenal gland**
   a. Supplied by **superior suprarenal arteries** arising from **inferior phrenic artery, middle suprarenal artery** arising from **abdominal aorta**, and **inferior suprarenal arteries** arising from **renal artery**
   b. Drained by single **suprarenal vein** that terminates on right in **inferior vena cava** and on left in **left renal vein**

The suprarenal medulla functions as a collection of postganglionic sympathetic neurons.

Acute adrenocortical insufficiency (adrenal crisis) may result from hemorrhagic necrosis of both suprarenal glands caused by **meningococcal infection** in **Waterhouse-Friderichsen syndrome.**

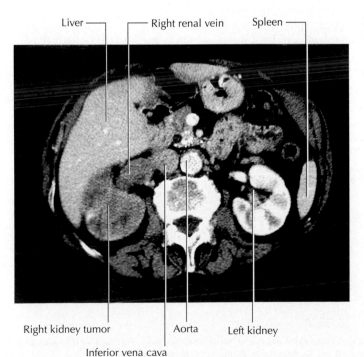

Liver — | — Right renal vein | Spleen —

Right kidney tumor | Aorta | Left kidney

Inferior vena cava

3-37: Axial CT of right kidney carcinoma spreading along renal vein to inferior vena cava. *(From Drake, R, Vogl, W A, Mitchell, A: Gray's Anatomy for Students, 2nd ed. Philadelphia, Churchill Livingstone, 2010, Figure 4.143.)*

D. **Respiratory Diaphragm** (see Figures 3-2, 3-10, and 3-35; see Chapter 2, Section VI)

E. **Muscles of the Posterior Abdominal Wall** (see Figures 3-33 and 3-35)

IX. **Development of the Kidney and Suprarenal Gland**

- Kidney and suprarenal cortex develop from **mesoderm,** but suprarenal medulla develops from **neural crest cells**

A. **Kidney (Figure 3-38)**

1. Overview
   a. On each side develops from **intermediate mesoderm** that forms **nephrogenic cord** in longitudinal **urogenital ridge**
   b. Develops from last of three sets of kidneys—pronephros, mesonephros, and metanephros—that appear in human embryo

2. **Pronephros**
   - Appears early in week 4 but is **nonfunctional** and disappears

3. **Mesonephros**
   a. Appears late in week 4 and functions as **interim kidney** until about week 9
   b. Largely degenerates except for **mesonephric (wolffian) duct**

4. **Metanephros**
   a. Appears early in week 5 and starts to function about week 9 as **permanent kidney**
   b. **Ureteric bud** repeatedly divides to form the ureter, renal pelvis, major and minor calyces, and collecting tubules.
   c. **Metanephrogenic (metanephric) mesoderm** forms **nephrons** of adult kidney (glomerulus, Bowman capsule, convoluted tubules, and loop of Henle)

5. **Ascent of kidneys**
   a. From pelvis to adult position accompanied by 90° medial rotation
   b. Accompanied by **change in blood supply** as nearby vessels change

B. **Suprarenal Gland**

1. **Suprarenal cortex**
   a. Develops by two waves of mesodermal proliferation, resulting in **fetal cortex** that is later enclosed by **adult cortex**
   b. Still includes fetal cortex at birth, but it regresses during first year
   c. Includes **zona glomerulosa** and **zona fasciculata** of adult cortex at birth with **zona reticularis** formed during third year

2. **Suprarenal medulla**
   a. Develops from **sympathetic ganglion cells of neural crest origin**
   b. Location of **chromaffin cells** in adults

C. **Anomalies of Kidney and Suprarenal Gland Development**

1. **Unilateral renal agenesis**
   a. Relatively common, usually involving left kidney in males
   b. Compensated for by hypertrophy of other kidney
   c. More common than **bilateral renal agenesis,** which is incompatible with life

Metanephros is the last of the three embryonic kidneys and forms the permanent kidney.

The kidney develops from metanephric mesoderm and the ureteric bud of the mesonephric duct.

The developing kidney ascends from the pelvis to the adult position due to differential growth and decreased body curvature.

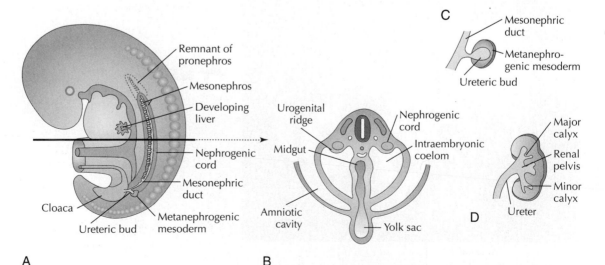

3-38: Development of the kidney. **A,** Lateral view of the early embryo showing mesonephros and metanephric primordia. **B,** Transverse section of the embryo from *panel A.* **C** and **D,** Successive stages of metanephros.

Bilateral renal agenesis is incompatible with postnatal survival. Fetal anuria results in decreased amniotic fluid (oligohydramnios), and the neonate exhibits Potter sequence, with a flattened face, hypoplastic lungs, limb deformities, and other defects.

Oligohydramnios in bilateral renal agensis results in fatal lung hypoplasia.

2. **Horseshoe kidney**
    a. Results from fusion of inferior poles of right and left kidneys in pelvis
    b. Trapped in its ascent by **inferior mesenteric artery** but usually functions normally
        • There is a slight increased risk for developing infection (pyelonephritis).
    c. Increased incidence in **Turner syndrome**
3. **Ectopic kidneys**
    a. Result from **abnormal ascent of embryonic kidneys**
    b. Usually located in pelvis and may fuse to form **pancake (discoid) kidney**
    c. Receive variable blood supply from closest vessels
4. **Polycystic kidney disease**
    • Relatively common **hereditary disease** in which kidney contains multiple cysts that cause renal insufficiency
    a. **Autosomal recessive (childhood) polycystic kidney disease** forms cysts from **collecting tubules** and requires early postnatal dialysis or kidney transplantation for survival.
        • May produce **Potter sequence** (see clinical correlation above)
    b. **Autosomal dominant (adult) polycystic kidney disease forms** cysts from **parts of nephron** with **renal failure in adulthood.**
5. **Bifid or double ureter**
    • Results from **abnormal division** of ureteric bud
6. **Congenital adrenal hyperplasia (adrenogenital syndrome)**
    a. Group of autosomal recessive disorders that cause **excessive androgen production** by cells of cortex during fetal period
    b. Causes **masculinization of external genitalia in females** (female pseudohermaphroditism) and precocious puberty in males.
X. **Abdominal Aorta, Inferior Vena Cava, Hepatic Portal Venous System, and Portocaval Anastomoses**
    A. **Abdominal Aorta (Figures 3-35 and 3-39, A)**

Autosomal dominant polycystic kidney patients are often asymptomatic into adulthood when hypertension precedes renal failure.

Female pseudohermaphroditism results from congenital adrenal hyperplasia.

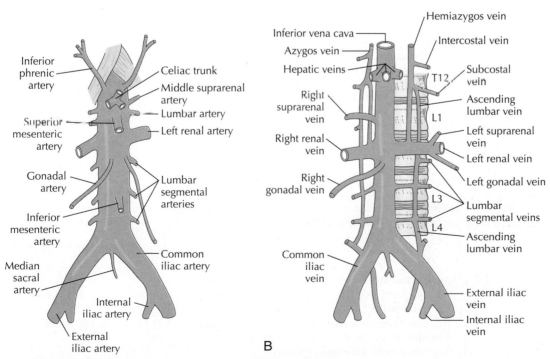

3-39: A, Abdominal aorta. **B,** Inferior vena cava and tributaries. Note that the right gonadal vein drains into the inferior vena cava, whereas the left gonadal vein drains into the higher pressure left renal vein.

1. Enters abdomen through **aortic hiatus** of diaphragm anterior to body of **T12** vertebra
2. Bifurcates over **L4 vertebra** (supracristal plane near level of umbilicus) into right and left **common iliac arteries**

Abdominal aorta may be compressed against L4 in children and thin adults to control pelvic or lower-extremity bleeding.

Abdominal aortic aneurysms occur mainly between the aortic bifurcation and the origin of the renal arteries. There is a genetic susceptibility to aneurysm development associated with **atherosclerosis** and **hypertension. Age** and **smoking** are risk factors. The aneurysm, which usually pulsates, can be palpated in the umbilical region. Leaking or ruptured aneurysms produce severe abdominal or lower back pain and may be rapidly fatal; many aneurysms are asymptomatic. Aneurysms may be surgically repaired by a **prosthetic tube graft** or endovascular **stent** placement. A prosthetic graft is wrapped by the wall of the opened aorta to prevent development of an **aortoenteric fistula** and fatal hemorrhage.

Abdominal aneurysms develop most commonly in the infrarenal aorta of white male smokers over 50 with atherosclerosis.

Gradual occlusion of the aortic bifurcation from **atherosclerosis** diminishes blood flow and can cause **intermittent claudication.**

B. **Inferior Vena Cava (see Figures 3-35 and 3-39, *B*)**
   • Receives blood from lower extremities, pelvis and perineum, and **abdomen excluding GI tract**

Collateral venous return in IVC obstruction occurs via ascending lumbar-azygos, superior-inferior epigastric, and thoracoepigastric veins.

The **inferior vena cava** (IVC) anastomoses via the **ascending lumbar vein** with the **azygos system** in the thorax, providing communication between the inferior and superior vena caval systems in **vena caval obstruction.** Other collateral routes for abdominal venous return to the heart include the **inferior-superior epigastric veins,** and the **thoracoepigastric veins.**

The portal vein drains the abdominal digestive tract to the liver.

C. **Hepatic Portal Venous System (see Figure 3-26)**
   1. **Portal vein**
      a. Formed by **union of superior mesenteric and splenic veins** behind neck of pancreas
      b. **Drains the abdominal part of the digestive tract** and **spleen** to the liver
      c. Ascends behind first part of duodenum and reaches liver within hepatoduodenal ligament

Portal hypertension may result from prehepatic, intrahepatic, or posthepatic obstruction.

In **portal hypertension,** pressure in the portal vein is elevated because of obstructed blood flow to or through the liver. **Obstruction may be intrahepatic** if caused by **cirrhosis, prehepatic** if caused by **portal vein thrombosis,** or **posthepatic** if the hepatic veins are involved, as in **Budd-Chiari syndrome.** Increased portal pressure reverses blood flow through tributaries that anastomose with vena caval systems (portocaval or portosystemic anastomoses).

   2. **Splenic vein**
      a. Forms at hilum of spleen and enters splenorenal ligament
      b. Courses posterior to pancreas to join superior mesenteric vein

Progressive **splenomegaly** caused by venous congestion in **portal hypertension** or **thrombosis of the portal or splenic vein** may cause **hypersplenism,** resulting in a decreased number of circulating formed elements.

   3. **Superior mesenteric vein**
      • Ends behind neck of pancreas by joining splenic vein to form portal vein
   4. **Inferior mesenteric vein**
      a. Receives terminations of left colic, sigmoidal, and superior rectal veins
      b. Usually drains into splenic or superior mesenteric vein
   5. **Left gastric vein (coronary vein)**
      • Has esophageal tributaries anastomosing with those of azygos system of veins

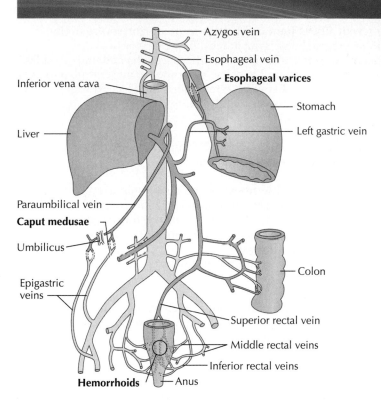

Inferior vena cava

Liver

Paraumbilical vein

Caput medusae

Umbilicus

Epigastric veins

Hemorrhoids

Azygos vein

Esophageal vein

Esophageal varices

Stomach

Left gastric vein

Colon

Superior rectal vein

Middle rectal veins

Inferior rectal veins

Anus

3-40: Portocaval anastomoses. Reversed blood flow in portal hypertension may cause development of esophageal varices, caput medusae, and hemorrhoids.

D. **Portocaval (Portosystemic) Anastomoses (Figure 3-40)**
  • Anastomoses between tributaries of portal vein and superior or inferior vena cava
  1. **Lower end of esophagus** between esophageal tributaries of **left gastric vein** (portal) and **azygos system** (systemic); engorgement of these veins may cause **esophageal varices**
  2. **Anal canal** between **superior rectal** (portal) and **inferior rectal** (systemic) veins; engorgement of these veins may cause **hemorrhoids**
  3. **Umbilicus** between **paraumbilical veins** (portal) and **superficial veins of anterior abdominal wall** (systemic); **caput medusae** is pattern formed by engorged veins radiating from umbilicus

In portal hypertension, esophageal varices, hemorrhoids, and caput medusae form from portocaval anastomoses.

XI. **Autonomic Nerves of the Abdomen**
  A. **Vagus Nerves**
  1. Supply **parasympathetic innervation** to gastrointestinal tract as far distally as **left colic (splenic) flexure**
  2. Enter abdomen on esophagus as **anterior and posterior vagal trunks**
  3. Distributed through **celiac and superior mesenteric plexuses**

Surgically sectioning the anterior and posterior vagal trunks **(truncal vagotomy)** decreases gastric acid production by over 50% but also impairs gastric emptying because vagal fibers relax the **pyloric sphincter.** Therefore, truncal vagotomy must be accompanied by a drainage procedure (e.g., pyloroplasty) and is rarely done anymore. **Highly selective vagotomy** reduces gastric acid output but spares fibers that relax the pyloric sphincter.

Vagus nerves supply the GI tract proximal to the left colic flexure.

Vagus nerve fibers relax the pyloric sphincter to allow gastric emptying.

  B. **Pelvic Splanchnic Nerves**
  • Supply **parasympathetic innervation** to GI tract caudal to **left colic flexure** (descending and sigmoid colon, rectum, upper anal canal)
  C. **Lumbar Sympathetic Trunk**
  1. Descends from thorax behind medial arcuate ligament of diaphragm and lies on bodies of lumbar vertebrae
  2. Typically has four segmentally arranged ganglia
  D. **Thoracic and Lumbar Splanchnic Nerves (T5-L2)**
  1. Overview
    a. Contain mostly **preganglionic sympathetic fibers** that synapse in abdominal **prevertebral ganglia**

Thoracic splanchnic nerve spinal cord levels: greater T5-9; lesser T10-11; least T12

Pain from abdominal viscera travels on GVA fibers accompanying sympathetic fibers.

GI visceral pain (e.g., in appendicitis) may start in the midline because of the original embryonic position of the organs.

   b. Contain **visceral afferent fibers** from cell bodies in **posterior root ganglia** at same level of origin as preganglionic sympathetic fibers
2. **Greater splanchnic** nerve arises from **T5-T9** sympathetic ganglia and ends in **celiac ganglion**; postganglionic fibers distributed in celiac and superior mesenteric plexuses
3. **Lesser splanchnic** nerve arises from **T10-T11** sympathetic ganglia and usually ends in **superior mesenteric ganglion** or **aorticorenal ganglion**
4. **Least splanchnic** nerve arises from **T12** sympathetic ganglion and enters **aorticorenal ganglion**
5. **Lumbar splanchnic** nerves arising from **L1 and L2** sympathetic ganglia end in superior mesenteric and **inferior mesenteric ganglia.**

E. **Autonomic Plexuses of Abdomen**
1. **Sympathetic** and **vagal parasympathetic fibers** of the autonomic nervous system are contained along with accompanying general visceral afferent fibers.
2. **Postganglionic sympathetic fibers** from cell bodies in **prevertebral ganglia** are distributed via plexuses around blood vessel supplying organ (i.e., **celiac, superior mesenteric,** and **inferior mesenteric plexuses**)
3. **Visceral afferent fibers** accompanying **sympathetic fibers** conduct **pain** impulses.

F. **Pain from Abdominal Viscera**
1. **Visceral pain**
   a. Results from **distention, spasm, inflammation,** or **ischemia** of walls of hollow abdominal viscera or of **stretched capsules** of solid abdominal organs
   b. **Aching or burning pain** that is poorly localized to a midline abdominal region (epigastric, umbilical, or hypogastric)
2. **Referred pain (see Table 3-8)**
   • Produced by visceral afferent fibers having cell bodies in **same posterior root ganglion** at same spinal cord level as somatic afferent nerve fibers that carry pain from a dermatome
   a. **Foregut derivatives**
      • Liver, gallbladder and bile ducts, pancreas, stomach, first and second parts of duodenum
         (1) Receive innervation via **greater splanchnic nerves** and **celiac plexus** from cell bodies in posterior root ganglia at **T5-T9**
         (2) Refer to **T5-T9 dermatomes** of lower thoracic and **epigastric** regions
   b. **Midgut derivatives**
      • Second and third parts of duodenum, jejunum, ileum, cecum and appendix, ascending and transverse colons
         (1) Receive innervation via **greater and lesser splanchnic nerves** and **superior mesenteric plexus** from cell bodies in posterior root ganglia at **T8-T11**
         (2) Refer mainly to **T8-T11 dermatomes** of **umbilical region**
   c. **Hindgut derivatives**
      • Descending colon, sigmoid colon, rectum, and upper part of anal canal rectum
         (1) Receive innervation via lumbar splanchnic nerves and inferior mesenteric plexus from cell bodies in posterior root ganglia at L1-L2
         (2) Refer pain to **T12-L2 dermatomes** of **hypogastric region,** inguinal region, scrotum, or labia
   d. **Retroperitoneal structures**
      • Kidneys, upper ureters, gonads, and aorta
         (1) Receive innervation via **lesser and least splanchnic nerves** (T11-12) and **lumbar splanchnic nerves** (L1-L2) and aortic plexus from cell bodies in posterior root ganglia at **T11-L2**
         (2) Refer to **T11-L2 dermatomes** of lumbar and inguinal regions

CHAPTER 4
THE PELVIS AND THE PERINEUM

I. **Bony Pelvis (Figure 4-1)** (see also Chapter 5)
   A. **Overview**
     1. Composed of paired **hip bones, sacrum,** and **coccyx**
     2. Oriented in anatomical position so **anterior superior iliac spines (ASIS)** and **pubic tubercles** lie in same vertical plane
   B. **Pelvic brim**
     1. Surrounds **superior pelvic aperture** or **pelvic inlet**
     2. Formed by **sacral promontory, arcuate line of ilium, pecten and crest of pubis,** and **pubic symphysis**
     3. Divides bony pelvis into superior **greater or false pelvis** and inferior **lesser or true pelvis**
   C. **Greater pelvis** (false pelvis)
     1. Expanded portion of bony pelvis **superior to pelvic brim**: deep in male; shallow in female
     2. Lowest part of **abdominal cavity** with superior part of bony pelvis providing protection to lower abdominal viscera
   D. **Lesser pelvis** (true pelvis)
     1. Bony pelvis **inferior to pelvic brim**
     2. Open to abdominal cavity superiorly but closed inferiorly by **pelvic diaphragm**
     3. Has inferior part of bony pelvis protecting pelvic organs and providing skeletal framework for perineum
   E. **Pelvic outlet**
     • Diamond-shaped area bounded by coccyx, sacrotuberous ligaments, ischial tuberosities, ischiopubic rami, and pubic symphysis

> Because the **pelvis** functions as a rigid ring of bone, traumatic injury frequently causes a **fracture in two places:** a site where traumatic force is applied and 180° opposite that site. If an individual falls on the **greater trochanter** or falls from a height and lands on his feet, the **head of the femur** may be driven through the **acetabulum** into the pelvic cavity. **Pelvic fractures** may injure pelvic organs, including the urinary bladder and reproductive organs, and cause **hemorrhage** from pelvic blood vessels and resultant **shock.** The majority of bleeding often results from venous plexus injury. A **full bladder** is more likely to rupture than an empty one, and **urethral injuries** are more likely in males. During surgical repair, screws must be carefully placed to avoid injuring the **internal iliac artery and vein** lying against the inner surface of the bone.

> In skeletally immature individuals, **avulsion fractures** at the sites of muscle attachments are common. Frequent sites of avulsion fractures include the **anterior superior iliac spine** (sartorius), **anterior inferior iliac spine** (rectus femoris), and **ischial tuberosity** (hamstrings).

II. **Pelvic Measurements (Figures 4-2 and 4-3)**
   A. **Overview**
     1. In a female, **dimensions of pelvic inlet, midpelvis, and pelvic outlet** are important determinants of successful vaginal birth.
     2. In a female, **pelvic deformities** and some individual variations may cause difficult labor **(dystocia).**
   B. **Measurements of Obstetrical Significance (Table 4-1)**

The pelvis has the ASIS and the pubic tubercle in the same vertical plane.

The greater pelvis is part of the abdominal cavity.

Traumatic pelvic fractures often occur in two places with pelvic organ injury and hemorrhage.

Avulsion fractures occur at muscle attachments in skeletally immature patients.

Fetal head rotates 90° during birth as maximum diameter changes from transverse at pelvic inlet to anteroposterior at pelvic outlet.

The midpelvic diameter is the narrowest point of the birth canal and the point of greatest difficulty during labor.

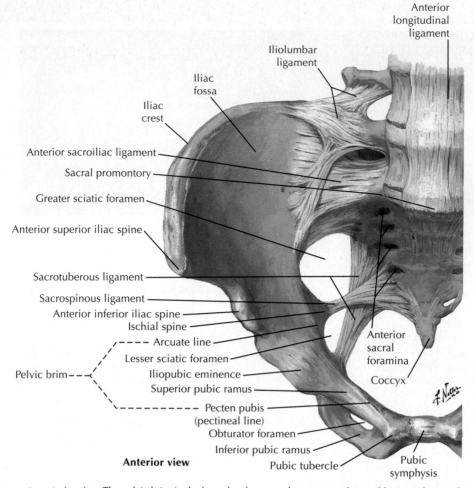

Anterior view

4-1: Bony pelvis and ligaments, anterior view. The pelvic brim is the boundary between the greater pelvis and lesser pelvis. In the anatomical position, the pubic tubercle and anterior superior iliac spine lie in the same vertical plane. *(From Netter, F H: Atlas of Human Anatomy, 4th ed. Philadelphia, Saunders, 2006, Plate 353.)*

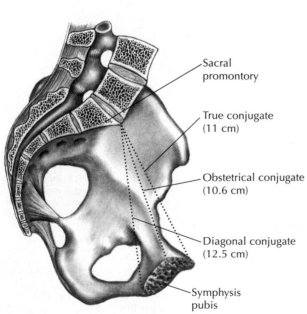

4-2: Pelvic measurements with obstetrical significance. Obstetrical conjugate is estimated as diagonal conjugate minus 1.5-2.0 cm. *(From Seidel, H M, Ball, J W, Dains, J E, Benedict, G W: Mosby's Guide to Physical Examination, 6th ed. St. Louis, Mosby Elsevier, 2006, Figure 18-28.)*

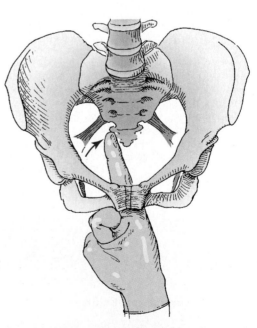

4-3: Interspinous diameter between ischial spines is narrowest transverse diameter of midpelvis. Measurement is estimated by moving examining fingers in vagina from side to side between spines. *(From Lowdermilk, D L, Perry, S E: Maternity and Women's Health Care, 8th ed. St. Louis, Mosby, 2004.)*

TABLE 4-1. PELVIC MEASUREMENTS OF OBSTETRICAL SIGNIFICANCE

MEASUREMENT	DISTANCE	COMMENTS
Pelvic Inlet		
True conjugate diameter	AP distance between sacral promontory and upper border of pubic symphysis	
Diagonal conjugate diameter	AP distance between sacral promontory and lower border of pubic symphysis	Measured during vaginal exam
Transverse diameter	Greatest distance between right and left arcuate lines	
Oblique diameter	Distance between one sacroiliac joint and contralateral iliopubic eminence	
Midpelvis		
Interspinous (midpelvic) diameter	Distance between ischial spines	Narrowest point of birth canal; estimated during vaginal exam
Pelvic Outlet		
Anteroposterior diameter	Distance between tip of coccyx and lower border of pubic symphysis	
Intertuberous (transverse) diameter	Distance between medial surfaces of ischial tuberosities	Smallest diameter of pelvic outlet

AP, anteroposterior.

TABLE 4-2. DIFFERENCES BETWEEN MALE AND FEMALE BONY PELVIS

FEATURE	MALE	FEMALE
False pelvis	Deep	Shallow
Pelvic inlet	Narrow and heart-shaped	Wide and almost oval
Pelvic cavity	Longer, tapered, cone-shaped	Shorter, cylindrical, roomier
Pelvic outlet	Smaller	Larger because of eversion of ischial tuberosities and wider subpubic angle
Subpubic angle	$<70°$	$>80°$
Shape of sacrum	Longer, narrower, and more curved	Shorter, wider, and flatter
Anterior pelvic wall	Longer	Shorter

III. Differences between Male and Female Bony Pelvis (Table 4-2)
   A. Android
      1. Typical funnel shape of **male pelvis**
      2. Heart-shaped pelvic inlet with maximum transverse diameter close to sacrum
   B. Gynecoid
      1. Typical shape of **female pelvis** with straight side walls and wide interspinous diameter
      2. Oval pelvic inlet with maximum transverse diameter well anterior to sacrum
IV. Joints of Pelvis
   A. Sacroiliac Joint (see Figure 4-1)
      1. Only joint between **axial skeleton** and **pelvic girdle**
      2. Transfers weight of upper body to lower extremity
      3. Reinforced by strong ligaments and so stable that bone on either side of joint is more likely to fracture than joint is to dislocate
   B. Pubic Symphysis
      1. Midline joint between bodies of two pubic bones
      2. **Fibrocartilaginous disc** connecting surfaces covered by hyaline cartilage
      3. Reinforced by **superior pubic** and **inferior (arcuate) pubic ligaments**
      4. Relatively **immovable** except in latter stages of **pregnancy,** when hormones cause ligaments to loosen
V. Pelvic Cavity
   A. Boundaries
      1. **Pelvic brim**
      2. **Lateral walls:** hip bone below pelvic brim, obturator membrane, obturator internus muscle and fascia, sacrotuberous and sacrospinous ligaments
      3. **Posterior wall:** sacrum and coccyx and piriformis muscle
      4. **Floor:** pelvic diaphragm

Sacroiliac joints transfer weight from the axial to the lower-extremity skeleton.

Sacroiliac joints and pubic symphysis allow limited mobility, more during pregnancy.

Hormonal changes during pregnancy relax the pelvic ligaments and pubic symphysis, allowing enlargement of the birth canal.

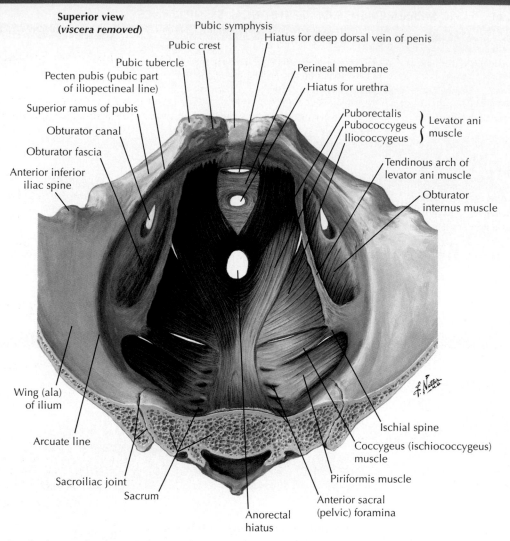

Superior view
(viscera removed)

Pubic symphysis

Hiatus for deep dorsal vein of penis

Pubic crest

Pubic tubercle

Perineal membrane

Pecten pubis (pubic part of iliopectineal line)

Hiatus for urethra

Superior ramus of pubis

Puborectalis
Pubococcygeus
Iliococcygeus } Levator ani muscle

Obturator canal

Tendinous arch of levator ani muscle

Obturator fascia

Obturator internus muscle

Anterior inferior iliac spine

Wing (ala) of ilium

Arcuate line

Ischial spine

Coccygeus (ischiococcygeus) muscle

Sacroiliac joint

Piriformis muscle

Sacrum

Anterior sacral (pelvic) foramina

Anorectal hiatus

4-4: Pelvic diaphragm of male, superior view. The levator ani and coccygeus muscles and their fasciae form the pelvic diaphragm. The urogenital hiatus is an anterior gap between the medial borders of the two levator ani muscles, which is filled by the urogenital diaphragm (including the perineal membrane) except for passage of the urethra in both sexes and the vagina in females. *(From Netter, F H: Atlas of Human Anatomy, 4th ed. Philadelphia, Saunders, 2006, Plate 358.)*

B. **Pelvic Diaphragm (Figure 4-4)**
  1. Overview
    a. **Muscular hammock** formed by **levator ani** and **coccygeus muscles** and their fasciae
    b. **Supports pelvic organs** and raises pelvic floor
    c. Incomplete anteriorly at **urogenital hiatus** to allow passage of **urethra** in both sexes and **vagina** in female
    d. Pierced posteriorly by **anal canal**
    e. Innervated by anterior rami of **S4** spinal nerves and **pudendal nerves** (S2-4)
  2. **Coccygeus (ischiococcygeus) muscle**
    • Parallels and blends inferiorly with **sacrospinous ligament**
  3. **Levator ani muscle**
    a. Overview
      (1) Funnel-shaped layer consisting of **iliococcygeus** and **pubococcygeus muscles**
      (2) Aids in **maintaining urinary and fecal continence** and **preventing prolapse** of pelvic organs
      (3) **Susceptible to damage during childbirth**
    b. **Iliococcygeus muscle**
      • Arises from **tendinous arch of levator ani** (arcus tendineus) and ischial spine and inserts into coccyx and **anococcygeal ligament**

The pelvic diaphragm provides dynamic support for pelvic organs.

Levator ani injury during childbirth may cause urinary or fecal incontinence and pelvic organ prolapse.

c. **Pubococcygeus muscle**
   (1) Arises from dorsal surface of pubis and fuses posteriorly with opposite muscle at **anococcygeal ligament**
   (2) Anteriorly surrounds base of prostate (**puboprostaticus,** levator prostatae) or inferior end of vagina (**pubovaginalis**)

d. **Puborectalis muscle**
   (1) Thicker inferomedial part of pubococcygeus muscle; joins opposite muscle to form **sling around anorectal junction,** maintaining **anorectal (perineal) flexure**
   (2) Relaxes only during **defecation**

VI. **Other Features of Pelvic Walls and Floor**
   A. **Obturator Membrane**
      1. Closes **obturator foramen** except superiorly at **obturator canal** where obturator nerve and vessels pass into thigh
      2. Surfaces provide attachment for **obturator internus** and **obturator externus muscles.**
   B. **Sacrotuberous Ligament (see Figure 4-1)**
      1. Extends from posterior iliac spines, sacrum, and coccyx to **ischial tuberosity**
      2. Forms inferior boundary of **lesser sciatic foramen**
      3. **Stabilizes sacroiliac joint**
   C. **Sacrospinous Ligament (see Figure 4-1)**
      1. Extends from sacrum and coccyx to **ischial spine,** separating **greater** and **lesser sciatic foramina**
      2. **Stabilizes sacroiliac joint**
   D. **Pelvic Fascia**
      1. **Parietal pelvic fascia** lines pelvic walls and is continuous with **transversalis and iliopsoas fasciae** of the abdomen.
      2. **Visceral pelvic fascia** covers and supports pelvic viscera; condensations form **fascial ligaments** extending from pelvic walls to viscera.

> **Pelvic fascial ligaments** and the **pelvic diaphragm** support the pelvic viscera, especially when intraabdominal pressure is increased. **Injury** to the pelvic floor **during childbirth** or laxity associated with **advancing age** causes loss of support with **prolapse of pelvic organs,** particularly the uterus and rectum. Other risk factors include genetic predisposition, nerve lesions, connective tissue disorders, and chronically increased intraabdominal pressure (e.g., from coughing or strenuous physical activity).

   E. **Pelvic Ligaments (Figure 4-5)**
      • Fibrous condensations of pelvic fascia containing variable amounts of smooth muscle
      1. **Puboprostatic (male) or pubovesical/pubocervical (female) ligament**
         a. Condensation of superior fascia of pelvic diaphragm
         b. Attaches **prostate** (male) or **neck of bladder and cervix** (female) to posterior surface of **pubis**
      2. **Transverse cervical ligament (female)**
         a. **Cardinal** (Mackenrodt) **ligament**
         b. Fascial condensation with embedded smooth muscle in base of **broad ligament**

The puborectalis produces anorectal flexure and maintains anal continence.

The sacrospinous ligament separates greater and lesser sciatic foramina, and the sacrotuberous ligament forms the inferior boundary of the lesser.

Risk factors for pelvic organ prolapse include childbirth, age, obesity, neurogenic dysfunction, and connective tissue disorders.

4-5: Female pelvic ligaments, superior view.

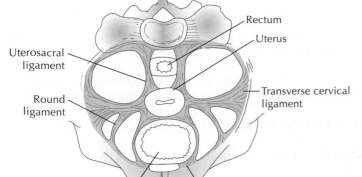

Uterosacral ligament

Round ligament

Bladder

Rectum

Uterus

Transverse cervical ligament

Pubovesical ligament

   c. Extends from lateral pelvic wall to **cervix of uterus** and **lateral fornix of vagina** with **uterine artery** running medially in it
   d. Most important ligament **supporting uterus and vagina**
3. **Sacrogenital ligament**
   a. Also called **rectoprostatic** in male; extends from prostate to sacrum
   b. Also called **uterosacral/rectouterine** in female; forms posterior continuation of transverse cervical ligament from cervix and vagina to sacrum
   c. **Stabilizes and supports pelvic organs**

VII. **Pelvic Organs in Both Male and Female (Figures 4-6 and 4-7)**
   A. **Ureter**
      1. Constricted at **ureteropelvic junction, pelvic brim,** and entrance into **bladder**
      2. Crosses pelvic brim near bifurcation of **common iliac artery**
      3. In male, crossed **superiorly** by **ductus deferens** near bladder
      4. In female, crossed **anteriorly and superiorly** by **uterine artery** in base of **broad ligament**

> **Renal calculi** (kidney stones) typically obstruct the **ureter** at its three **sites of constriction.** Most calculi are too small to be seen on plain radiographs, so an **intravenous pyelogram** is required **(Figure 4-8).**
>
> The **ureter** can be **damaged** during a **hysterectomy** or **surgical repair** of a **prolapsed uterus** because it lies posterior and inferior to the **uterine artery.** This relationship, easily remembered as "water flows under the bridge," is an important one for surgeons.

   B. **Urinary Bladder**
      1. **External features**
         a. **Apex**
            • Attached to umbilicus by **median umbilical ligament,** a remnant of the fetal **urachus**
         b. **Fundus (base)**
            (1) Related to **seminal vesicles and rectum** in male and **uterus and vagina** in female
            (2) Receives **ureters;** internally features **trigone**
         c. **Superior surface**
            • Completely covered by **peritoneum** and domes into abdominal cavity as bladder fills
         d. **Neck**
            • Surrounds urethra; relatively immobile, especially in male where attached to **prostate**

> The full adult **urinary bladder** may be **palpated** through the **anterior abdominal wall** above the pubic symphysis. The empty adult bladder occupies the lesser pelvis but may be palpated when one hand is placed over the bladder with a finger from the other hand placed in the rectum of the male or in the vagina of the female. In a child, the empty or full bladder can always be palpated because it extends above the pubic symphysis into the abdomen.

      2. **Muscle of bladder wall**
         a. Interlacing layers of smooth muscle known as **detrusor muscle**
         b. Surrounds urethra at bladder neck as circularly arranged **internal urethral sphincter**
      3. **Internal features of urinary bladder**
         a. **Trigone**
            • Small triangular area of fundus defined by two **ureteric orifices** and **internal urethral orifice** where mucosa remains smooth whether bladder is empty or filled
         b. **Ureteric orifices**
            • Slitlike openings at superolateral angles of trigone
         c. **Interureteric fold**
            • **Landmark** for **introducing catheter into ureter**
         d. **Internal urethral orifice**
            • Lies at inferior angle of **trigone**

The transverse cervical and uterosacral ligaments passively support the uterus.

Obstruction of a ureter by a calculus usually occurs at sites of constriction.

Uterine artery passes anterior and above ureter ("water flows under the bridge").

A young child's bladder is always an abdominal organ, but an adult's empty bladder is pelvic.

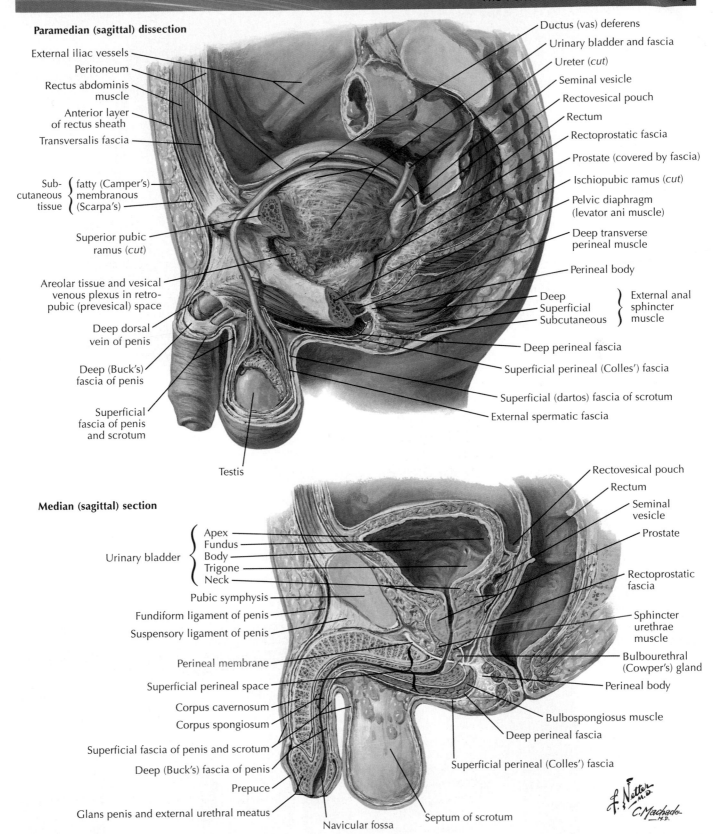

Paramedian (sagittal) dissection

- External iliac vessels
- Peritoneum
- Rectus abdominis muscle
- Anterior layer of rectus sheath
- Transversalis fascia
- Subcutaneous tissue { fatty (Camper's) / membranous (Scarpa's)
- Superior pubic ramus (cut)
- Areolar tissue and vesical venous plexus in retropubic (prevesical) space
- Deep dorsal vein of penis
- Deep (Buck's) fascia of penis
- Superficial fascia of penis and scrotum
- Testis

- Ductus (vas) deferens
- Urinary bladder and fascia
- Ureter (cut)
- Seminal vesicle
- Rectovesical pouch
- Rectum
- Rectoprostatic fascia
- Prostate (covered by fascia)
- Ischiopubic ramus (cut)
- Pelvic diaphragm (levator ani muscle)
- Deep transverse perineal muscle
- Perineal body
- Deep / Superficial / Subcutaneous } External anal sphincter muscle
- Deep perineal fascia
- Superficial perineal (Colles') fascia
- Superficial (dartos) fascia of scrotum
- External spermatic fascia

Median (sagittal) section

- Urinary bladder { Apex / Fundus / Body / Trigone / Neck
- Pubic symphysis
- Fundiform ligament of penis
- Suspensory ligament of penis
- Perineal membrane
- Superficial perineal space
- Corpus cavernosum
- Corpus spongiosum
- Superficial fascia of penis and scrotum
- Deep (Buck's) fascia of penis
- Prepuce
- Glans penis and external urethral meatus
- Navicular fossa
- Septum of scrotum

- Rectovesical pouch
- Rectum
- Seminal vesicle
- Prostate
- Rectoprostatic fascia
- Sphincter urethrae muscle
- Bulbourethral (Cowper's) gland
- Perineal body
- Bulbospongiosus muscle
- Deep perineal fascia
- Superficial perineal (Colles') fascia

4-6: Male pelvic organs in paramedian and median sagittal sections. *(From Netter, F H: Atlas of Human Anatomy, 4th ed. Philadelphia, Saunders, 2006, Plate 361.)*

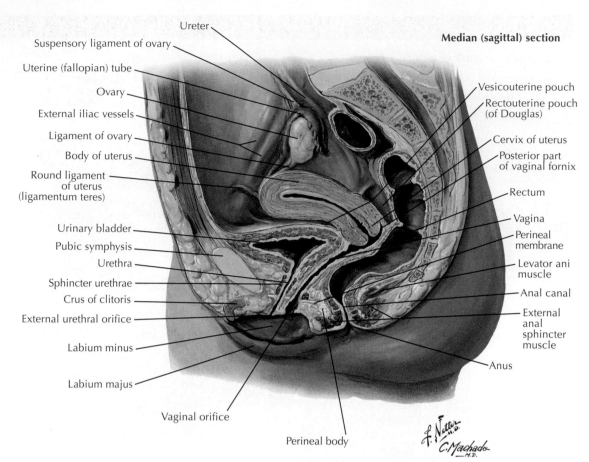

Ureter

Suspensory ligament of ovary

Uterine (fallopian) tube

Ovary

External iliac vessels

Ligament of ovary

Body of uterus

Round ligament
of uterus
(ligamentum teres)

Urinary bladder

Pubic symphysis

Urethra

Sphincter urethrae

Crus of clitoris

External urethral orifice

Labium minus

Labium majus

Vaginal orifice

Perineal body

Vesicouterine pouch

Rectouterine pouch
(of Douglas)

Cervix of uterus

Posterior part
of vaginal fornix

Rectum

Vagina

Perineal
membrane

Levator ani
muscle

Anal canal

External
anal
sphincter
muscle

Anus

4-7: Median sagittal section of female pelvic organs. Note close relationship of rectouterine pouch to posterior fornix of vagina. (*From Netter, F H: Atlas of Human Anatomy, 4th ed. Philadelphia, Saunders, 2006, Plate 360.*)

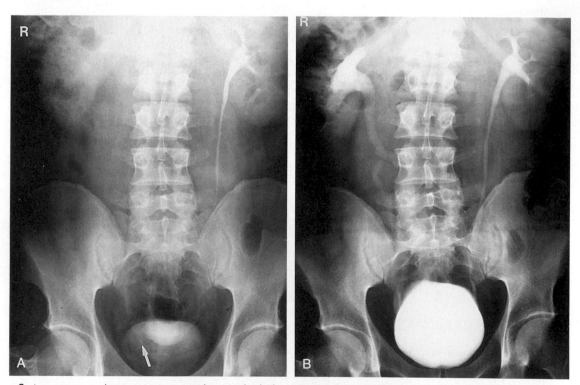

4-8: Intravenous pyelograms in patient with ureteral calculus. Images taken at 5 minutes and 25 minutes following contrast agent injection in young male with intense right flank pain and hematuria. **A,** Small calculus is shown at the entrance of the right ureter into the bladder (*arrow*). **B,** Delayed image shows right renal collecting system and ureter dilated due to the distal obstruction. (*From Mettler, F A: Essentials of Radiology, 2nd ed. Philadelphia, Saunders, 2004, Figure 7-12.*)

The **uvula** is a small elevation in the male at the inferior angle of the **trigone,** just above the **internal urethral orifice.** It enlarges with age due to enlargement of the underlying **median lobe of the prostate** and may inhibit complete bladder emptying. Stagnation of retained urine results in development of **urinary tract infections.** There also may be hesitancy starting urination, diminished force and size of stream, terminal dribbling, and hematuria.

Obstruction of the oblique course of the ureter through the bladder wall (e.g., due to **detrusor muscle hypertrophy, invasion by cervical cancer**) or **vesicoureteral reflux** due to trigonal muscle weakness may cause backup of urine. The result is **hydroureter** and **hydronephrosis.** The **ureter** becomes **elongated and tortuous** due to smooth muscle that hypertrophies to increase peristaltic force **(see Figure 4-8, B).**

Ninety percent of **bladder cancers** are **transitional cell carcinomas.** They are most common in males over the age of 50. **Cigarette smoking** is the most important risk factor, although occupational exposure to chemicals such as aniline dyes may account for one-third of cases. **Painless hematuria** is the most common presenting symptom, but frequency, urgency, and dysuria also may be present.

An enlarging uvula in the lower trigone may inhibit bladder emptying and predispose to infections.

4. **Blood supply: superior vesical branches of umbilical arteries;** inferior **vesical arteries** in males and **vaginal arteries** in females
5. **Venous drainage:** internal iliac veins by **vesical** and **prostatic venous plexuses;** connections with the **vertebral venous plexus** provide a route for cancer metastases
6. **Innervation: vesical** and **prostatic plexuses**
7. **Micturition reflex**
   a. **Sympathetic fibers** inhibit detrusor muscle and stimulate internal urethral sphincter contraction, **inhibiting emptying.**
   b. **Parasympathetic fibers** stimulate detrusor muscle contraction and inhibit the internal sphincter, **facilitating emptying.**
   c. **Somatic motor fibers** (pudendal nerve) cause **voluntary relaxation** of external urethral sphincter (sphincter urethrae).
8. **Retropubic space**
   • Potential space containing extraperitoneal connective tissue separating pubic bones and symphysis from anterior surface of bladder

Drainage from vesical to vertebral venous plexus provides a route for cancer metastasis to the vertebral column and spinal cord.

Sympathetic fibers stimulate internal urethral sphincter contraction to prevent retrograde ejaculation in males.

Sympathetic nerve fibers inhibit and parasympathetic fibers facilitate micturition, with pudendal nerve providing voluntary control.

Retropubic space allows extraperitoneal access to the urinary bladder and prostate gland.

If a urethral catheter can't be inserted in a patient with obstruction or to provide drainage in patients with spinal cord injuries, **urine can be removed from the bladder** without penetrating the peritoneum by **inserting a needle or catheter just above the pubic symphysis (suprapubic cystotomy).** The catheter passes successively through skin, fatty and membranous layers of superficial abdominal fascia, linea alba, transversalis fascia, extraperitoneal connective tissue, and the wall of the bladder.

C. Rectum
1. Overview
   a. Large intestine connecting sigmoid colon and anal canal
   b. Has complete outer longitudinal layer of smooth muscle and therefore lacks teniae coli and haustra; also lacks omental appendices
   c. Peritoneal covering on anterior and lateral sides in **proximal third;** anterior surface in **middle third;** none in **distal third**
   d. Transverse rectal folds (Houston valves) may serve to support fecal matter.
2. **Blood supply: superior rectal artery** from inferior mesenteric artery with contributions from **middle and inferior rectal arteries** from internal iliac artery
3. **Venous drainage: superior rectal vein** (inferior mesenteric vein), which anastomoses with **middle and inferior rectal veins** (internal iliac vein) in a **portocaval anastomosis**
4. **Innervation:** preganglionic parasympathetic innervation from **pelvic splanchnic nerves** and postganglionic sympathetic innervation from **inferior hypogastric plexus**

The rectum lacks teniae coli, haustra, and omental appendices that are characteristic of the rest of the large intestine.

A **sigmoidoscope** or other rigid object **can perforate the wall of the rectum.** Any object that penetrates the middle third anteriorly or the upper third anteriorly or laterally enters the peritoneal cavity.

Cancer from midgut and hindgut derivatives metastasizes to the liver through the portal vein.

4-9: Radiograph of ulcerative colitis following double-contrast barium enema showing small irregular, confluent ulcers extending from the rectum to the right colic flexure. *(From Mettler, F A: Essentials of Radiology, 2nd ed. Philadelphia, Saunders, 2004, Figure 6-75.)*

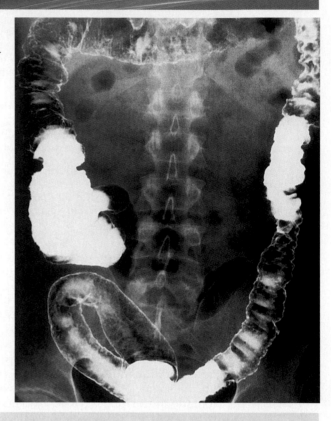

Ulcerative colitis is a chronic inflammatory bowel disease that begins in the rectum and spreads proximally.

Ulcerative colitis: continuous mucosal-submucosal ulcerations of the rectum and colon. Crohn disease: transmural inflammation with skip lesions involving ileum ± colon

Carcinoma of the rectum is relatively common. Initially it remains localized, but then it spreads along lymphatic vessels and through the venous system. Because the superior rectal vein is a tributary of the portal vein, **metastasis to the liver is common.** A tumor may penetrate the rectal wall posteriorly and invade the **sacral plexus,** producing sciatica. Laterally, the tumor may invade the **ureter.** Anterior spread may involve the **vagina and uterus** in the female and the **prostate, seminal vesicles, or bladder** in the male.

Ulcerative colitis is the **most common inflammatory disease of the bowel** and is limited to the colon. It is mainly a disease of **young adults** that **begins in the rectum and spreads proximally,** involving only the **mucosa and submucosa** with **continuous ulcerations (Figure 4-9).** Islands of residual mucosa produce **pseudopolyps.** The patient experiences recurrent left-sided abdominal cramping with bloody mucoid diarrhea. In the most severe cases, **toxic damage to parasympathetic ganglia stops bowel function,** and the colon progressively swells and becomes gangrenous **(toxic megacolon).** Patients have an increased risk of **adenocarcinoma.**

D. Development of Urinary Bladder, Rectum, and Anal Canal (Figure 4-10)
1. **Cloaca**
   a. Dilated common chamber of allanois and hindgut that gives rise to urinary bladder, rectum, and anal canal
   b. Contacts surface ectoderm at **cloacal membrane**
2. **Urorectal septum**
   a. Mesenchymal wedge that divides cloaca into **urogenital sinus** ventrally and **rectum** and **anal canal** dorsally
   b. Fuses with cloacal membrane at future site of **perineal body**
3. **Urinary bladder**
   • Develops mainly from upper, vesical part of **urogenital sinus**
4. **Allantois**
   a. Initially diverticulum of yolk sac into connecting stalk continuous with cloaca
   b. Continuous with vesical part of urogenital sinus but constricts into fibrous **urachus,** extending to umbilicus

The cloaca is the dilated common chamber of the allantois and the embryonic hindgut that is divided into the ventral urinary bladder and the dorsal rectum and anal canal.

A urachal fistula causes urine to leak from the neonatal umbilicus.

Usually the embryonic **allantois** is obliterated to form the fibrous **urachus** connecting the apex of the bladder to the umbilicus. In the adult it is known as the **median umbilical ligament.** If the **lumen remains patent in a newborn (urachal fistula),** this connection causes **urine to leak from the umbilicus.** Midline urachal cysts also may occur.

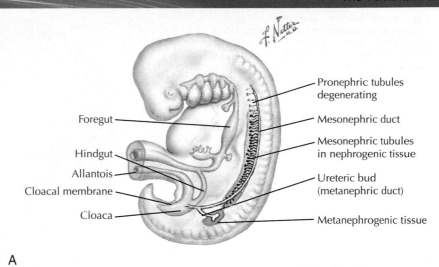

A

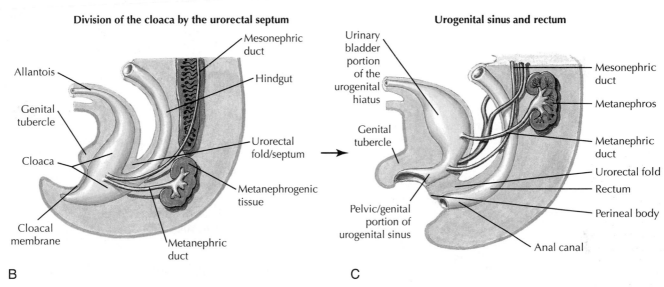

Division of the cloaca by the urorectal septum

Allantois

Genital
tubercle

Cloaca

Cloacal
membrane

Mesonephric
duct

Hindgut

Urorectal
fold/septum

Metanephrogenic
tissue

Metanephric
duct

B

Urogenital sinus and rectum

Urinary
bladder
portion
of the
urogenital
hiatus

Genital
tubercle

Pelvic/genital
portion of
urogenital sinus

Mesonephric
duct

Metanephros

Metanephric
duct

Urorectal fold

Rectum

Perineal body

Anal canal

C

4-10: A, Orientation view of developing urinary and gastrointestinal systems. **B-C,** Progressive development of urinary bladder, rectum, and anal canal. Urorectal septum grows toward cloacal membrane to divide cloaca into ventral urogenital sinus (urinary bladder) and dorsal rectum and superior part of anal canal. Perineal body develops at site of fusion of urorectal septum with cloacal membrane **(C).** *(From Cochard, L: Netter's Atlas of Human Embryology, Icon Learning Systems. Philadelphia, Saunders, 2002, Figures 7.2 and 7.4.)*

5. **Rectum and anal canal above pectinate line**
   a. Develop from endoderm of **hindgut**
   b. Supplied by **superior rectal artery** and drained by **superior rectal vein** and by lymphatic vessels to **inferior mesenteric and internal iliac lymph nodes**
   c. Innervated by **visceral afferent fibers**
6. **Anal canal below pectinate line**
   a. Develops from ectoderm of **proctodeum**
   b. Supplied by **inferior rectal arteries** and drained by **inferior rectal veins** and by lymphatic vessels to **superficial inguinal lymph nodes**
   c. Innervated by **somatic afferent fibers** of pudendal nerve

VIII. **Male Pelvic Structures (Figure 4-11; see also Figures 4-6 and 4-12)**
   A. **Seminal Vesicle**
   1. Coiled, blind-ending tube **posterior to fundus of bladder,** lateral to ampulla of ductus deferens, and **anterior to rectum,** through which it normally can be palpated
   2. Joins **ductus deferens** near base of prostate to form **ejaculatory duct**
   3. Produces **seminal fluid** but does *not* store spermatozoa

The hepatic portal and inferior vena caval systems anastomose at the pectinate line.

The anal canal below the pectinate line drains to the superficial inguinal lymph nodes.

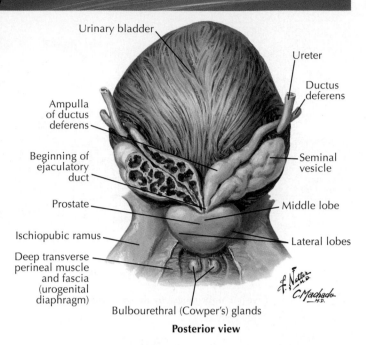

4-11: Urinary bladder and pelvic organs unique to male, posterior view. Note formation of ejaculatory ducts, position of lateral and middle lobes of prostate, and relationship of ureter to ductus deferens. *(From Netter, F H: Atlas of Human Anatomy, 4th ed. Philadelphia, Saunders, 2006, Plate 384.)*

Urinary bladder

Ureter

Ductus deferens

Ampulla of ductus deferens

Seminal vesicle

Beginning of ejaculatory duct

Prostate

Middle lobe

Ischiopubic ramus

Lateral lobes

Deep transverse perineal muscle and fascia (urogenital diaphragm)

Bulbourethral (Cowper's) glands

Posterior view

B. Ductus Deferens
  1. Thick-walled muscular tube that begins as continuation of **epididymis** and carries sperm to ejaculatory duct
  2. Traverses **inguinal canal** as part of **spermatic cord**
  3. Becomes dilated posterior to bladder to form **ampulla**

C. Ejaculatory Duct
  1. Formed by union of **ductus deferens** and **duct of seminal vesicle**
  2. Passes through **prostate** to open into **prostatic urethra**

D. Prostate Gland
  1. Overview
    a. Pyramidal gland surrounding **prostatic urethra** with its **base** at neck of bladder and its **apex** resting on superior fascia of urogenital diaphragm
    b. Enclosed by fibrous **capsule** that is separated from visceral pelvic fascia **(prostatic sheath)** by **prostatic venous plexus**
    c. Supported laterally by **pubococcygeus** muscles and bound anteriorly to pubic bones by **puboprostatic ligaments**
  2. **Internal features of prostatic urethra (Figure 4-12)**
    a. **Urethral crest**
      • Longitudinal ridge in posterior wall
    b. **Seminal colliculus (verumontanum)**
      • Enlargement of **urethral crest** that receives openings of paired **ejaculatory ducts** and median **prostatic utricle**
    c. **Prostatic utricle**
      (1) Blind pouch opening at summit of **seminal colliculus**
      (2) **Homologue** of **uterus and proximal vagina** because it is considered remnant of fused **paramesonephric** (müllerian) **ducts**
    d. **Prostatic sinus**
      • Depression on each side of urethral crest that receives openings of **prostatic ducts**
  3. **Lobes of prostate gland**
    a. **Anterior lobe**
      • Anterior to urethra and consists of fibromuscular tissue
    b. **Posterior lobe**
      • Posterior to urethra and inferior to plane of ejaculatory ducts; referred to clinically as peripheral zone

The prostatic venous plexus is a potential source of hemorrhage during prostate surgery.

Benign prostatic hyperplasia usually involves the median lobe, and prostate cancer involves the posterior lobe.

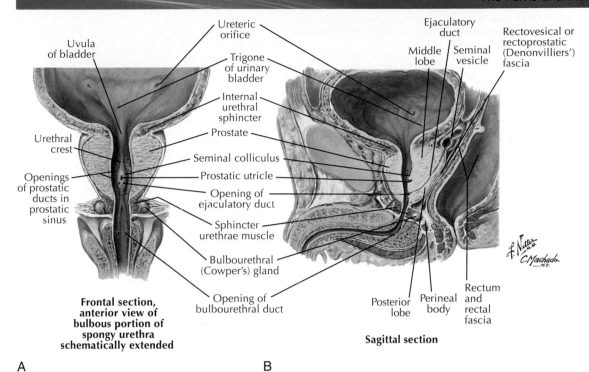

4-12: Sections through prostate gland and urethra. **A,** Frontal section showing posterior wall of prostatic, membranous, and proximal spongy urethra. Note seminal colliculus with prostatic utricle and openings of ejaculatory ducts. **B,** Median sagittal section through bladder, prostate, and proximal penis. *(From Netter, F H: Atlas of Human Anatomy, 4th ed. Philadelphia, Saunders, 2006, Plate 384.)*

Prostate cancer usually begins in the periphery of the gland in a region that corresponds to the anatomical **posterior lobe (Figure 4-13),** so early stages are often asymptomatic. Later, in advanced disease, prostate cancer can occlude the prostatic urethra, causing obstruction. After age 50, primary methods of detection include an annual **digital rectal examination (Figure 4-14)** and blood tests for **prostate-specific antigen** (PSA).

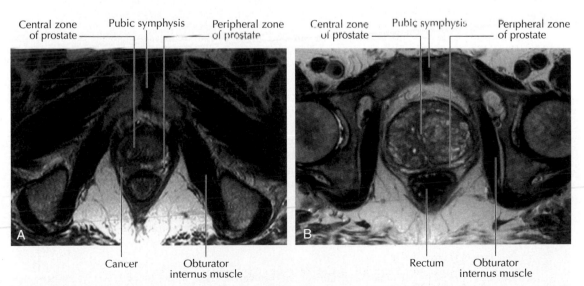

4-13: Axial T-2 weighted MR images of prostate gland pathology. **A,** Small prostatic cancer in peripheral zone of a normal-sized prostate. **B,** Benign prostatic hypertrophy involving central zone of prostate and compressing prostatic urethra. Compressed peripheral zone provides cleavage plane for surgical enucleation of hyperplastic tissue. *(From Drake, R, Vogl, W A, Mitchell, A: Gray's Anatomy for Students, 2nd ed. Philadelphia, Churchill Livingstone, 2010, Figure 5.48.)*

4-14: Digital rectal examination allows evaluation of size and texture of the prostate gland and seminal vesicles through the anterior wall of the rectum.

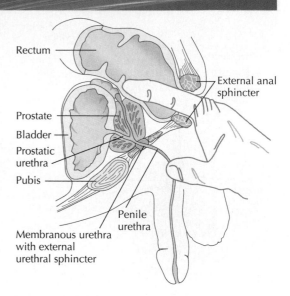

Rectum

External anal sphincter

Prostate

Bladder

Prostatic urethra

Pubis

Penile urethra

Membranous urethra with external urethral sphincter

c. Median (middle) lobe
- Posterior to urethra and superior to plane of ejaculatory ducts; includes regions referred to clinically as **central zone + transitional zone**

BPH causes increased frequency, urgency, and nocturia.

> In middle age, the **median lobe** of the prostate develops **benign prostatic hyperplasia (BPH)** with resulting enlargement of the **uvula** and **obstruction of the internal urethral orifice.** Signs of obstructive uropathy include increased **frequency, urgency,** difficulty in fully emptying the bladder, the need to void at night **(nocturia).** In advanced cases, bladder diverticula may develop and bilateral hydronephrosis resulting in renal failure. The most commonly used medical therapy for benign hyperplasia are **α-blockers,** which decrease prostate smooth muscle tone via inhibition of α₁-adrenergic receptors, and **5 α-reductase inhibitors,** which shrink the prostate.

d. Lateral lobes
- Paired **lateral lobes** comprise most of the gland.

> A **prostatectomy** may be performed through a **suprapubic or perineal incision** or **transurethrally.** Because damage to the nerves in the capsule of the prostate and around the urethra **(cavernous nerves)** can cause **impotence,** procedures to spare nerves have been developed. **Urinary incontinence** also may follow prostatectomy. **External beam radiotherapy** or **interstitial radiotherapy** implanting radioactive seeds (brachytherapy) are alternative treatments for localized prostate cancer.

> **Prostatic malignancies** tend to **metastasize to vertebrae** (osteoblastic metastases) and the **brain** because the **prostatic venous plexus** has numerous connections with the **vertebral venous plexus.**

Erectile tissue is supplied by parasympathetic fibers traversing cavernous nerves, not pudendal nerves.

IX. Female Pelvic Structures (Figure 4-15; see Figure 4-7)
A. Ovary
1. Overview
   a. Suspended from **posterior** aspect of **broad ligament** by **mesovarium** and from lateral pelvic wall by **suspensory ligament of ovary,** which conveys **ovarian vessels**
   b. Joined to uterine body inferior to uterine tube by **ovarian ligament**
2. **Blood supply: ovarian artery** from abdominal aorta and through anastomotic ovarian branch of **uterine artery**
3. **Venous drainage: ovarian vein,** which joins **inferior vena cava** on right and **left renal vein** on left

Accessory ovary may occur in mesovarium or adjacent area and show tumor or cyst formation

The ureter may be cut during oophorectomy because it lies near ovarian vessels in suspensory ligament.

> The **ureter** lies immediately behind the peritoneum of the **ovarian fossa** on the lateral pelvic wall, where it **may be cut or ligated** while transecting or suturing the suspensory ligament of the ovary.

> Although **ovarian tumors** are common and usually benign, malignant tumors are the leading cause of **gynecologic cancer deaths.** Unfortunately, most neoplasms are either asymptomatic or are associated

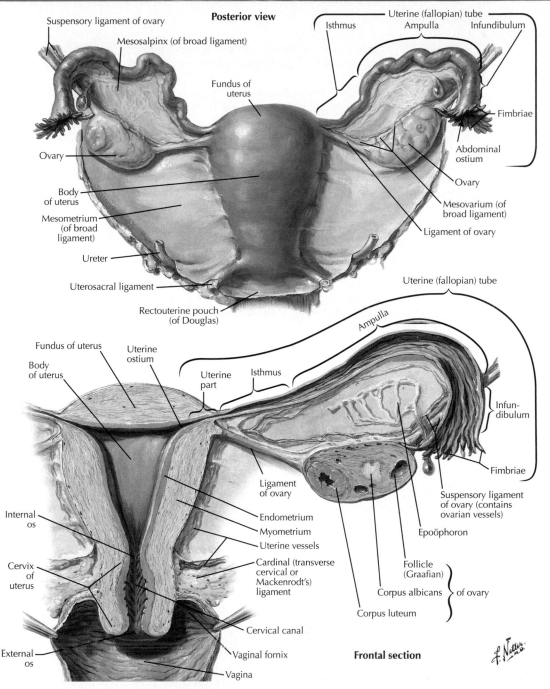

Posterior view

Suspensory ligament of ovary

Mesosalpinx (of broad ligament)

Uterine (fallopian) tube

Isthmus   Ampulla   Infundibulum

Fundus of uterus

Fimbriae

Abdominal ostium

Ovary

Ovary

Body of uterus

Mesovarium (of broad ligament)

Mesometrium (of broad ligament)

Ligament of ovary

Ureter

Uterosacral ligament

Rectouterine pouch (of Douglas)

Uterine (fallopian) tube

Ampulla

Fundus of uterus   Uterine ostium

Body of uterus

Uterine part   Isthmus

Infundibulum

Ligament of ovary

Endometrium

Myometrium

Uterine vessels

Fimbriae

Internal os

Suspensory ligament of ovary (contains ovarian vessels)

Cervix of uterus

Cardinal (transverse cervical or Mackenrodt's) ligament

Epoöphoron

Follicle (Graafian)

External os

Corpus albicans   } of ovary

Cervical canal

Corpus luteum

Vaginal fornix   **Frontal section**

Vagina

f. Netter

4-15: A, Pelvic organs unique to female covered by broad ligament, posterior view. **B,** Coronal section of uterus, uterine tube, and ovary. (*From Netter, F H: Atlas of Human Anatomy, 4th ed. Philadelphia, Saunders, 2006, Plate 371.*)

with nonspecific symptoms until in advanced stages. **Accessory ovaries** are uncommon but probably underreported because their presence isn't discovered until they develop symptomatic tumors or cysts.

Streak gonads consisting mainly of fibrous connective tissue and **lacking oocytes** are a form of **gonadal dysgenesis.** They are characteristic of **Turner syndrome** (45,X) but also may result from genetic mutations. Ovarian dysgenesis causes increased risk of **ovarian cancer.**

Postpartum loss of ligamentous support may allow **prolapse of an ovary** into the **rectouterine pouch,** resulting in painful intercourse **(dyspareunia).** The prolapsed ovary can be palpated through the posterior vaginal fornix.

The ovary may prolapse into the rectouterine pouch following childbirth.

B. Uterine Tube (oviduct)
  1. Overview
     a. Draped by upper border of **broad ligament** between ovary and uterus
     b. Connects **uterine cavity** to **peritoneal cavity** near ovary
  2. **Infundibulum**
     a. Funnel-shaped expansion of lateral end, fringed with **fimbriae**
     b. Abdominal ostium overlies ovary and receives oocyte at ovulation.
  3. **Ampulla**
     a. Medial continuation of infundibulum comprising about half of uterine tube
     b. Usual **site of fertilization**
  4. **Isthmus**
     • Narrowest part of tube just lateral to uterus
  5. **Intramural part**
     • Pierces **uterine wall** to open into uterine cavity

The fimbriae of infundibulum sweep a discharged oocyte from the peritoneal cavity into the uterine tube for fertilization.

The uterine tube transports the conceptus to the uterine cavity for implantation.

Tubal scarring from pelvic inflammatory disease causes infertility or ectopic pregnancy.

Most ectopic pregnancies are tubal pregnancies ending with tubal rupture and intraperitoneal hemorrhage.

Symptoms from ruptured right tubal pregnancy may be confused with acute appendicitis.

Anteverted, anteflexed position resting atop urinary bladder provides passive support for the uterus.

Sexually transmitted disease can spread from the vagina to the uterus and the uterine tubes, causing **pelvic inflammatory disease.** The resulting **salpingitis** produces scarring, which often causes infertility or ectopic pregnancy. In **tubal pregnancy,** the most common form of **ectopic pregnancy,** the **uterine tube ruptures** and causes potentially fatal **intraperitoneal hemorrhage** with intense abdominal pain. The close relationship of the **appendix** to the uterine tube and ovary on the right side mean that a ruptured tubal pregnancy may be mistaken for **acute appendicitis.**

C. Uterus
  1. **Fundus**
     • Rounded **upper part of body** above entrances of uterine tubes
  2. **Body**
     a. Main part of uterus between fundus and cervix
     b. Contains triangular **uterine cavity** continuous superiorly with lumina of uterine tubes and inferiorly with internal os

The adult uterus is usually tilted anteriorly relative to the vagina **(anteverted)** with the body flexed anteriorly on the cervix **(anteflexed) (Figure 4-16).** This position places the body of the uterus above the empty bladder, providing **passive support** to supplement that provided by the **pelvic fascial ligaments**

4-16: T2-weighted sagittal MRI in a young female showing the usual anteverted, anteflexed position of the uterus when the bladder is empty. The band labeled the junctional zone is the inner portion of the myometrium. *(From Standring, S: Gray's Anatomy: The Anatomical Basis of Clinical Practice, 39th ed. London, Churchill Livingstone, 2005, Figure 104.2.)*

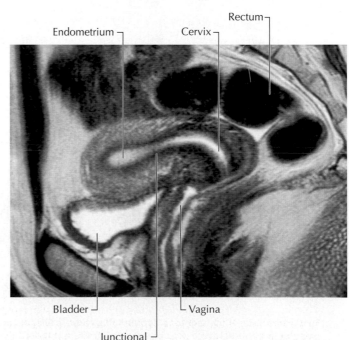

Endometrium — Cervix — Rectum —

Bladder — — Vagina

Junctional zone

(e.g., transverse cardinal ligament), **perineal body,** and **perineal membrane. Dynamic support** for the uterus is provided by the **pelvic diaphragm.** If the uterus assumes a **retroverted** positon, increased intraabdominal pressure tends to push it down into or through the vagina **(prolapse of the uterus).**

Other types of pelvic organ prolapse include herniation of the bladder **(cystocele)** or urethra **(urethrocele)** into the anterior vaginal wall and the small intestine **(enterocele)** or rectum **(rectocele)** into the posterior vaginal wall. Factors contributing to pelvic organ prolapse include **pregnancy and childbirth,** connective tissue disorders, denervation of the pelvic diaphragm, obesity, chronically increased intraabdominal pressure (e.g., chronic pulmonary disease, strenuous physical activity), and **menopause.**

> The rectouterine pouch is the lowest point in the female peritoneal cavity, and pathological fluids collect there.

The peritoneum covers only the fundus and body of the uterus anteriorly, but posteriorly it descends to also cover the supravaginal cervix and posterior fornix of the vagina. Therefore, a shallow peritoneal recess, the **vesicouterine pouch,** separates the uterus from the **bladder** anteriorly, while posteriorly the deep **rectouterine pouch** intervenes between the uterus and **rectum.** The rectouterine pouch is the **lowest point in the peritoneal cavity** in the female and thus is a site for pathological fluids to collect.

> Pregnancy and childbirth, estrogen deficiency, and chronic increases in intraabdominal pressure contribute to pelvic organ prolapse.

3. **Cervix**
   a. Cylindrical **lower third** of uterus projecting inferiorly into **vagina**
   b. **Cervical canal** communicates with uterine cavity at **internal os** and with cavity of vagina at **external os**

> Placenta previa with painless vaginal bleeding follows blastocyst implantation close to internal os.

Until the 1940s **cervical cancer** was the leading cause of cancer deaths in North American women. **Papanicolaou (Pap) smears** leading to the detection of premalignant conditions (called dysplasia) and regular examinations have greatly decreased the incidence to the point that it is now the least common gynecologic cancer. A vaccine is now available for the **human papillomavirus (HPV),** which should even further decrease the risk for developing cervical cancer.

The **external os** is circular in the nulliparous female and slitlike transversely in the multiparous female. If a blastocyst implants close to the **internal os,** the placenta bridges the opening **(placenta previa)** and causes **painless vaginal bleeding** late in pregnancy. If the **decidua basalis is absent** from the placenta, as may occur in a pregnancy following a cesarean section or other source of uterine scarring, villi of the **chorion frondosum** attach directly to the myometrium **(placenta accreta).** The condition is clinically important both because placenta previa often is associated with it and because **life-threatening postpartum hemorrhage** occurs due to failure of placental separation. A **hysterectomy** frequently is necessary, but **embolization** of the arterial supply may be attempted.

> The placenta is formed by maternal decidua basalis and fetal chorion frondosum.
>
> Placenta accreta causes life-threatening postpartum hemorrhage.

4. **Uterine artery**
   a. Crosses pelvic floor in base of **broad ligament** and ascends along lateral wall of uterus
   b. Near uterus passes **superior and anterior to ureter**
   c. **Vaginal branch** anastomoses with vaginal artery
   d. **Ovarian branch** anastomoses with ovarian artery
5. **Round ligament of uterus**
   • Attaches to labium majus, traverses **inguinal canal,** and is joined to uterine body near **ovarian ligament,** with which it shares an origin from the **gubernaculum**
6. **Bimanual examination of uterus (Figure 4-17)**

> Endometriosis is functioning endometrial tissue outside the uterus.

The **round ligament** is **stretched** as the uterus enlarges **during pregnancy.** Its attachment in the labium accounts for the sensation some patients describe as a "pulling" in the groin. **Uterine prolapse** may occur from damage to the pelvic floor during **childbirth** or **after menopause** because of atrophied pelvic structures.

> A leiomyoma is a common benign tumor of the uterus.

Endometriosis is aberrant growth of endometrial tissue outside the uterus, often in the ovaries and in adjacent parts of the pelvis. Symptoms include dyspareunia, dysmenorrhea, and infertility. It is the most common cause of chronic pelvic pain. Endometrial tissue in the **rectouterine pouch** may form a palpable mass and cause painful defecation during menses due to rectal wall involvement.

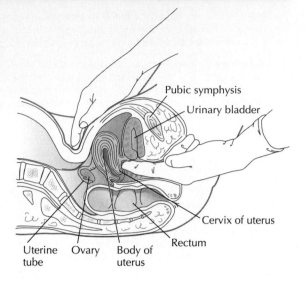

4-17: Bimanual examination of uterus. By placing one hand on the lower abdominal wall and one or two fingers of other hand in the vagina, the examiner can palpate the cervix and body of uterus, bladder base, urethra, and abnormal pelvic masses. Ovaries can be felt through the lateral fornices and rectal masses through the posterior wall.

> **Leiomyomas (uterine fibroids)** are the **most common benign tumors** of the female genital tract. They may be asymptomatic or may cause urinary frequency, abnormal uterine bleeding, pain, impaired fertility, or spontaneous abortion. **Hysterectomy** is surgical removal of the uterus through the anterior abdominal wall or vagina.

    D. **Broad Ligament (see Figures 4-15 and 4-18)**
      1. Overview
        a. Double **layer of peritoneum** extending from lateral border of **uterine body** to **pelvic wall**
        b. Prolonged superiorly over ovarian vessels at lateral pelvic wall as **suspensory ligament of ovary**
      2. **Mesosalpinx**
        • Covers uterine tube and extends inferiorly to base of mesovarium
      3. Mesovarium
        • Shelflike posterior extension suspending ovary
      4. **Mesometrium**
        • Inferior to base of mesovarium extending to uterine wall
    E. **Vagina (see Figures 4-7, 4-16, and 4-17)**
      1. Overview
        a. Distensible fibromuscular tube usually collapsed in an H-shape with its anterior and posterior walls in contact
        b. Superior three-fourths in **pelvis** and inferior fourth in **perineum**
        c. Recess around uterine cervix divided into **anterior, posterior,** and **lateral fornices**
        d. Opening into **vestibule** may be partially closed by thin, crescentic **hymen** in virgins
      2. **Blood supply:** vaginal branch of uterine artery, vaginal artery, and internal pudendal artery
      3. **Venous drainage:** vaginal tributaries of internal iliac veins
      4. **Lymphatic drainage:** superior to hymen drains to **external and internal iliac nodes;** inferior to hymen follows perineal drainage to **superficial inguinal nodes**
      5. **Vaginal supports**
        a. **Inferior part:** perineal body
        b. **Middle part:** urogenital diaphragm
        c. **Superior part:** levator ani and transverse cervical, uterosacral, and pubocervical ligaments

The posterior fornix of the vagina provides access to the rectouterine pouch.

> Because the **rectouterine pouch** is the lowest part of the peritoneal cavity in females, it can **collect fluid.** Access for aspiration **(culdocentesis)** is through the **posterior fornix of the vagina.** The needle passes successively through the mucous membrane, muscle, and connective tissue of the vaginal wall;

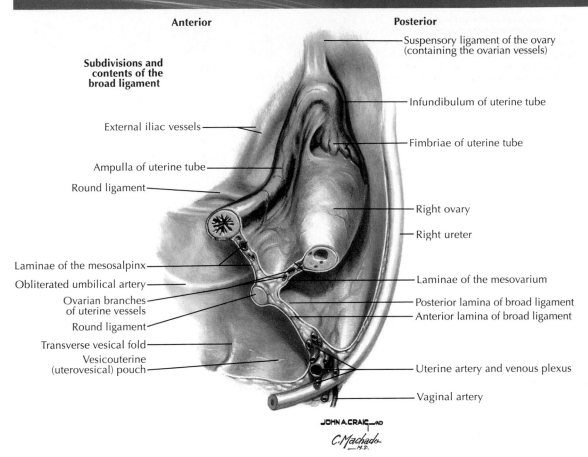

Anterior   **Posterior**

Subdivisions and
contents of the
broad ligament

Suspensory ligament of the ovary
(containing the ovarian vessels)

External iliac vessels

Infundibulum of uterine tube

Ampulla of uterine tube

Fimbriae of uterine tube

Round ligament

Right ovary

Right ureter

Laminae of the mesosalpinx

Obliterated umbilical artery

Ovarian branches
of uterine vessels

Laminae of the mesovarium

Round ligament

Posterior lamina of broad ligament
Anterior lamina of broad ligament

Transverse vesical fold

Vesicouterine
(uterovesical) pouch

Uterine artery and venous plexus

Vaginal artery

JOHN A. CRAIG—MD

C. Machado
—M.D.

4-18: Subdivisions and contents of the broad ligament in sagittal section. The uterine artery runs medially toward the cervix in the transverse cervical (cardinal) ligament at the base of the broad ligament. Note the ureter passing below the uterine artery. *(From Netter, F H: Atlas of Human Anatomy, 4th ed. Philadelphia, Saunders, 2006, Plate 372.)*

visceral pelvic fascia; and peritoneum. If the **vaginal wall** is **pierced** by a misdirected instrument used to abort a fetus, life-threatening **peritonitis** and uncontrollable **hemorrhage** can occur.

The close relationship of other pelvic organs to the vagina facilitates development of some conditions. **Cystocele** or **urethrocele** may cause the anterior wall of the vagina to bulge, and **rectocele** or **enterocele** may cause the posterior wall to bulge. Cancer, trauma, or necrosis due to prolonged labor can result in **fistula formation** with the bladder (**vesicovaginal**) or urethra (**urethrovaginal**) anteriorly or with the rectum (**rectovaginal**) posteriorly. Consequently, urine or fecal matter may enter the vagina.

Cancer may cause a vesicovaginal or urethrovaginal fistula with urine escaping from the vagina.

Vaginismus is involuntary spasm of the muscles surrounding the lower vagina, causing inability to engage in coitus and often making pelvic examinations difficult. It may have an organic basis, be caused by past sexual abuse or trauma, or be entirely psychological in origin.

X. Vessels of Pelvis
A. Internal Iliac (Hypogastric) Artery (Figure 4-19; Table 4-3)
- Arises from bifurcation of **common iliac artery** at pelvic brim and descends into pelvis anterior to **sacroiliac joint**

Peripheral vascular disease commonly affects the **internal and external iliac arteries,** requiring **surgical bypass** to restore blood flow. If only the external iliac artery is occluded, collateral circulation via the inferior gluteal artery to the **cruciate anastomosis** may maintain the lower extremity (see Chapter 5).

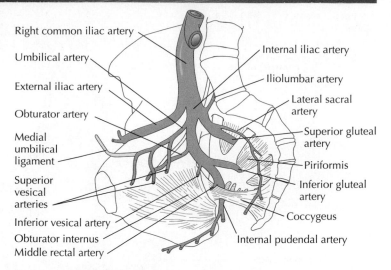

4-19: Branches of internal iliac artery in male, medial view. Note that the internal pudendal artery leaves the pelvis through the greater sciatic foramen, winds around the sacrospinous ligament, and enters the perineum through the lesser sciatic foramen.

Right common iliac artery
Umbilical artery
External iliac artery
Obturator artery
Medial umbilical ligament
Superior vesical arteries
Inferior vesical artery
Obturator internus
Middle rectal artery

Internal iliac artery
Iliolumbar artery
Lateral sacral artery
Superior gluteal artery
Piriformis
Inferior gluteal artery
Coccygeus
Internal pudendal artery

TABLE 4-3. BRANCHES OF INTERNAL ILIAC ARTERY

BRANCH	AREAS SUPPLIED
Posterior Division	
Iliolumbar	Iliacus, psoas major, and quadratus lumborum muscles
Lateral sacral	Branches into anterior sacral foramina
Superior gluteal	Gluteal region including hip joint
Anterior Division	
Obturator	Hip joint; adductor thigh
Umbilical	Bladder via superior vesical branches
Inferior gluteal	Gluteal region including hip joint
Internal pudendal	Perineum
Inferior vesical	Fundus of bladder, prostate, ductus deferens, and seminal vesicle; present only in males
Middle rectal	Lower rectum and anal canal
Uterine	Uterus, vagina, ovaries, and uterine tube
Vaginal	Vagina and base of bladder; corresponds to inferior vesical artery of males

    B. Ovarian Artery
       1. Branch of **abdominal aorta** descending retroperitoneally to enter **suspensory ligament of ovary** at pelvic brim
       2. Anastomoses with **ovarian branch of uterine artery**
    C. Superior Rectal Artery (Figure 4-20)
       1. Direct continuation of **inferior mesenteric artery** supplying **rectum** and upper half of **anal canal**

Pelvic veins damaged in pelvic fractures may cause a fatal hemorrhage.

       2. Anastomoses with **middle rectal artery** (internal iliac artery) and **inferior rectal artery** (internal pudendal artery)
    D. Veins of Pelvis
      • Generally correspond to arteries

> **Tumor cells can metastasize from pelvic organs** (e.g., prostate) to the **vertebral column, spinal cord, and brain** via connections of the **pelvic veins** with the **vertebral venous plexus.** Osteoblastic (bone-forming) lesions in older males are characteristic of metastatic prostate cancer and often involve the lumbar spine, proximal femur, and pelvis. Prostatic carcinoma also may spread to the lungs and other organs via the internal and common iliac veins into the inferior vena cava.

Lymphatic drainage of ovary and testis follows blood supply to aortic nodes

    E. Lymphatic Drainage of Pelvis
       1. Mostly follows internal iliac vessels to **internal iliac nodes** and then to **common iliac** and **aortic (lumbar) nodes;** some lymph goes first to **sacral nodes**
       2. From **upper rectum** is largely along superior rectal vessels first to **inferior mesenteric nodes** and then to **aortic nodes**

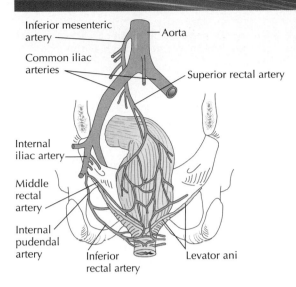

4-20: Arteries supplying rectum and anal canal, posterior view. Main blood supply is from the superior rectal branch of the inferior mesenteric artery with contributions from middle and inferior rectal branches of the internal iliac system.

Labels: Inferior mesenteric artery, Aorta, Common iliac arteries, Superior rectal artery, Internal iliac artery, Middle rectal artery, Internal pudendal artery, Inferior rectal artery, Levator ani

TABLE 4-4. NERVES OF PELVIS AND THEIR DISTRIBUTION

NERVE	DISTRIBUTION AND COMMENTS
Femoral nerve (L2-4)	Skin of anterior and medial thigh, medial leg; iliacus, psoas major, sartorius and quadriceps femoris muscles
Obturator nerve (L2-4)	Muscles of medial (adductor) compartment of thigh and overlying skin
Sciatic nerve (L4, L5, S1-3)	Common fibular and tibial nerves distributed to posterior thigh, leg, and foot
Superior gluteal nerve (L4, L5, S1)	Gluteus medius, gluteus minimus, and tensor fasciae latae muscles and hip joint
Inferior gluteal nerve (L5, S1, S2)	Gluteus maximus muscle
Posterior femoral cutaneous nerve (S1-3)	Skin of buttock, posterior thigh, popliteal fossa, and external genitalia
Nerve to obturator internus (L5, S1, S2)	Obturator internus and superior gemellus muscles
Nerve to quadratus femoris (L4, L5, S1)	Quadratus femoris and inferior gemellus muscles
Pudendal nerve (S2-4)	Perineum

XI. Nerves of Pelvis (Table 4-4)
A. Sacral Plexus

Cancer from adjacent organs can invade the **sacral roots and plexus**, causing **severe pain in late-stage malignancy.** The sacral plexus may be damaged in **pelvic fractures** or the resulting hemorrhage. Temporary lesions can occur from a **difficult delivery** (e.g., forceps delivery of a large baby).

Sacral plexus injury may occur from cancer, pelvic fracture, or difficult delivery.

In **caudal epidural anesthesia,** the needle is inserted into the **sacral hiatus** using the **cornua** as guides, and anesthetic is injected into the extradural space to numb the sacral nerve roots. The birth canal, pelvic floor, and most of the perineum are anesthetized, but pain from the body of the uterus is unaffected (see clinical correlation under D.2. following). The anterior perineum, which is innervated by the ilioinguinal and genitofemoral nerves, is unaffected.

B. Branches of Lumbar Plexus in Pelvis
1. Lumbosacral trunk (L4-5)
  • Forms in psoas major and descends into pelvis to contribute to **sacral plexus**
2. Obturator nerve (L2-4)
  a. Forms in psoas major and enters pelvis
  b. Enters **medial thigh** through **obturator canal** with **obturator vessels**

Tumors of adjacent viscera may compress or invade the obturator nerve. An inflamed appendix hanging inferiorly across the pelvic brim may irritate the nerve. Pain in the medial thigh and/or weakness occurs when adducting the thigh (e.g., crossing legs).

C. **Autonomic Nerves of Pelvis**
1. **Sacral sympathetic trunk**
   a. **Four** paravertebral ganglia **joined by gray rami communicantes** to corresponding spinal nerve
   b. Contains **preganglionic sympathetic** and **general visceral afferent fibers** derived from L1 and L2 spinal nerves
2. **Sacral splanchnic nerves**
   a. Visceral branches of **sacral sympathetic ganglia**
   b. Contain **postganglionic sympathetic** and visceral afferent fibers
   c. Join inferior hypogastric plexus
3. **Pelvic splanchnic nerves (nervi erigentes)**
   a. Only "**splanchnic**" nerves containing **parasympathetic** fibers
   b. **Preganglionic parasympathetic** cell bodies in **sacral parasympathetic nucleus** of **S2-4** with fibers branching from anterior rami; postganglionic cell bodies in terminal ganglia in inferior hypogastric plexus *or* in wall of organ innervated
   c. Source of parasympathetic innervation to **descending colon, sigmoid colon, pelvic organs,** and **external genitalia**

D. **Autonomic Plexus of Pelvis**
1. **Inferior hypogastric plexus (pelvic plexus)**
   a. Supplies pelvic organs and gastrointestinal tract **distal to left colic (splenic) flexure**
   b. Formed by contributions from hypogastric nerves, pelvic splanchnic nerves, and sacral splanchnic nerves
   c. Divided into parts named according to **organ** to which it is related (thus **vesical, prostatic, rectal,** and **uterovaginal plexuses**)
2. **Hypogastric nerves**
   • Left and right nerves connect **superior** and **inferior hypogastric plexuses**

> **S2-4 are the only spinal nerves carrying parasympathetic nerve fibers.**

> **Pelvic splanchnic nerves mediate parasympathetic influences on defecation, micturition, and erection.**

> **Visceral afferent fibers carrying pain from thoracic, abdominal, and upper pelvic viscera accompany sympathetic fibers.**

Sympathetic fibers in the **hypogastric plexuses** originate in spinal cord segments T10-L2 and are accompanied by visceral afferent fibers from nerve cell bodies in posterior root ganglia at the same levels. Consequently, pain from the pelvic viscera may be referred to dermatomes of these segments lying at and inferior to the umbilicus. **Unlike the rest of the trunk,** visceral **pain from pelvic organs inferior to and not in contact with peritoneum** (e.g., uterine cervix and upper vagina) probably travels with sacral **parasympathetic fibers** to enter spinal cord segments **S2-4.** The boundary at which visceral afferent fibers carrying pain impulses start accompanying parasympathetic rather than sympathetic fibers is known as the "**pelvic pain line.**"

XII. **Perineum**
A. **Overiew**
1. **Diamond-shaped** area below pelvic diaphragm with same boundaries as inferior pelvic aperture: **pubic symphysis, ischiopubic rami, ischial tuberosities, sacrotuberous ligaments,** and **coccyx**
2. **Roof** formed **by pelvic diaphragm,** and **floor** formed by **skin and fascia**
3. Divided by line connecting **ischial tuberosities** into anterior **urogenital triangle** and posterior **anal triangle**

B. **Anal Triangle**
1. **Anal canal (Figures 4-21 and 4-22)**
   a. Overview
      (1) Continuous with **rectum** at **pelvic diaphragm** and opens externally at **anus**
      (2) Bends posteriorly at junction with rectum (**perineal or anorectal flexure**) because of forward pull of **puborectalis muscle**
      (3) Kept closed by **puborectalis** and **internal and external anal sphincters** except during defecation
   b. **Internal anal sphincter**
      (1) Circular **smooth muscle** surrounding superior two-thirds of anal canal

> **The perineum is the region below the pelvic diaphragm, which is divided into urogenital and anal triangles.**

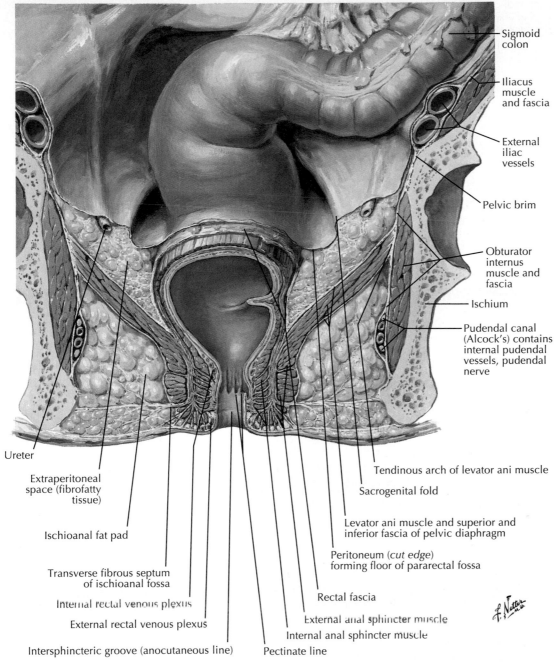

Labels on figure:
- Sigmoid colon
- Iliacus muscle and fascia
- External iliac vessels
- Pelvic brim
- Obturator internus muscle and fascia
- Ischium
- Pudendal canal (Alcock's) contains internal pudendal vessels, pudendal nerve
- Ureter
- Extraperitoneal space (fibrofatty tissue)
- Ischioanal fat pad
- Transverse fibrous septum of ischioanal fossa
- Internal rectal venous plexus
- External rectal venous plexus
- Intersphincteric groove (anocutaneous line)
- Pectinate line
- Internal anal sphincter muscle
- External anal sphincter muscle
- Rectal fascia
- Peritoneum (*cut edge*) forming floor of pararectal fossa
- Levator ani muscle and superior and inferior fascia of pelvic diaphragm
- Sacrogenital fold
- Tendinous arch of levator ani muscle

4-21: Rectum and anal canal, coronal section. Note relationship of anal canal to ischioanal fossae. *(From Netter, F H: Atlas of Human Anatomy, 4th ed. Philadelphia, Saunders, 2006, Plate 392.)*

(2) Controlled **reflexly** and **involuntarily,** with parasympathetic nervous system promoting relaxation and sympathetic nervous system promoting contraction

c. **External anal sphincter**

(1) Three adjacent rings of **skeletal muscle** surrounding inferior two-thirds of anal canal as **subcutaneous, superficial,** and **deep parts**

(2) Attaches anteriorly to **perineal body** (central tendon of perineum)

(3) Controlled **voluntarily** by inferior rectal branches of **pudendal nerve**

d. **Internal features of anal canal (Table 4-5)**

e. **Characteristics of rectum and anal canal (Table 4-6)**

The parasympathetic nervous system relaxes and the sympathetic system contracts the internal anal sphincter.

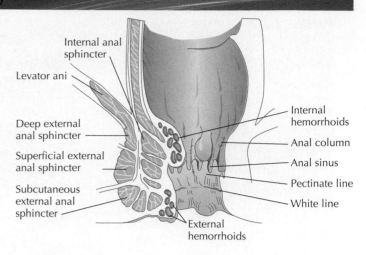

4-22: Anal canal, coronal section. Note relationship of internal and external hemorrhoids to pectinate line.

TABLE 4-5. INTERNAL FEATURES OF ANAL CANAL

FEATURE	DESCRIPTION	COMMENTS
Anal columns	Longitudinal ridges of mucosa in upper half of anal canal	Related to underlying rectal veins
Anal valves	Crescentic mucosal folds joining bases of adjacent anal columns	
Anal sinuses	Pocket-like recesses above anal valves	Receive openings of anal glands; obstruction and infection of anal glands can produce fistulae and painful abscesses
Pectinate (dentate) line	Serrated line joining lower margins of anal valves	Marks junction of embryonic hindgut and proctodeum; divides visceral and somatic arterial supply, venous drainage, lymphatic drainage, and innervation

TABLE 4-6. CHARACTERISTICS OF RECTUM AND ANAL CANAL

CHARACTERISTIC	RECTUM	ANAL CANAL
Epithelium	Columnar (endodermal origin)	Above pectinate line: columnar (endodermal origin) Below pectinate line: stratified squamous (ectodermal origin)
Innervation	Visceral	Above pectinate line: visceral Below pectinate line: somatic (from pudendal nerve)
Arterial supply	Superior rectal from inferior mesenteric artery and middle rectal from internal iliac artery	Above pectinate line: superior rectal from inferior mesenteric artery Below pectinate line: inferior rectal from internal iliac artery
Venous drainage	Superior rectal to portal system and middle rectal to vena caval system	Above pectinate line: superior rectal to portal system Below pectinate line: inferior rectal to inferior vena cava
Lymphatic drainage	Inferior mesenteric and internal iliac nodes	Above pectinate line: inferior mesenteric nodes Below pectinate line: superficial inguinal nodes

Internal hemorrhoids develop above the pectinate line and external hemorrhoids below.

Internal hemorrhoids usually cause painless bleeding but become painful if prolapsed and strangulated.

Internal hemorrhoids are dilated tributaries of the **superior rectal veins** above the pectinate line and typically are **not painful** because the mucosa is supplied by visceral afferent fibers. Internal hemorrhoids frequently develop during pregnancy because of pressure on the abdominal and pelvic veins. **External hemorrhoids** are dilated tributaries of the **inferior rectal veins** below the pectinate line and are **painful** because the mucosa is supplied by somatic afferent fibers of the inferior rectal nerves. Hemorrhoids are commonly associated with constipation, extended sitting and straining at the toilet, pregnancy, and disorders that hinder venous return **(see Figure 4-22).**

Anal fissures are vertical slitlike lesions in the anal mucosa, usually in the posterior midline just inferior to the anal valves. They often result from traumatic tearing by a hard stool in chronic constipation and are among the most common causes of **anal pain.**

Carcinomas developing **above the pectinate line** tend to be **painless,** whereas those developing **below the pectinate line** are painful because of the transition from visceral to somatic innervation. The pectinate line is a site of dilation of **portocaval anastomoses in portal hypertension.**

Ulcerative colitis and adenocarcinomas occur above the pectinate line, and squamous cell carcimomas occur below.

Venous drainage above the pectinate line: hepatic portal system. Venous drainage below the pectinate line: inferior vena cava

The ischioanal fat pad is one of the last fat reserves to disappear with starvation, which favors rectal prolapse.

2. **Ischioanal (ischiorectal) fossa (Figure 4-21; see also Figures 4-23 and 4-24)**
   a. **Wedge-shaped** space on each side bounded by **anal canal** medially, **obturator internus muscle and fascia** laterally, **pelvic diaphragm** superiorly, and **skin** inferiorly
   b. Has **anterior recess** above urogenital diaphragm and **posterior recess** above gluteus maximus
   c. Filled with **ischioanal fat pad,** which cushions perineum and allows distension of rectum
   d. Contains **inferior rectal nerves and vessels**

Infection commonly spreads laterally from the anal mucosa into the **ischioanal fossa. An ischioanal infection may spread to the opposite ischioanal fossa** by tracking behind the anal canal. An **abscess** may become localized in the **anterior or posterior recesses** or open onto the surface of the anal canal or skin **(anal sinus)** or open onto both surfaces **(anal fistula).**

3. **Pudendal (Alcock) canal (see Figure 4-21)**
   a. Tunnel formed by split in **obturator internus fascia** on lateral wall of **ischioanal fossa**
   b. Gives passage to **pudendal nerve** and **internal pudendal vessels,** which supply perineum

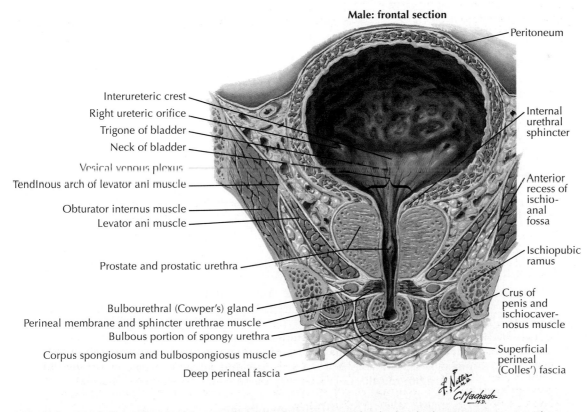

Male: frontal section

- Peritoneum
- Interureteric crest
- Right ureteric orifice
- Trigone of bladder
- Neck of bladder
- Vesical venous plexus
- Tendinous arch of levator ani muscle
- Obturator internus muscle
- Levator ani muscle
- Prostate and prostatic urethra
- Bulbourethral (Cowper's) gland
- Perineal membrane and sphincter urethrae muscle
- Bulbous portion of spongy urethra
- Corpus spongiosum and bulbospongiosus muscle
- Deep perineal fascia
- Internal urethral sphincter
- Anterior recess of ischioanal fossa
- Ischiopubic ramus
- Crus of penis and ischiocavernosus muscle
- Superficial perineal (Colles') fascia

4-23: Male urogenital triangle and pelvis, coronal section, showing urogenital and pelvic diaphragms, anterior view. The urogenital diaphragm is represented by the perineal membrane and sphincter urethrae (external urethral sphincter) muscle. *(From Netter, F H: Atlas of Human Anatomy, 4th ed. Philadelphia, Saunders, 2006, Plate 366.)*

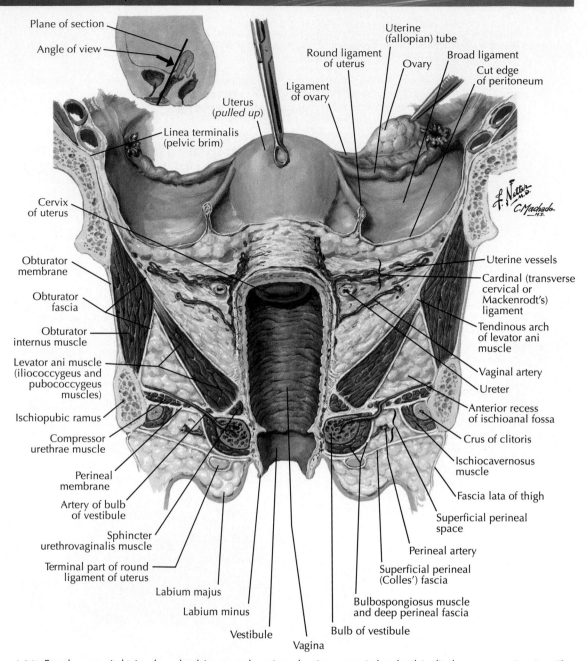

Plane of section
Angle of view
Uterus (*pulled up*)
Ligament of ovary
Round ligament of uterus
Uterine (fallopian) tube
Ovary
Broad ligament
Cut edge of peritoneum
Linea terminalis (pelvic brim)
Cervix of uterus
Obturator membrane
Obturator fascia
Obturator internus muscle
Levator ani muscle (iliococcygeus and pubococcygeus muscles)
Ischiopubic ramus
Compressor urethrae muscle
Perineal membrane
Artery of bulb of vestibule
Sphincter urethrovaginalis muscle
Terminal part of round ligament of uterus
Labium majus
Labium minus
Vestibule
Vagina
Bulb of vestibule
Bulbospongiosus muscle and deep perineal fascia
Superficial perineal (Colles') fascia
Perineal artery
Superficial perineal space
Fascia lata of thigh
Ischiocavernosus muscle
Crus of clitoris
Anterior recess of ischioanal fossa
Ureter
Vaginal artery
Tendinous arch of levator ani muscle
Cardinal (transverse cervical or Mackenrodt's) ligament
Uterine vessels

4-24: Female urogenital triangle and pelvis, coronal section, showing urogenital and pelvic diaphragms, anterior view. The urogenital diaphragm is represented by the perineal membrane, compressor urethrae muscle, and sphincter urethrovaginalis muscle in this section. *(From Netter, F H: Atlas of Human Anatomy, 4th ed. Philadelphia, Saunders, 2006, Plate 370.)*

The perineal membrane and the perineal body provide passive support for pelvic organs.

C. **Urogenital triangle (see Figures 4-12, 4-23, and 4-24)**
  1. **Urogenital diaphragm** (Note: traditional concept is now controversial but still used clinically)
     a. Connects **ischiopubic rami** inferior to pelvic diaphragm
     b. Composed of **deep transverse perineal** and **external urethral sphincter muscles** sandwiched between **superior and inferior fasciae of urogenital diaphragm;** female urogenital diaphragm contains additional muscles **(Figure 4-25, *B*)**
     c. Inferior fascia is tough **perineal membrane**
     d. Penetrated by **membranous urethra** in male and **membranous urethra and vagina** in female

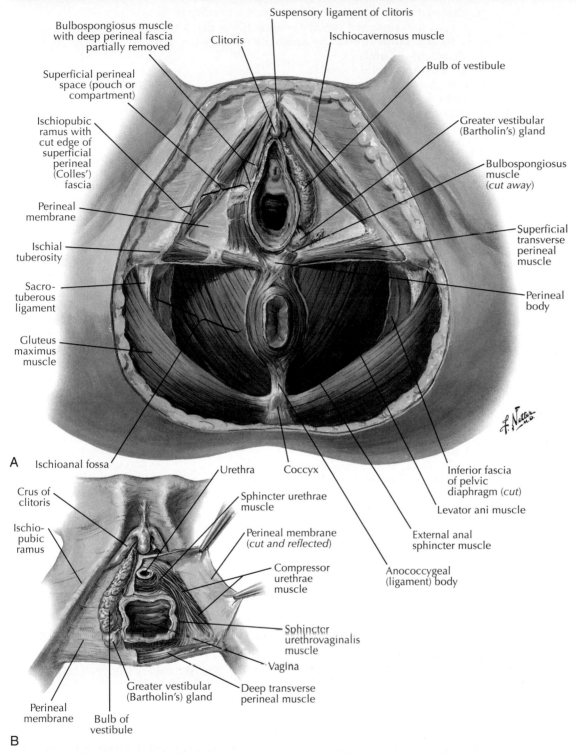

Bulbospongiosus muscle
with deep perineal fascia
partially removed

Clitoris

Suspensory ligament of clitoris

Ischiocavernosus muscle

Bulb of vestibule

Superficial perineal
space (pouch or
compartment)

Greater vestibular
(Bartholin's) gland

Ischiopubic
ramus with
cut edge of
superficial
perineal
(Colles')
fascia

Bulbospongiosus
muscle
(cut away)

Perineal
membrane

Superficial
transverse
perineal
muscle

Ischial
tuberosity

Sacro-
tuberous
ligament

Perineal
body

Gluteus
maximus
muscle

A   Ischioanal fossa

Urethra

Coccyx

Inferior fascia
of pelvic
diaphragm (cut)

Levator ani muscle

External anal
sphincter muscle

Anococcygeal
(ligament) body

Crus of
clitoris

Ischio-
pubic
ramus

Sphincter urethrae
muscle

Perineal membrane
(cut and reflected)

Compressor
urethrae
muscle

Sphincter
urethrovaginalis
muscle

Vagina

Perineal
membrane

Bulb of
vestibule

Greater vestibular
(Bartholin's) gland

Deep transverse
perineal muscle

B

4-25: Muscles and erectile tissues of female perineum. **A,** Muscles of superficial perineal pouch. **B,** Muscles of urogenital diaphragm (deep perineal pouch) are dissected on cadaver's left side and erectile tissues in superficial perineal pouch are shown on right side. *(From Netter, F H: Atlas of Human Anatomy, 4th ed. Philadelphia, Saunders, 2006, Plate 379.)*

2. **Deep perineal pouch**
   - Closed space lying **between superior fascia and inferior fascia of urogenital diaphragm** (Note: Some authors describe the superior boundary of the deep pouch as the pelvic diaphragm.)
   a. **Deep transverse perineal muscle**
      - Joins contralateral muscle to help support pelvic viscera and stabilize **perineal body**

b. **External urethral sphincter (sphincter urethrae)**
- Circularly arranged skeletal muscle fibers that surround and compress **membranous urethra** to provide **voluntary control** of micturition

c. **Membranous urethra**
d. **Internal pudendal vessels**
e. **Dorsal nerve of penis or clitoris**
f. **Bulbourethral glands in male**
g. **Portion of vagina in female**

3. **Superficial perineal pouch**
   a. Overview
      (1) Space between inferior fascia of urogenital diaphragm and membranous layer of superficial perineal fascia containing erectile bodies in both sexes
      (2) Closed, except anteriorly, where pouch communicates over pubis with potential space deep to membranous layer of superficial abdominal fascia (Scarpa fascia)
   b. **Ischiocavernosus muscle**
      (1) Arises from **ischiopubic ramus** and **ischial tuberosity** and inserts into and covers **crus** of penis or clitoris
      (2) Helps **maintain erection** of penis or clitoris by compressing crus and impeding venous return
   c. **Bulbospongiosus muscle**
      - Paired muscle joining in midline in males, remaining separate in females
      (1) In male, arises from **central tendon** and **median raphe**, invests **bulb of penis**, and inserts into **dorsum of penis** and **perineal membrane**
      (2) In female, arises from **perineal body**, invests **bulb of vestibule**, and inserts into **dorsum of clitoris** and **pubic arch (Figure 4-25, A)**
      (3) In male, compresses bulb of penis to help **maintain erection** and to expel urine and semen from urethra
      (4) In female, compresses bulb of vestibule and greater vestibular gland
   d. **Bulb of vestibule, crus of clitoris, and greater vestibular (Bartholin) gland in female**
   e. **Bulb and crus of penis in male**
   f. **Branches of internal pudendal vessels**
   g. **Perineal branches from pudendal nerves**
   h. **Superficial transverse perineal muscle**
      (1) Often poorly developed paired muscle arising near ischial tuberosity and inserting into **perineal body**
      (2) Helps **stabilize** perineal body
   i. **Superficial perineal (Colles) fascia (Figure 4-26)**
      - Membranous layer continuous with **dartos** layer of scrotum, superficial fascia of penis, and deep layer of superficial abdominal fascia

> After a crushing blow or a penetrating injury, the **spongy urethra** commonly **ruptures** within the bulb of the penis, and **urine leaks** into the **superficial perineal pouch**. Attachments of the **superficial perineal fascia** keep urine from passing into the thigh or the anal triangle, but after distending the scrotum and penis, urine can pass upward over the pubis into the anterior abdominal wall deep to the deep layer of superficial abdominal fascia **(see Figure 4-26).**

D. **Perineal Body (Central Tendon of Perineum)**
1. Median **fibromuscular mass** at posterior edge of **urogenital diaphragm** midway between vagina or bulb of penis and **anal canal**
2. Provides support for pelvic organs through attachments for pelvic diaphragm, perineal membrane, and perineal muscles of urogenital and anal triangles

> **During childbirth,** the **perineal body** is **susceptible to stretching or tearing,** which may cause permanent weakness of the pelvic floor. To **prevent tearing** and to control damage, an **episiotomy** may be performed either through the posterolateral vaginal wall or through the vaginal wall and the perineal body in the posterior midline. Because the perineal body anchors perineal structures, an injury may affect urination, defecation, and sexual function.

Margin notes (left column):

Extravasated urine may pass from the superficial perineal pouch into the lower abdominal wall.

Greater vestibular glands are nonpalpable except following infection or cyst formation.

Colles, dartos, superficial penile, and Scarpa fascia are one continuous layer.

Bulbospongiosus, superficial and deep transverse perineal, external anal sphincter, and levator ani muscles attach to the perineal body.

Episiotomy prevents uncontrolled tearing of the perineal body and external anal sphincter.

The pudendal nerve is the principal motor and sensory nerve supply to the perineum.

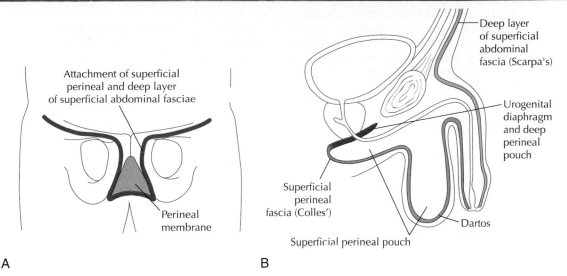

4-26: Attachments of superficial perineal fascia and extent of superficial perineal pouch. **A,** Anterior view. **B,** Midsagittal view. Deep perineal pouch is defined by urogenital diaphragm.

E. Pudendal Nerve (S2-4) (Figure 4-27)

- Lies against **ischial spine** as it passes through **lesser sciatic foramen** to traverse **pudendal canal** on lateral wall of **ischioanal fossa**

> To **relieve pain** for the mother and to prepare for an episiotomy, a **pudendal nerve block** may be administered during **early labor.** The nerve may be blocked either by piercing the vaginal wall posterolaterally near the **ischial spine** or percutaneously along the medial side of the ischial tuberosity. **Complete anesthesia of the perineal skin requires additional injections** to block the perineal branches of the ilioinguinal, genitofemoral, and posterior femoral cutaneous nerves. Pain from uterine contractions is unaffected because uterine body pain is carried by visceral afferent fibers accompanying sympathetic nerve fibers in the pelvic plexus.

The pudendal nerve gives the inferior rectal, perineal, and dorsal nerve of penis/clitoris branches.

The pudendal nerve can be readily blocked at the ischial spine as it enters the perineum.

1. **Inferior rectal nerve**
   a. Arises from pudendal nerve proximal to or in **pudendal canal**
   b. Supplies **external anal sphincter muscle** and **skin** around anus
2. **Perineal nerve**
   a. **Deep branch** is **motor nerve** to muscles of urogenital triangle
   b. **Superficial branch** gives cutaneous **posterior scrotal or labial branches.**
3. **Dorsal nerve of penis or clitoris**
   a. Runs on dorsal surface with dorsal artery and deep dorsal vein
   b. Supplies body, prepuce, and glans of penis or clitoris

The deep perineal nerve supplies the muscles of the superficial and deep perineal pouches.

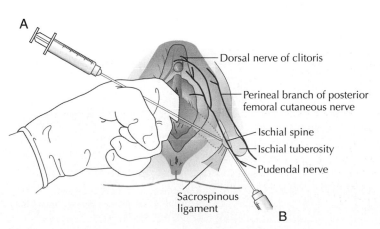

4-27: Two approaches for pudendal nerve block. Needle can be inserted through the posterolateral vaginal wall near the ischial spine **(A)** or percutaneously along the medial side of the ischial tuberosity **(B).**

Dorsal nerve of clitoris
Perineal branch of posterior femoral cutaneous nerve
Ischial spine
Ischial tuberosity
Pudendal nerve
Sacrospinous ligament

The deep artery of the penis or clitoris supplies the erectile tissue of the corpus cavernosum.

F. **Internal Pudendal Artery (see Figure 4-19)**
   1. Arises from **internal iliac artery** and traverses greater and lesser sciatic foramina to become principal blood supply to perineum
   2. Traverses **pudendal canal** with **pudendal nerve**
   3. **Branches (Table 4-7)**
G. **Veins of Perineum**
   1. Correspond mostly to branches of internal pudendal artery and follow **internal pudendal vein** to **internal iliac vein**
   2. **Superficial dorsal vein of penis** drains into **external pudendal vein,** a tributary of the great saphenous vein
   3. **Deep dorsal vein of penis** enters pelvis to drain into **prostatic venous plexus** (male)
   4. **Deep dorsal vein of clitoris** enters pelvis to drain into **vesical venous plexus** (female)

The deep dorsal vein of the penis or clitoris drains directly into pelvic veins.

H. **Lymphatic Drainage of Perineum**
   1. Is mostly to **superficial inguinal nodes** along external pudendal vessels, including drainage of **lower parts of vagina and anal canal**
   2. Deep perineal pouch, membranous urethra, and most of vagina drain to **internal iliac nodes** along internal pudendal vessels
   3. Glans and body of the penis drain to **deep inguinal** and **internal iliac nodes.**
   4. Lymph from **testis** drains along testicular vessels to **aortic (lumbar) nodes.**

Enlarged superficial inguinal lymph nodes may be the first sign of superficial perineal cancer or infection.

XIII. **Male External Genitalia and Associated Structures**
   A. **Penis (Figures 4-28 and 4-29)**
      1. **Root of penis**
         a. **Crus of penis**
            (1) **Erectile tissue** attached to **ischiopubic ramus** and adjacent **perineal membrane;** continues onto body of penis as **corpus cavernosum**
            (2) Covered by **ischiocavernosus muscle**
         b. **Bulb of penis**
            (1) Midline body of **erectile tissue** firmly attached to **perineal membrane** that continues onto body of penis as **corpus spongiosum**
            (2) Pierced by **spongy urethra** and **ducts of bulbourethral glands**
            (3) Covered by **bulbospongiosus muscle**
      2. **Body of penis**
         a. Overview
            (1) Two dorsal **corpora cavernosa** and one ventral **corpus spongiosum,** each enclosed in **tunica albuginea**
            (2) Capped distally by **glans of penis**
         b. **Glans**

The external urethral orifice is the narrowest and least distensible part of the male urethra during catheterization.

            (1) Expanded distal portion of corpus spongiosum having **external urethral orifice** at its tip

TABLE 4-7. **BRANCHES OF INTERNAL PUDENDAL ARTERY**

ARTERY	DESCRIPTION	COMMENTS
Inferior rectal	Supplies skin and muscle of lower anal canal	Arises proximal to or within pudendal canal
Perineal artery	Supplies perineal body and posterior scrotal or labial branches	
Artery of bulb of penis or clitoris	Supplies bulb of penis and bulbourethral gland (males) or bulb of vestibule and greater vestibular gland (females)	Arises in deep perineal space and pierces perineal membrane to enter bulb
Deep artery of penis or clitoris	Runs in crus of penis or clitoris to supply erectile tissue of corpus cavernosum	Terminal branch of internal pudendal in deep perineal space; pierces perineal membrane to enter crus
Dorsal artery of penis or clitoris	Supplies body and glans of penis or clitoris	Terminal branch of internal pudendal in deep perineal space; pierces perineal membrane to run with dorsal nerve

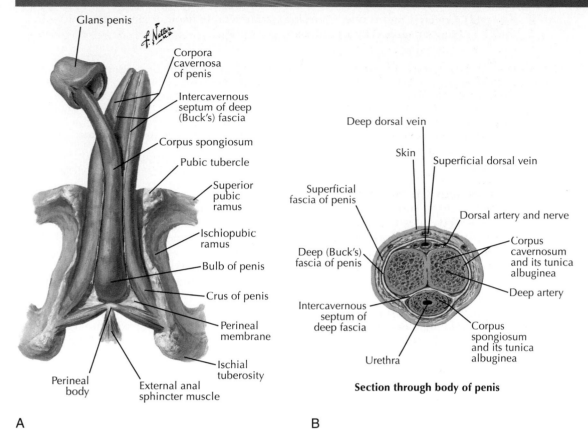

Section through body of penis

A

B

4-28: A, Penis with fascia removed, inferior view. **B,** Cross section through body of penis. The body of the penis is formed by two dorsal corpora cavernosa and the ventral corpus spongiosum. The spongy urethra is within the corpus spongiosum. The glans is the distal expansion of the corpus spongiosum. *(From Netter, F H: Atlas of Human Anatomy, 4th ed. Philadelphia, Saunders, 2006, Plates 381 and 382.)*

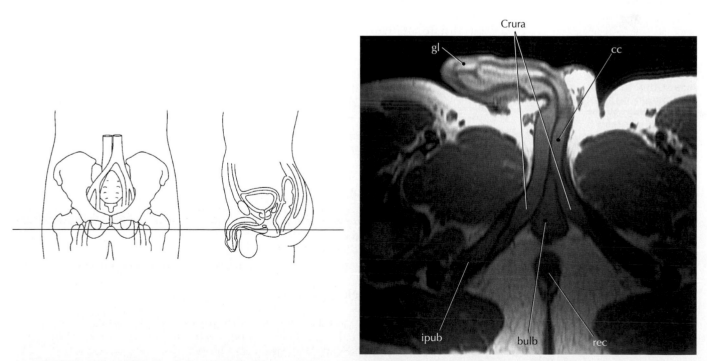

4-29: Axial, T1-weighted MRI at level of penis. Bulb of penis = bulb; crura = crura of penis; corpus cavernosum = cc; glans of penis = gl; rectum = rec; inferior pubic ramus = ipub. *(From Kelley, L, Petersen, C: Sectional Anatomy for Imaging Professionals, 2nd ed. St Louis, Mosby, 2007, Figure 8.96.)*

(2) Covered by **prepuce** (foreskin), a retractable hood of skin connected to ventral surface by **frenulum**

Phimosis is the inability to retract the prepuce and may result from repeated infections.

> **Circumcision** is the **removal** of the **prepuce.** The procedure is usually performed on newborn males and may reduce the incidence of infection. The incidence of **cervical cancer** may be lower in females whose sexual partners are circumcised, and human papillomavirus (HPV) and human immunodeficiency virus (HIV) transmission rates are reduced. Circumcision is also performed to correct either the inability to retract the prepuce over the glans **(phimosis)** or the inability to move the retracted foreskin forward over the glans **(paraphimosis).** Phimosis may be congenital or result from scarring after repeated infections.

    c. **Spongy (penile) urethra**
      (1) Distal continuation of **membranous urethra**
      (2) Traverses **bulb** and **corpus spongiosum** to become dilated in glans as **navicular fossa** just proximal to external urethral orifice
   3. **Erection and ejaculation**
    a. **Erection: parasympathetic fibers** from the **pelvic splanchnic nerves** dilate arteries supplying erectile bodies of the penis, allowing them to fill with blood.

Sympathoinhibitory drugs, diabetic neuropathy, or transurethral prostate resection may cause male infertility due to retrograde ejaculation.

    b. **Ejaculation: sympathetic fibers** cause contraction of smooth muscle of epididymis, ductus deferens, seminal vesicles, and prostate; sympathetic nerve fibers also stimulate **internal urethral sphincter** to prevent semen from entering bladder **(retrograde ejaculation)**
    c. **Note:** some authors separate delivery of semen into the prostatic urethra **(emission)** under sympathetic control from expulsion from the urethra through the external urethral orifice **(ejaculation)** under combined autonomic and somatic control
 B. **Scrotum, Testis, and Epididymis**
   • See Chapter 3, I.G.
 C. **Bulbourethral (Cowper) Glands**
   • Lie on either side of **membranous urethra** embedded in muscle in **deep perineal pouch** with ducts opening into bulbous part of **spongy urethra**

The clitoris has no corpus spongiosum and does not contain a urethra.

XIV. **Female External Genitalia and Associated Structures (Figures 4-30 and 4-31)**
 A. **Clitoris**
   1. **Erectile organ** formed by fusion of two **crura** as **corpora cavernosa** in **body of clitoris**
   2. Ends distally in highly sensitive **glans**
   3. Attached to pubic symphysis by **suspensory ligament of clitoris**
 B. **Labia Majora**

The pudendal cleft between the labia majora contains the labia minora and the vestibule with the openings of the urethra and vagina.

   1. Two prominent fatty folds of skin that extend inferiorly and posteriorly from **mons pubis** separated by median **pudendal cleft**
   2. Unite anteriorly at **anterior labial commissure**
   3. Contain terminations of **round ligaments of uterus**
 C. **Labia Minora**
   1. Skin folds lying between labia majora and extending posteriorly from clitoris on either side of **vestibule**
   2. Divide anteriorly into laminae that fuse above clitoris to form **prepuce** and below clitoris to form **frenulum**
 D. **Vestibule**

Because the female urethra is short and opens directly into the vestibule, females are prone to cystitis.

   • Cleft between labia minora containing openings of **urethra, vagina,** and **ducts of greater vestibular glands**
 E. **Bulb of Vestibule**
   1. Homologue of **bulb of penis,** a paired mass of **erectile tissue** on each side of **vaginal orifice**
   2. Covered by **bulbospongiosus muscle**
 F. **Greater Vestibular Glands**
   1. Paired **mucus-secreting glands** homologous to **bulbourethral glands**
   2. Lie in **superficial perineal pouch** deep to posterior part of bulbs of vestibule and open into **vestibule** to provide lubrication for coitus

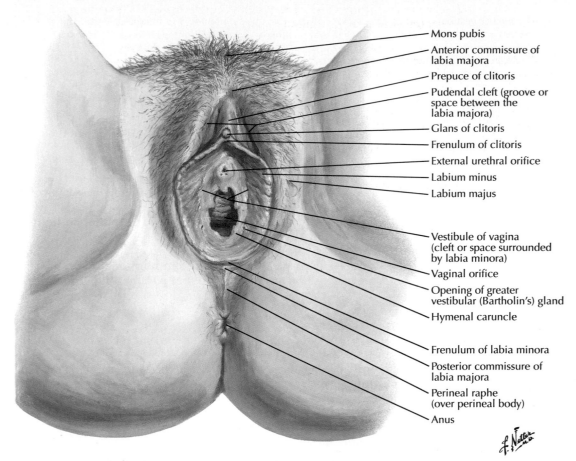

Mons pubis

Anterior commissure of labia majora

Prepuce of clitoris

Pudendal cleft (groove or space between the labia majora)

Glans of clitoris

Frenulum of clitoris

External urethral orifice

Labium minus

Labium majus

Vestibule of vagina (cleft or space surrounded by labia minora)

Vaginal orifice

Opening of greater vestibular (Bartholin's) gland

Hymenal caruncle

Frenulum of labia minora

Posterior commissure of labia majora

Perineal raphe (over perineal body)

Anus

4-30: Female external genitalia (vulva, pudendum). *(From Netter, F H: Atlas of Human Anatomy, 4th ed. Philadelphia, Saunders, 2006, Plate 377.)*

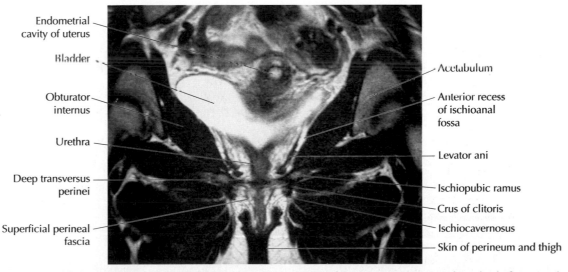

Endometrial cavity of uterus

Bladder

Obturator internus

Urethra

Deep transversus perinei

Superficial perineal fascia

Acetabulum

Anterior recess of ischioanal fossa

Levator ani

Ischiopubic ramus

Crus of clitoris

Ischiocavernosus

Skin of perineum and thigh

4-31: Coronal, T2-weighted MRI of female pelvis and perineum. Section of deep transverse perinei shows level of urogenital diaphragm closing midline urogenital hiatus between right and left levator ani muscles. Crura of clitoris and overlying ischiocavernosus muscles are shown in superficial perineal pouch. *(Provided by Dr J Lee and Ms K Wimpey, Chelsea and Westminster Hospital, London.)*

The **greater vestibular glands** are usually not palpable unless **infected and inflamed (Bartholinitis).** An **abscess** may develop and hamper pelvic examination or sexual relations due to pain and swelling. Most infections are due to *Neisseria gonorrhoeae.* Occlusion of the gland's duct may result in a **Bartholin gland cyst. Vulvar carcinoma** occasionally arises in the gland.

XV. **Development of Genital System**
    A. **Determination of Sex (Figure 4-32)**
        • Genetic basis of maleness and femaleness depends on fertilization of ovum by sperm containing X or Y chromosome.
        1. **Development of maleness**
            a. Differentiation of **mesonephric** (wolffian) **ducts** induced by **testosterone** secreted by testicular **interstitial (Leydig) cells** under stimulation of human chorionic gonadotropin
            b. Development of paramesonephric ducts suppressed by **antimüllerian hormone** produced by **sustentacular (Sertoli) cells**
        2. **Development of femaleness**
            • **Absence** of testicular **testosterone** and **antimüllerian hormone** results in regression of mesonephric ducts and development of **paramesonephric ducts,** respectively
    B. **Development of Gonads**
        1. **Indifferent gonads**
            a. **Gonadal (genital) ridges** develop from mesothelium and mesoderm of dorsal body wall medial to mesonephros
            b. **Primary sex (gonadal) cords** form by epithelial proliferation into underlying mesenchyme of gonadal ridges.
            c. **Indifferent gonad** consists of epithelial **cortex** and underlying **medulla** of mesenchyme.
            d. **Primordial germ cells** migrate from **yolk sac** to gonadal ridges and are incorporated into primary sex cords.
        2. **Testis (Figure 4-33)**
            a. Overview
                (1) Testis differentiation depends on presence of *SRY* **gene on Y chromosome** responsible for **testis-determining factor**

The *SRY* gene on the Y chromosome encodes for testis-determining factor.

Mesonephric ducts: male genital system.
Paramesonephric ducts: female genital system

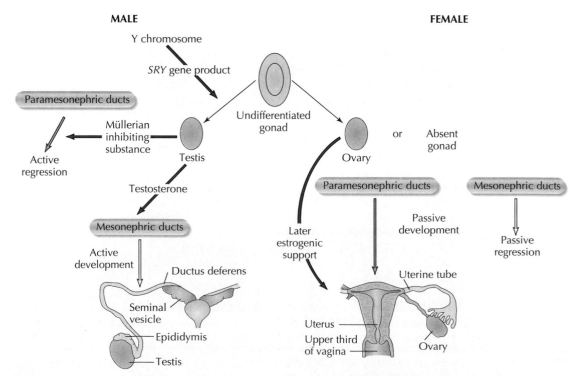

4-32: Factors involved in determination of an embryo's sex. Testosterone and antimüllerian hormone are required for development of normal male phenotype.

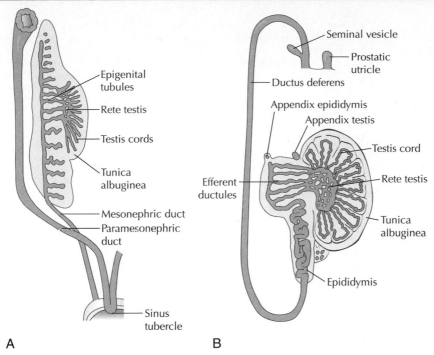

4-33: Progressive development of testis and male genital ducts (**A** and **B**). Epididymis, ductus deferens, and ejaculatory duct develop from mesonephric ducts in response to testosterone, and paramesonephric ducts degenerate in response to antimüllerian hormone. *(Adapted from Carlson, B M: Human Embryology and Developmental Biology, 2nd ed. St. Louis, Mosby, 1999, p 383.)*

(2) Develops mostly from **medulla** of indifferent gonad; cortex largely disappears
  b. **Tunica albuginea** separates sex cords from surface epithelium and foreshadows testicular development.
  c. **Interstitial cells** develop from mesenchyme separating sex cords.
  d. **Sustentacular cells** develop from sex cords.
  e. **Spermatogonia** develop from primordial germ cells of seminiferous cords; **seminiferous tubules** develop a lumen at puberty.

3. **Ovary (Figure 4-34)**
  • Requires **two X chromosomes**; individuals with only one X chromosome (Turner syndrome) exhibit **ovarian dysgenesis**
  a. **Primary sex cords** disappear; **secondary sex (cortical) cords** arise from surface epithelium and incorporate primordial germ cells.
  b. **Primordial follicles** (each containing **oogonium** derived from primordial germ cell surrounded by follicular cells) arise from secondary sex cords.
  c. **Primary oocytes** before birth become arrested in **prophase of first meiotic division** and may remain in arrested stage for decades, until first meiotic division is completed shortly before ovulation.

C. **Development of Genital Ducts and Accessory Sex Glands**
  • **Weeks 5 and 6** are an indifferent stage in which both male and female genital ducts are present.
  1. **Male genital ducts (see Figure 4-33)**
    a. **Epididymis, ductus deferens,** and **ejaculatory duct**
    b. Develop from **mesonephric ducts** in response to testosterone; paramesonephric ducts degenerate in response to antimüllerian hormone.
  2. **Male accessory sex glands**
    a. **Seminal vesicles** develop as outgrowth from caudal end of mesonephric duct.
    b. **Prostate** and **bulbourethral glands** arise as endodermal outgrowths of prostatic and spongy urethra, respectively.
  3. **Female genital ducts (see Figure 4-34)**
    a. **Uterus, uterine tubes,** and **upper vagina** develop from **paramesonephric ducts** in absence of antimüllerian hormone secreted by testes
    b. **Mesonephric ducts** regress in absence of testosterone secreted by testes.

The ovary differentiates from the cortex of the indifferent gonad in an XX embryo, and the testis from the medulla in an XY embryo.

Primary oocytes are arrested in the prophase of the first meiotic division until near ovulation.

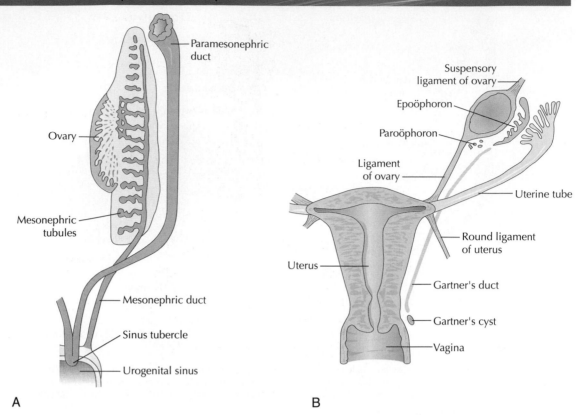

4-34: Progressive development of ovary and female genital ducts. **A,** Contact of uterovaginal primordium (sinus tubercle) with urogenital sinus induces sinovaginal bulbs that fuse to form vaginal plate. It canalizes to form lumen of vagina. **B,** Uterus, uterine tubes, and upper vagina develop from paramesonephric ducts while mesonephric ducts regress.

    c. **Uterovaginal primordium** induces endodermally derived **sinovaginal bulbs** from urogenital sinus that fuse to form **vaginal plate,** which canalizes to form **lumen of vagina**

    d. Membranous **hymen** separates lumen of vagina from urogenital sinus until rupture during perinatal period

<table>
<tr>
<td>Fetal compression in a bicornuate uterus may cause deformities.</td>
<td>**Incomplete fusion of the paramesonephric ducts** can cause a **double uterus and vagina** or a **bicornuate uterus.** Pregnancy in a bicornuate uterus may result in premature delivery or compression of the fetus, causing deformities (e.g., club foot or craniosynostosis). **Failure of the sinovaginal bulbs to develop** can cause **absence of the vagina; failure of the lower end of the vaginal plate to complete canalization** can produce an **imperforate hymen.**</td>
</tr>
</table>

    D. Development of External Genitalia (Figure 4-35)
- Distinguishing sexual characteristics begin to appear during **week 9.**

    1. **Indifferent external genitalia**
      a. Mesenchymal proliferation produces **genital tubercle** that elongates to form **phallus**
      b. **Labioscrotal swellings** and **urogenital folds** develop on each side of the **cloacal membrane.**
      c. **Anal membrane** and **urogenital membrane** separated by fusion of **urorectal septum** with cloacal membrane; rupture produces anus and urogenital orifice

Cellular resistance to testosterone causes feminization of male external genitalia.

    2. **Development of male external genitalia**
      a. **Phallus** enlarges to become penis with **urethral groove** on ventral surface bounded by **urogenital folds** on each side, which subsequently fuse to form **spongy urethra**
      b. Ectodermal ingrowth from tip of glans **(ectodermal cord)** meets spongy urethra and canalizes as **navicular fossa** and **external urethral meatus**
      c. **Prepuce** is formed as peripheral ingrowth of ectoderm around glans penis that later breaks down.
      d. **Labioscrotal swellings** fuse in midline to form **scrotum** at **scrotal raphe**

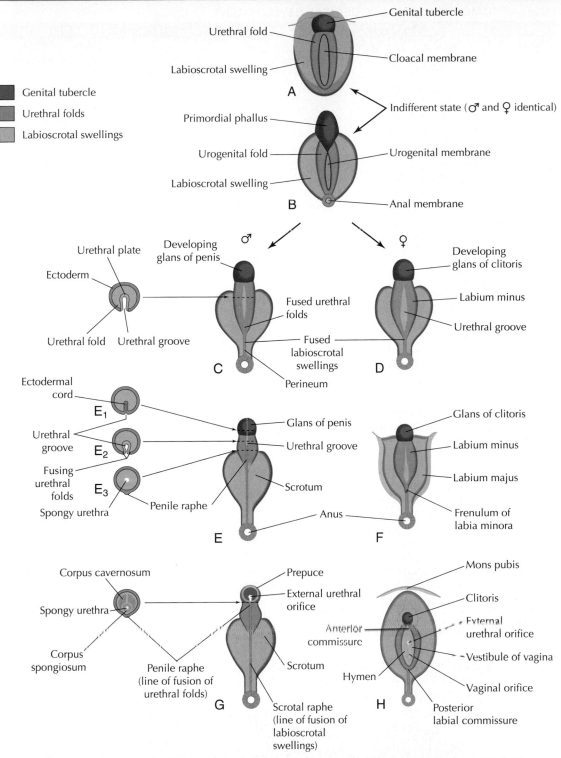

4-35: Development of the external genitalia. **A** and **B,** Appearance of the genitalia during the indifferent state (fourth to seventh weeks). **C, E,** and **G,** Stages in the development of the male external genitalia at 9, 11, and 12 weeks, respectively. On the left are schematic transverse sections of the developing penis, showing the formation of the spongy urethra. **D, F,** and **H,** Stages in the development of the female external genitalia at 9, 11, and 12 weeks, respectively. *(From Moore, K L, Persaud, T V N: Before We Are Born: Essentials of Embryology and Birth Defects, 7th ed. Philadelphia, Saunders, 2008, Figure 13-24.)*

The **spongy urethra** may open onto the dorsal surface **(epispadias)** or the ventral surface **(hypospadias)** of the penis. Hypospadias is the most frequent developmental anomaly of the penis. **Recurrent urinary tract infection** may be associated with these two **developmental defects.**

In hypospadias, the most common anomaly of the penis, abnormal openings of the urethra occur on the ventral surface.

TABLE 4-8. HOMOLOGUES IN UROGENITAL DEVELOPMENT

INDIFFERENT STRUCTURE	MALE DERIVATIVE	FEMALE DERIVATIVE
Genital ridge	Testis	Ovary
Mesonephric duct	Epididymis Ductus deferens Ejaculatory duct	Appendix of ovary* Gartner duct*
Paramesonephric duct	Appendix of testis* Prostatic utricle*	Uterine tubes Uterus Upper vagina
Upper urogenital sinus	Urinary bladder Prostatic urethra	Urinary bladder Urethra
Lower urogenital sinus	Spongy urethra	Lower vagina Vaginal vestibule
Genital tubercle	Penis	Clitoris
Urogenital folds	Spongy urethra (base)	Labia minora
Labioscrotal swellings	Scrotum	Labia majora

*Vestigial structures of potential medical significance.

3. **Development of female external genitalia**
   a. **Phallus** ceases to grow and becomes **clitoris**
   b. **Urogenital folds** become **labia minora** and fuse anteriorly to form **prepuce** and **frenulum of clitoris** and posteriorly to form **frenulum of labia minora**
   c. **Labioscrotal folds** become **labia majora** and fuse only posteriorly and anteriorly to form **labial commissures** and **mons pubis.**
   d. Anomalies include **clitoral hypertrophy** and **partial fusion of labia majora.**

E. **Homologues in Urogenital Development (Table 4-8)**

F. **Abnormalities of Sexual Differentiation**
   1. **Gonadal dysgenesis (Turner syndrome)**
      a. **45,X** karyotype usually results from **meiotic nondisjunction of chromosomes** but sometimes occurs in **mosaicism** due to **mitotic nondisjunction of chromosomes.**
      b. Primordial **germ cells degenerate,** and gonadal differentiation fails, leaving a **streak gonad.**
         • **"Menopause before menarche"**
      c. Immature female genitalia caused by absence of gonadal hormones
      d. Short stature, broad chest, short webbed neck, and lymphedema of hands and feet; preductal coarctation of aorta are common associations
   2. **Hermaphroditism (intersexuality)**
      • Discrepancy between gonad and appearance of external genitalia
      a. **True hermaphrodites**
         (1) **Rare,** most with **46,XX** genotype
         (2) Both **testicular and ovarian tissue** present with female or ambiguous external genitalia
      b. **Female pseudohermaphrodites**
         (1) **46,XX** genotype
         (2) Female internal genitalia with variable **masculinization** of external genitalia, including clitoral hypertrophy and partial fusion of labia majora
         (3) Results from **excessive androgen production** with most common cause being **congenital adrenal hyperplasia**
      c. **Male pseudohermaphrodites**
         (1) **46,XY** genotype
         (2) Variable genitalia caused by **inadequate testosterone and antimüllerian hormone** production by fetal testes
   3. **Testicular feminization (androgen insensitivity syndrome)**
      a. **46,XY** genotype and internal testes but **female phenotype**
      b. Often discovered at puberty because of **amenorrhea**
      c. Results from **receptor insensitivity** to testosterone and dihydrotestosterone
      d. **Upper vagina, uterus, and uterine tubes absent** or rudimentary because of **antimüllerian hormone** produced by testis

Excess androgen production causes masculinization of female external genitalia.

Turner syndrome is only monosomy compatible with life with 1-2% survival.

Hermaphrodites have characteristics of both sexes.

Excessive androgen production in congenital adrenal hyperplasia (adrenogenital syndrome) causes a female pseudohermaphrodite.

Testicular feminization patients are 46,XY with testes but a female phenotype.

CHAPTER 5
THE LOWER EXTREMITY

I. Skeleton of Lower Extremity
A. Pelvic Girdle
1. Overview
   a. **Transmits weight** of upper body from axial skeleton to lower extremities
   b. **Fusion of pubis, ilium, and ischium** at **acetabulum** to form **coxal or hip bone**
   c. Joins sacrum and coccyx to form **bony pelvis**
2. **Pubis**
   a. **Body** articulates with opposite pubic bone at **pubic symphysis**
   b. **Superior ramus** articulates laterally with **ilium and ischium** at acetabulum
   c. **Inferior ramus** fuses posteroinferiorly with ramus of ischium
3. **Ilium**
   a. **Body** forms superior portion of acetabulum
   b. **Wing** (ala) gives origin to gluteal and iliacus muscles and articulates with sacrum

Because of its subcutaneous location, the **iliac crest** is particularly susceptible to injury in contact sports. A **hip pointer** is a **contusion** of the iliac crest usually caused by a direct blow or a fall on the hip.

A hip pointer is a contusion of the iliac crest.

4. **Ischium**
   a. **Ischial tuberosity** gives origin to **hamstring muscles** and provides attachment for the **sacrotuberous ligament.**
   b. **Ischial spine** provides attachment for the **sacrospinous ligament.**

The **origin of the hamstrings** may be **avulsed** from the **ischial tuberosity** in skeletally immature athletes. When sitting, the ischial tuberosity is not covered by the **gluteus maximus muscle;** therefore, one sits on the ischial tuberosities, not the gluteus maximus. **Repetitive movement** against a bicycle seat may **inflame the ischial bursa** (ischial bursitis), which covers the ischial tuberosity. In debilitated or sensory-impaired individuals (e.g., spinal cord injury patients), compression and ischemia in skin and subcutaneous tissues overlying the ischial tuberosities caused by unrelieved sitting or lying down in one position may result in **pressure sores,** or **decubitus ulcers.**

The hamstring origin from the ischial tuberosity is often avulsed before skeletal maturity.

Pressure ulcers may develop over ischial tuberosities from unrelieved pressure.

5. **Acetabulum**
   a. Cup-shaped depression that articulates with head of femur to form **hip joint**
   b. Articular **lunate surface** around central nonarticular **acetabular fossa**
   c. Margin is deficient inferiorly, forming the **acetabular notch.**
B. Femur (Figure 5-1)
1. **Head**
   a. Articulates with acetabulum
   b. Covered by **hyaline cartilage** except at **fovea capitis** for attachment of **ligament of the head**

The main blood supply to the femoral head in adults is the medial femoral circumflex artery.

Traumatic injury or systemic conditions such as sickle cell disease may cause **avascular necrosis of bone.** In children, the avascular necrosis is often **idiopathic** and involves epiphyseal ossification centers **(osteochondrosis)** of the lower extremity. The most common and serious example is osteochondrosis of the femoral head **(Legg-Calvé-Perthes disease).** The condition is painful and causes

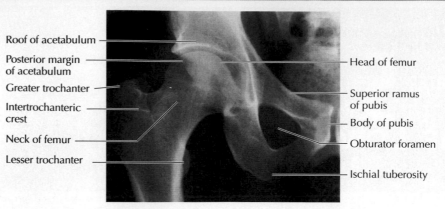

Roof of acetabulum

Posterior margin
of acetabulum

Greater trochanter

Intertrochanteric
crest

Neck of femur

Lesser trochanter

Head of femur

Superior ramus
of pubis

Body of pubis

Obturator foramen

Ischial tuberosity

5-1: Anteroposterior radiograph of the right hip.

Legg-Calvé-Perthes
disease is idiopathic
avascular necrosis of a
child's femoral head.

an **antalgic** (protective) **limp** but usually is self-limiting and may heal completely. **Pain** may be felt in the hip or **referred to the knee.** In adults, **osteonecrosis of the femoral head** is a form of avascular necrosis frequently seen in **alcoholics** or following long-term use of **corticosteroids.** The adult form doesn't heal spontaneously, and severe pain may accompany collapse of the femoral head.

Fractures involving the **epiphyseal plate** may cause **growth disturbance** (e.g., causing a discrepancy in leg length) and/or bony deformity. Prognosis is based on the relationship of the fracture line to the epiphyseal plate **(Salter-Harris classification).**

2. **Neck**
   • Typically forms **angle of inclination** of about 125° with shaft

A common fracture in elderly women with **osteoporosis** is the **fracture of the femoral neck.** Femoral neck fractures in younger individuals are usually due to high-energy trauma but can be stress fractures from unaccustomed strenuous activity (e.g., in military recruits). The **angle of inclination** is decreased in **coxa vara** (e.g., femoral neck fracture) and increased in **coxa valga** (e.g., developmental dysplasia of the hip) **(Figure 5-2).** Both may congenital or acquired conditions.

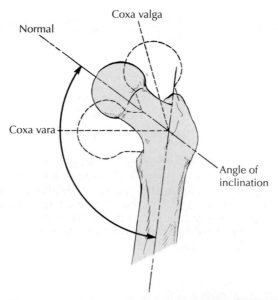

Normal

Coxa valga

Coxa vara

Angle of
inclination

5-2: Angle of inclination is formed by line drawn longitudinally through center of femoral shaft and line bisecting femoral head and neck. Angle is decreased in coxa vara and increased in coxa valga. *(From Chung, S M K: Hip Disorders in Infants and Children. Philadelphia, Lea & Febiger, 1981, p 85.)*

3. **Junction of neck and shaft**
    a. **Greater trochanter**
        - Insertions for **hip abductors and rotators**
    b. **Lesser trochanter**
        - Insertion for **iliopsoas muscle**

A fall or direct blow can easily fracture the **greater trochanter** because it is relatively superficial, being covered only by skin, fascia, and tendinous fibers of the gluteus maximus. **Trochanteric bursitis,** which affects the bursa separating the greater trochanter from the gluteus maximus at its insertion into the iliotibial tract, causes tenderness over the greater trochanter and pain that may radiate along the **iliotibial tract** to the tibia. It is a type of **friction bursitis** that frequently follows episodes of repeatedly carrying heavy objects up stairs or a steep incline.

The **lesser trochanter** is unlikely to fracture after a fall or direct blow because it is well protected by muscles. In contrast, **avulsion fractures** of the lesser trochanter from the pull of the **iliopsoas** are common in adolescents. Lesser trochanteric avulsions may occur in adults due to **metastatic or,** less commonly, **primary carcinoma.**

Traumatic lesser trochanter avulsion in adults requires screening for metastatic carcinoma.

4. **Linea aspera**
    - Prominent longitudinal ridge on **posterior** surface of **shaft** for attachment of thigh muscles and **intermuscular septa**
5. **Medial and lateral condyles**
    a. Covered on articular surface by **hyaline cartilage** for articulation with **tibial condyles** at knee joint
    b. Have roughened convex prominences called medial and lateral **epicondyles,** respectively
6. **Popliteal surface**
    - Floor of **popliteal fossa,** against which **popliteal artery** lies

Although less common than those of the clavicle or humerus, **birth fractures of the femur** may occur during the difficult delivery of a large infant, especially during a breech presentation. Multiple birth fractures, including the femur, usually occur in **osteogenesis imperfecta** (brittle bone disease) caused by **mutations of type I collagen genes.** Patients often also have a **blue sclera** (reflection of underlying choroidal veins) and develop **deafness. Type II** osteogenesis imperfecta is fatal in the prenatal or early postnatal period. Transmission is **autosomal dominant.**

Osteogenesis imperfecta is a defect in type I collagen synthesis resulting in multiple fractures.

Fracture of the femoral shaft causes substantial shortening of the femur from contraction of the powerful longitudinally oriented muscles **(Figure 5-3, A).**

When a long bone fractures, fatal fat emboli may travel to the lungs and/or brain.

C. **Patella**
    1. Sesamoid bone in **quadriceps femoris tendon**
    2. Covered by **hyaline cartilage** on its posterior surface for articulation with patellar surface of femur

A **patellar fracture** from a **direct blow** often leaves small undisplaced fragments. **Transverse fractures** caused by sudden quadriceps contraction usually result in the fragments being pulled apart. The articular cartilage on the patella is frequently the initial site of degenerative joint disease (osteoarthritis) of the knee. It involves softening (malacia), fissuring, and uneven erosion of the cartilage **(chondromalacia patellae)** with retropatellar pain that is worse walking up or down stairs and running. Patellectomy may be required if conservative treatment fails.

The patellar articular cartilage is often the initial site of knee osteoarthritis.

The tibia is the medial weight-bearing bone of the leg, and the fibula is the lateral non-weight-bearing bone.

D. **Tibia**
    1. Overview
        a. Medial **weight-bearing** bone of leg
        b. Articulates with **femur** at knee joint, with **talus** at ankle joint, and with **head and distal end of fibula** at superior and inferior tibiofibular joints

The tibia helps to form the knee and ankle joints, and the fibula helps to form the ankle but not the knee joint.

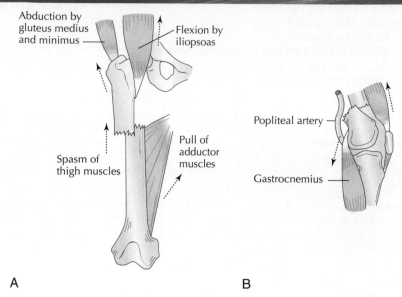

Abduction by gluteus medius and minimus

Flexion by iliopsoas

Spasm of thigh muscles

Pull of adductor muscles

Popliteal artery

Gastrocnemius

A   B

5-3: Femoral fractures. **A,** Proximal fragment is flexed by the iliopsoas and abducted by the gluteus medius and minimus muscles; adductor muscles pull the distal fragment proximally and medially. **B,** In supracondylar fracture, the gastrocnemius muscle can rotate the distal fragment posteriorly, damaging the popliteal artery. *Arrows,* direction of force.

2. **Medial and lateral tibial condyles**
   a. Form expanded proximal end of tibia, each with slightly concave superior articular surface for corresponding femoral condyle
   b. Separated by **anterior intercondylar area, intercondylar eminence,** and **posterior intercondylar area**
3. **Tibial tuberosity**
   • Attachment of quadriceps femoris tendon (patellar ligament)
4. **Shaft**
   • Thinnest and most likely to fracture at junction of middle and inferior thirds

Osgood-Schlatter disease is adolescent knee pain and tibial tubercle enlargement ("knobby knees") from partial avulsion.	**Osgood-Schlatter disease** is the **partial avulsion of the tibial tuberosity** from the epiphyseal plate at the insertion of the patellar tendon. The resulting inflammation (apophysitis), knee pain, and enlargement of the tibial tubercle are frequent in male athletes 11-15 years of age. Alternatively, the tibial tubercle may be completely **avulsed** by forceful quadriceps contraction before closure of the epiphyseal plate.
Tibial shaft fractures often compound fractures and result in osteomyelitis.	**Tibial shaft fractures** are frequent and are often open **(compound fractures)** because of the tibia's extensive subcutaneous surface. Infection of the bone **(osteomyelitis)** is a serious complication. In adults, delayed union and nonunion are common in severely displaced fractures.
Tibial shaft fractures frequently cause compartment syndrome.	If inflammation or bleeding causes increased pressure within an osseofibrous compartment of the leg **(compartment syndrome),** a fasciotomy can prevent necrosis from ischemia of the muscles **(Volkmann ischemic contracture)** and nerves (see clinical correlation under VI.C.1. following). Anterior or medial leg pain **(shin splints)** is frequent in athletes who run on hard surfaces. The condition is probably a stress reaction of the tibial periosteum (or perhaps muscle attachments) to repetitive use. Shin splints must be distinguished from **stress (fatigue) fractures of the tibia** resulting from sudden increases in strenuous activity (e.g., daily marching in previously sedentary military recruits). These microscopic cracks in bone usually are not apparent in initial radiographs. Stress fractures can progress to complete fractures if overuse continues.

5. **Medial malleolus**
   a. **Subcutaneous prominence** at medial side of ankle
   b. Proximal attachment of **medial (deltoid) ligament** of ankle

E. Fibula
1. Overview
   a. Lateral **non-weight-bearing** bone serving mainly for **muscle attachments**
   b. Articulates proximally with lateral condyle of tibia and distally with tibia and talus, **participating in ankle joint but *not* knee joint**
   c. Often used for bone grafts
2. Head
   a. Forms synovial joint with lateral condyle of **tibia** and provides attachment to **fibular collateral** (lateral collateral) **ligament** at pointed apex
   b. Connected to shaft by slender **neck**, against which **common fibular nerve** lies in vulnerable subcutaneous position
3. Shaft
   a. Nonpalpable except distally where it continues as **lateral malleolus**
   b. **Interosseous border** connected to tibia by **interosseous membrane**
4. Lateral malleolus
   a. Palpable **subcutaneous prominence** at lateral side of ankle that articulates medially with trochlea of talus
   b. Gives attachment to **lateral ligaments** of ankle joint

> The fibula is often used for vascularized bone grafts.

F. Skeleton of Foot (Figure 5-4)
- Formed by 7 tarsals, 5 metatarsals, and 14 phalanges
1. **Tarsals**
   a. **Talus**
      (1) Transmits weight of body from leg to foot
      (2) Articulates with tibia, fibula, calcaneus, and navicular bones
      (3) Head is supported by **plantar calcaneonavicular** (spring) **ligament** in medial longitudinal arch of foot

Falling or jumping from a height may fracture the **body of the talus** and **calcaneus**. Violent dorsiflexion of the ankle joint (e.g., in motor vehicle accidents) may fracture the **neck of the talus (Figure 5-5),** which can interrupt the blood supply and lead to **avascular necrosis** of the body of the talus.

> A fracture of the talar neck may cause avascular necrosis of the talar body.

   b. **Calcaneus**
      (1) Largest and strongest bone of foot
      (2) **Tuberosity gives attachment to calcaneal tendon** and forms posterior end of longitudinal arch of foot, where it **transmits 50% of weight on that extremity to ground**

Avulsion or rupture of the **calcaneal** (Achilles) **tendon** disables the gastrocnemius-soleus so that the patient cannot plantar flex the foot. The **calcaneus** is the **most frequently fractured tarsal bone,** with the usual mechanism being a fall onto one or both heels from a height. There is a high incidence of associated **vertebral compression fractures** with that mechanism of injury, so the thoracolumbar spine should always be examined in these patients.

> Calcaneal fracture from a fall is often accompanied by vertebral compression fractures.

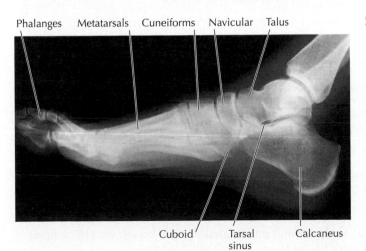

Phalanges Metatarsals Cuneiforms Navicular Talus

Cuboid Tarsal sinus Calcaneus

5-4: Radiograph of the right foot and ankle, lateral projection.

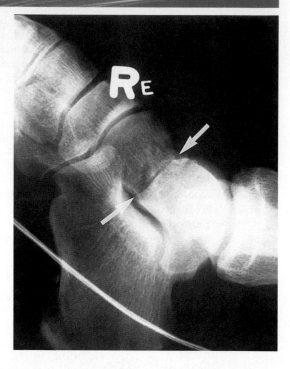

5-5: Radiograph of the proximal foot showing a fracture of the talar neck (*arrows*), which may interrupt the blood supply to the body of the talus to cause avascular necrosis. *(From Mettler, F A: Essentials of Radiology, 2nd ed. Philadelphia, Saunders, 2004, Figure 8-153.)*

c. **Navicular**
  • Palpable medial **tuberosity** for **tibialis posterior tendon**

An **accessory navicular bone** may develop from a secondary ossification center in the **navicular tuberosity** at the attachment site of the **tibialis posterior tendon**. It may be a source of **pain** that is **activity related** or caused by **pressure from a shoe.** An accessory navicular often is associated with flatfoot (pes planus) (see II.K.4 following).

> An accessory navicular bone may be a source of pain and is associated with flatfoot.

d. **Cuboid**
  • **Grooved** on plantar surface by **sulcus for fibularis longus tendon**
e. **Cuneiforms**
  • Medial, intermediate, and lateral
2. **Metatarsals**
  a. Overview
    (1) Numbered from one to five from great toe to small toe
    (2) Proximal **base,** curved **shaft** (convex dorsally), and distal **head**
    (3) Heads collectively form **anterior end of longitudinal arch** of foot, **transmitting 50% of weight on that extremity to ground**
  b. **First metatarsal**
    (1) **Shorter and stouter** than other metatarsals because its head bears twice the weight of any other metatarsal bone
    (2) **Tuberosity** on plantar surface of base for attachment of **fibularis longus tendon**
  c. **Fifth metatarsal**
    • Prominent **tuberosity** for attachment of **fibularis brevis**

> The toes are numbered 1 to 5 starting with the great toe.

> Fibularis brevis may avulse tuberosity of the fifth metatarsal in forced inversion.

The metatarsal bones are frequently fractured either by dropping a heavy object on the forefoot or by the foot being run over. **Stress fractures** in the distal third of the **second to fourth metatarsal bones** are common in joggers and hikers. The **tuberosity of the fifth metatarsal** may be **avulsed** by the tendon of the **fibularis brevis** during forced inversion of the foot.

3. **Phalanges**
  a. Miniature long bones with proximal **base, shaft,** and distal **head**
  b. Number **two in great toe** and **three each in toes 2-5**
II. **Joints of Lower Extremity**
  A. **Sacroiliac Joint**
    1. Paired joint between **axial skeleton** and **pelvic girdle,** transferring weight of upper body to lower extremity

> Foot skeleton: 7 tarsal, 5 metatarsal, and 14 phalangeal bones

> Sacroiliac joints transfer weight from the upper body to the lower extremities.

2. Synovial joint (at least early in life) between **auricular surfaces of sacrum and ilium,** allowing little movement
3. Stabilized by interosseous sacroiliac, ventral and dorsal sacroiliac, iliolumbar, sacrospinous, and sacrotuberous ligaments

Pain resulting from an inflamed **sacroiliac joint** is often referred to the inferior part of the buttock and to the thigh. The sacroiliac joint is often the initial source of pain in young men with **ankylosing spondylitis,** a seronegative (rheumatoid factor) spondyloarthropathy. This chronic inflammatory disease subsequently involves the vertebral column, causing fusion of vertebrae ("bamboo spine") and kyphosis. Aortitis with a diastolic murmur from aortic regurgitation may be present. Approximately 90% of patients possess the **HLA-B27 antigen.**

Sacroiliac joints are involved first in ankylosing spondylitis— the "bamboo spine" disease.

B. **Pubic Symphysis**
   - Anterior midline joint with **fibrocartilaginous interpubic disc** between bodies of two pubic bones

The **pubic symphysis** is relatively immovable except in the latter stages of **pregnancy,** when hormones cause ligaments to loosen.

C. **Hip Joint**
   1. Overview
      a. **Synovial ball-and-socket joint** between head of **femur** and **acetabulum of hip bone**
      b. **Stable,** while still allowing substantial movement, including flexion and extension, abduction and adduction, and medial and lateral rotation
      c. Receives blood supply from medial and lateral **femoral circumflex,** superior and inferior **gluteal,** and **obturator arteries**
      d. Innervated by femoral and obturator nerves, superior gluteal nerve, and nerve to quadratus femoris

      Pain may be referred to the hip from the lumbar spine.

   2. **Acetabular labrum**
      - Fibrocartilaginous rim that **deepens acetabulum** and continues across acetabular notch as **transverse acetabular ligament**
   3. **Articular capsule**
      - Extends from acetabulum and transverse acetabular ligament to intertrochanteric line anteriorly and distal neck of femur posteriorly
   4. **Iliofemoral ligament**
      a. Inverted Y-shaped ligament, strongest of hip joint, reinforcing capsule anteriorly
      b. **Limits extension** of hip joint and allows standing without muscular fatigue
   5. **Ischiofemoral ligament**
      a. Supports hip joint capsule posteriorly
      b. Limits extension and medial rotation of hip joint
   6. **Pubofemoral ligament**
      a. Reinforces anterior, inferior part of capsule
      b. Limits excessive abduction and helps limit extension of hip joint

      Hip joint ligaments: iliofemoral, ischiofemoral, and pubofemoral

   7. **Ligament of head of femur**
      - Transmits **artery to head of femur** (from obturator artery), an **important source of blood to femoral head in children** but usually small or absent in adults
   8. **Movements at hip joint**
      a. **Flexion:** iliopsoas, rectus femoris, tensor fasciae latae, sartorius, pectineus, adductor longus, adductor brevis
      b. **Extension:** gluteus maximus, hamstrings
      c. **Abduction:** gluteus medius, gluteus minimus, tensor fasciae latae, sartorius
      d. **Adduction:** adductor magnus, adductor longus, adductor brevis, pectineus, gracilis
      e. **Medial rotation:** gluteus minimus, gluteus medius, tensor fasciae latae
      f. **Lateral rotation:** obturator internus, obturator externus, piriformis, quadratus femoris, superior and inferior gemelli

      "Developmental dysplasia of the hip" is the new term for "congenital dislocation of the hip."

Femoral neck fractures
are common in
postmenopausal women
due to osteoporosis.

Osteoarthritis is the most common disease of the hip in adults. Severe joint degeneration may necessitate **total hip replacement.**

The hip frequently **fractures at the femoral neck** adjacent to the femoral head **(subcapital fracture)** and less frequently **between the trochanters (petrochanteric/intertrochanteric fracture).** Intracapsular fractures of the femoral neck may interrupt the blood supply to the femoral head, resulting in **avascular necrosis (Figures 5-6 and 5-7).** Fractures are more common in elderly females than males because the incidence of **osteoporosis** is increased after menopause.

Most traumatic hip
dislocations are posterior
with possible damage to
the sciatic nerve.

Traumatic hip dislocations are associated with automobile accidents and usually occur posteriorly from a blow to the knee while the hip is flexed and adducted (as when sitting in an automobile). The affected extremity will be shortened and will assume a **characteristic position of flexion, adduction, and internal rotation** in most cases. The posterior margin of the acetabulum may fracture, with damage to the **sciatic nerve.** Delayed reduction increases the risk of avascular necrosis of the femoral head.

Coronal section

Anterior view

A   B

5-6: Blood supply to head and neck of femur in anterior view and coronal section. In adults the blood supply to the head of the femur is mainly from the medial femoral circumflex artery. The artery to the head of the femur is usually small or absent in adults but is an important source of blood in children. *(From Netter, F H: Atlas of Human Anatomy, 4th ed. Philadelphia, Saunders, 2006, Plate 504.)*

5-7: Fractures of proximal femur. Intracapsular fracture of femoral neck, especially if displaced, may disrupt blood supply to femoral head via retinacular branches of medial femoral circumflex artery and cause avascular necrosis. Intertrochanteric fracture is extracapsular and does not compromise blood supply to femoral head (see Figure 5-6). *(From Greene, W B: Netter's Orthopaedics. Philadelphia, Saunders, 2006, Figure 17-21.)*

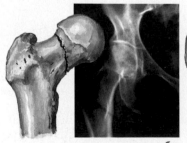

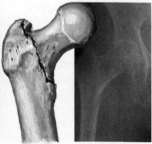

Nondisplaced femoral
neck fracture   Two-part, minimally displaced
                       intertrochanteric femur fracture

A **positive Trendelenburg sign** often indicates paralyzed or weak gluteus medius and minimus muscles on the **weight-bearing side** that cause inability to abduct the hip (i.e., keep the pelvis level) **(Figure 5-8).**

Avascular necrosis of the femoral head is common after a femoral neck fracture.

D. Knee Joint (Figure 5-9)

1. Overview
   a. **Synovial hinge joint** between **femoral and tibial condyles,** and including **patellofemoral joint**
   b. Permits **flexion** and **extension;** last part of extension is accompanied by **medial rotation** of femur on weight-bearing tibia
   c. Supplied by arteries forming genicular anastomosis **(see Figure 5-24)**
   d. Supplied by **femoral, obturator, tibial,** and common **fibular** nerves

Osteosarcoma (osteogenic sarcoma) is one of the most common primary malignant tumors of bone. It often occurs in the distal femur or proximal tibia, with 50% of the tumors involving the knee joint. Approximately 75% occur in patients under 20 years of age.

Fifty percent of osteosarcomas involve the knee joint.

2. **Articular capsule**
   a. Attaches to margins of femoral and tibial condyles
   b. Replaced anteriorly by **quadriceps tendon** and embedded **patella**

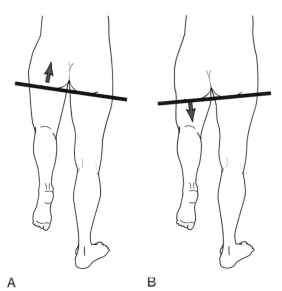

5-8: A, Normal right gluteus medius and minimus muscles. Left buttock does not sag when the left foot is raised from floor. **B,** Positive Trendelenburg sign. Left buttock drops when the left foot is raised as in walking or standing, indicating injury on the right side. *Arrows,* direction of pelvis movement.

A   B

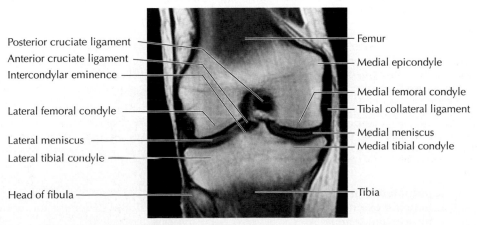

Posterior cruciate ligament — Femur
Anterior cruciate ligament — Medial epicondyle
Intercondylar eminence —
Medial femoral condyle
Lateral femoral condyle — Tibial collateral ligament
Lateral meniscus — Medial meniscus
Lateral tibial condyle — Medial tibial condyle
Head of fibula — Tibia

5-9: Magnetic resonance image of the right knee, coronal section.

3. **Tibial collateral ligament** (medial collateral ligament)
   a. Broad flat band extending from **medial epicondyle of femur** to **medial condyle and shaft of tibia**
   b. Blends with capsule and **firmly attaches to medial meniscus**
   c. **Limits extension** and **abduction of leg** at knee

The unhappy triad of knee injuries: tibial collateral ligament, medial meniscus, and ACL

Because the lateral side of the knee is struck more often (e.g., in a football tackle), the **tibial collateral ligament** is the **most frequently torn ligament at the knee.** Attachment to the **medial meniscus** means that the two structures usually are injured together. The **unhappy triad** of athletic knee injuries involves the **tibial collateral ligament, medial meniscus, and anterior cruciate ligament.**

4. **Fibular collateral ligament** (lateral collateral ligament)
   a. Rounded cord between **lateral epicondyle of femur** and **head of fibula**
   b. Does *not* blend with joint capsule and **does not attach to lateral meniscus**
   c. **Limits extension** and **adduction of leg** at knee
5. **Anterior and posterior cruciate ligaments**
   a. Overview
      (1) Located inside articular capsule but **outside synovial cavity**
      (2) Named for attachments to **intercondylar area of tibia**
      (3) Stabilize joint best when knee is **fully extended**
   b. Anterior cruciate ligament (ACL) limits anterior movement of tibia on femur
   c. Posterior cruciate ligament (PCL) limits posterior movement of tibia on femur

Ruptured anterior cruciate ligament: anterior drawer sign. Ruptured posterior cruciate ligament: posterior drawer sign

With a **rupture of the anterior cruciate ligament,** the tibia can be pulled forward excessively on the femur in the flexed knee, exhibiting **anterior drawer sign.** In the less common rupture of the **posterior cruciate ligament,** the tibia can be pulled backward excessively on the femur, exhibiting **posterior drawer sign.**

6. **Medial and lateral menisci**
   a. **Fibrocartilage wedges** anchored to anterior and posterior **intercondylar areas** of tibia
   b. Medial meniscus C-shaped but lateral meniscus almost circular

The medial meniscus is frequently injured with the attached tibial collateral ligament.

The **medial meniscus** is more frequently injured because it is firmly attached to the fibrous capsule and the **tibial collateral ligament,** whereas the **lateral meniscus** is *not* attached to the **fibular collateral ligament.** A displaced cartilage fragment from a **torn meniscus** may lock the knee and prevent full extension. Only the periphery of the meniscus has the potential to heal because it has a vascular supply.

7. **Synovial cavity**
   a. **Horseshoe-shaped,** with the two sides communicating anteriorly
   b. Does *not* contain **cruciate ligaments** (i.e., they are intracapsular, but extrasynovial)
   c. Frequently communicates with **synovial bursae** around knee

Increased joint fluid from knee injuries may not be obvious because of the **large synovial cavity** and **communication with the suprapatellar bursa,** where excess fluid may reside unless the bursa is "milked" downward. **Hemarthrosis** usually causes the knee joint to swell quickly; **inflammatory joint effusion** usually causes slow swelling.

Degenerative joint disease (osteoarthritis) of the knee may involve the lateral compartment between the lateral femoral and tibial condyles, the medial compartment **(Figure 5-10),** or both compartments. If the joint is irreparably damaged, **replacement arthroplasty** of the affected compartment or the entire joint may be required.

Rapid swelling of an injured joint indicates hemarthrosis.

8. **Suprapatellar bursa**
   a. Superior extension of synovial cavity between distal end of **femur** and **quadriceps** muscle and tendon

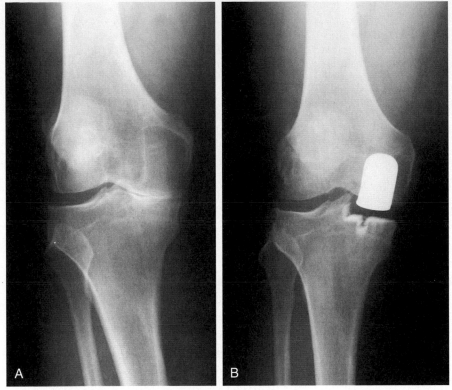

5-10: A, Preoperative radiograph showing severe osteoarthritis in medial compartment of right knee in 58-year-old male. Note the bone-on-bone contact due to destruction of articular cartilage. **B,** Postoperative radiograph following unicompartmental replacement arthroplasty. *(From Greene, W B: Netter's Orthopaedics. Philadelphia, Saunders, 2006, Figure 18-8.)*

  b. **Articularis genus muscle** pulls synovial membrane superiorly to protect it as leg is extended
9. **Prepatellar bursa**
  a. Between superficial surface of patella and skin
  b. May become inflamed and swollen (**prepatellar bursitis**)
10. **Infrapatellar bursae**
  • Superficial (**subcutaneous infrapatellar bursa**) and deep (**deep infrapatellar bursa**) to quadriceps femoris tendon
11. **Knee deformities (Figure 5-11)**
  • Common in very young children and usually correct spontaneously with growth; pathological in adolescents and adults
  a. **Genu valgum** (knock-knee): tibia is deviated laterally at knee, stretching medial side of joint and compressing lateral side; it predisposes to lateral dislocation of patella
  b. **Genu varum** (bowleg): tibia is deviated medially at knee, stretching lateral side and compressing medial side of knee
12. **Movements at knee joint**
  a. **Flexion:** hamstrings, sartorius, gracilis, and gastrocnemius; popliteus unlocks fully extended knee joint
  b. **Extension:** quadriceps femoris
  c. **Medial rotation (of leg):** popliteus, semitendinosus, and semimembranosus
  d. **Lateral rotation (of leg):** biceps femoris

The **patellar tendon reflex** ("knee-jerk" reflex) is tested by tapping the patellar tendon with a reflex hammer to elicit extension at the knee joint. Both afferent and efferent limbs of the reflex arc are in the **femoral nerve (L2-4).**

E. **Tibiofibular Joints**
  1. **Superior tibiofibular joint** is **synovial joint** between lateral condyle of tibia and head of fibula

Prepatellar bursitis is called "housemaid's knee."

Genu valgum: knock-knee.
Genu varum: bowleg

The popliteus muscle unlocks the fully extended knee joint at the beginning of flexion.

Knee-jerk reflex: tests spinal nerves L2-4

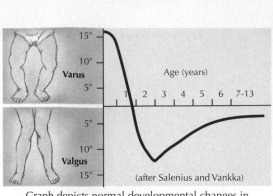

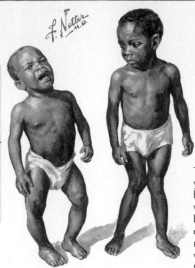

Graph depicts normal developmental changes in tibio-femoral angle. Substantial deviation suggests pathologic cause such as rickets, Blount's disease, or other disorders requiring specific treatment.

Two brothers, younger (left) with bowleg, older (right) with knock-knee. In both children, limbs eventually became normally aligned without corrective treatment

5-11: Bowleg and knock-knee deformities. In bowleg deformity the leg is angled medially at the knee (genu varum). In knock-knee the leg is angled laterally at the knee (genu valgum). These deformities are usually self-correcting in young children. *(From Greene, W B: Netter's Orthopaedics. Philadelphia, Saunders, 2006, Figure 3-5.)*

 2. **Interosseous membrane** connects shafts of tibia and fibula
 3. **Inferior tibiofibular joint** has strong **interosseous and inferior tibiofibular ligaments** that stabilize ankle joint
F. **Ankle (Talocrural) Joint (Figure 5-12)**
 1. Overview
  a. **Synovial hinge joint** formed by **tibia, fibula, and talus**
  b. Allows **dorsiflexion** and **plantar flexion**
  c. Most stable in **dorsiflexion** because **trochlea of talus** is wider anteriorly
 2. **Medial ligament (deltoid ligament)**
  a. Strong, triangular ligament with apex attached to **medial malleolus**
  b. Strongly resists **eversion** of foot
 3. **Lateral ligament** (lateral collateral ligament)
  a. Consists of three distinct ligaments—**anterior** and **posterior talofibular** and **calcaneofibular**—attached superiorly to **lateral malleolus**
  b. Resists **inversion** of foot
 4. **Movements at ankle joint**
  a. **Dorsiflexion:** tibialis anterior, extensor digitorum longus, extensor hallucis longus, and fibularis tertius muscles
  b. **Plantar flexion:** gastrocnemius, soleus, plantaris, tibialis posterior, flexor digitorum longus, flexor hallucis longus muscles

5-12: AP radiograph with ankle in 15-20° of medial rotation. The inferior surface of the tibia joins the medial and lateral malleoli to form a mortise (socket) for the upper part of the body of the talus. *(Frank, E D, Long, B W, Smith, B J: Merrill's Atlas of Radiographic Positioning and Procedures: 3-Volume Set, 11th ed. Mosby, 2007, Figure 6-102.)*

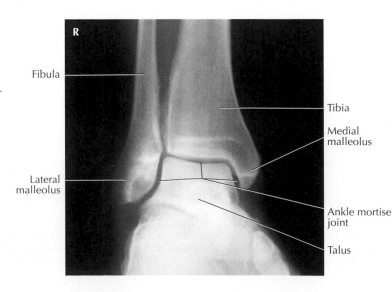

A **sprain** is an injury to a ligament. Sprains are the **most common ankle injuries** and are classified as **first, second, or third degree** according to the amount of ligament tearing. Most are **inversion sprains** because the **deltoid ligament** is strong and the lateral malleolus is long. Sprains occur most frequently when the foot is plantar flexed and involve the **anterior talofibular,** and sometimes calcaneofibular, **ligaments.**

An ankle sprain is most commonly an anterior talofibular ligament tear during forced inversion of the plantar flexed foot.

Injuries from excessive eversion or inversion may avulse the medial or lateral malleolus instead of tearing the collateral ligaments **(Figure 5-13).** The deltoid ligament is especially strong, so avulsion of the medial malleolus is more common.

The **Achilles tendon reflex** ("ankle-jerk" reflex) is tested by tapping the calcaneal tendon to elicit plantar flexion at the ankle joint. Both afferent and efferent limbs of the reflex arc are carried in S1-2 fibers of the tibial nerve.

Ankle-jerk reflex: tests spinal nerves S1 and S2.

G. **Talocalcaneal (Subtalar) Joint**
1. **Inversion:** tibialis anterior and tibialis posterior muscles
2. **Eversion:** fibularis longus and brevis, fibularis tertius muscles
H. **Transverse Tarsal Joint (Midtarsal Joint)**
- Contributes to movement between forefoot and hindfoot, most importantly **eversion** and **inversion,** allowing foot to compensate for uneven ground

Talipes (clubfoot) is a combination congenital deformity with several variations. The most common type, **talipes equinovarus,** involves the subtalar and transverse tarsal joints. The ankle is plantar flexed, the foot inverted, and the forefoot adducted **(Figure 5-14).** The condition may be unilateral or bilateral and is twice as common in males.

Talipes equinovarus—ankle plantar flexion, foot inversion, and forefoot adduction—is the most common form of clubfoot.

I. **Tarsometatarsal Joints**
- Stable synovial joints with strong plantar ligaments

Metatarsus adductus is a relatively common congenital anomaly characterized by adduction of all five metatarsals at the **tarsometatarsal joints.** A related condition involves adduction of only the first metatarsal accompanied by lateral deviation of the great toe **(hallux valgus).**

Hallux valgus is the lateral deviation of the great toe at the MP joint.

J. **Metatarsophalangeal (MP) and Interphalangeal (IP) Joints**
1. Overview
   a. Synovial joints (similar to those of hand) with articular capsules reinforced by collateral and plantar ligaments
   b. Toe 2 is the digit of reference for abduction and adduction.

The second toe is the digit of reference for the abduction and adduction of toes.

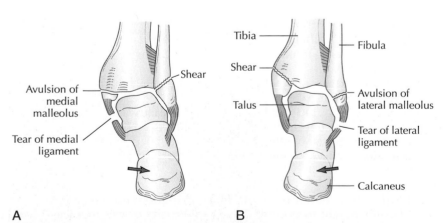

5-13: Fracture-dislocations of the right ankle, posterior view. **A,** Forced eversion (abduction) of the foot (Pott fracture). The medial ligament avulses the medial malleolus or the medial ligament tears, and the fibula fractures at a higher level. **B,** Forced inversion (adduction) avulses the lateral malleolus or tears the lateral ligament and fractures the tibia at a higher level. *Arrows,* direction of force.

5-14: Congenital clubfoot (talipes equinovarus). In this form of clubfoot the ankle is plantar flexed, the foot is inverted, and the forefoot is adducted. *(From Hansen, J T, Lambert, D R: Netter's Clinical Anatomy, Icon Learning Systems, 2005, p 279.)*

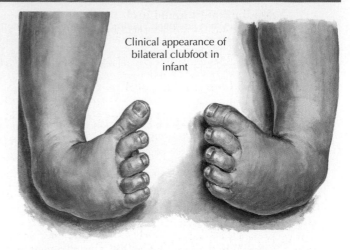

Clinical appearance of bilateral clubfoot in infant

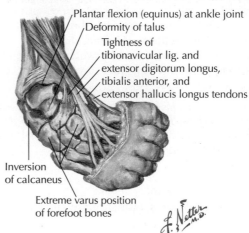

Plantar flexion (equinus) at ankle joint
Deformity of talus
Tightness of tibionavicular lig. and extensor digitorum longus, tibialis anterior, and extensor hallucis longus tendons
Inversion of calcaneus
Extreme varus position of forefoot bones

Hallux valgus is lateral deviation of the great toe at the **metatarsophalangeal joint** in association with an enlarged head of the first metatarsal bone. The condition is seen frequently in females who wear tight, narrow-toed shoes. A **bunion** is **friction bursitis** over the **first metatarsophalangeal joint.**

---

2. **Movements of metatarsophalangeal joints** of toes 2-5
   a. **Flexion:** lumbricals, interosseous muscles
   b. **Extension:** extensor digitorum longus and brevis muscles
   c. **Abduction:** dorsal interossei
   d. **Adduction:** plantar interossei
3. **Movements of interphalangeal joints** of toes 2-5
   a. **Flexion:** flexor digitorum longus and brevis muscles, flexor digiti minimi brevis muscle (toe 5)
   b. **Extension:** extensor digitorum longus and brevis, lumbricals, and interossei
4. **Movements of great toe**
   a. **Flexion:** flexor hallucis longus and brevis muscles
   b. **Extension:** extensor hallucis longus and brevis muscles
   c. **Abduction:** abductor hallucis muscle
   d. **Adduction:** adductor hallucis muscle
K. **Arches of Foot**
   1. Overview
      a. Function in weight distribution, support, and forward propulsion
      b. **Transmit weight to ground** only at **tuberosity of calcaneus** and **heads of metatarsals**
      c. **Stability** depends on bony conformation, plantar ligaments, short plantar muscles, and long leg muscles.
      d. **Plantar aponeurosis** functions as ligament, helping support longitudinal arches

Weight is transferred from the foot to the ground only at the calcaneal tuberosity and metatarsal heads.

2. **Medial longitudinal arch**
   a. Formed by calcaneus, talus, navicular, cuneiform bones, and first three metatarsal bones
   b. Highest at head of talus, which receives support from **plantar calcaneonavicular (spring) ligament**
3. **Lateral longitudinal arch**
   a. Formed by calcaneus, cuboid, and lateral two metatarsal bones
   b. Receives support from **long plantar** and **short plantar ligaments**
4. **Transverse arch**
   a. Formed by bases of metatarsal bones, cuboid, and three cuneiform bones
   b. Is actually a **half arch** formed in each foot when feet are planted and parallel

---

Pes planus (flatfoot), in which the **medial longitudinal arch is unusually low,** is common in a strong, stable foot and is not necessarily pathological. In most cases of acquired flatfoot, plantar ligaments stretch and the **tibialis posterior muscle** provides insufficient dynamic support. The absence of an arch may cause pain when bearing weight. The less common **pes cavus** exhibits an **unusually high arch** and is usually due to muscle imbalance from **neuromuscular diseases** (e.g., Charcot-Marie-Tooth disease, poliomyelitis).

Pes planus is a flat foot. Pes cavus is a high-arched foot.

III. Gluteal Region
A. Nerves of the Gluteal Region (Table 5-1)

Posterior dislocations of the hip joint or improperly placed gluteal intramuscular injections may damage the **sciatic nerve.** Lesions paralyze the posterior thigh muscles and all muscles below the knee. **Sciatica** is pain along the distribution of the sciatic nerve and is often caused by a **herniated or protruded intervertebral disc** that presses on the nerve roots of the lumbosacral plexus.

The sciatic nerve may be damaged by improperly placed gluteal injection or traumatic posterior hip dislocation.

A common fibular nerve that passes through the piriformis is vulnerable to compression.

B. Vessels of Gluteal Region
1. **Superior gluteal artery**
   - Passes above piriformis, supplying gluteus maximus, gluteus medius, and gluteus minimus muscles
2. **Inferior gluteal artery**
   a. Enters gluteus maximus with **inferior gluteal nerve**
   b. Supplies **gluteal and hamstring muscles** and **hip joint**, participating in **cruciate anastomosis**

A sciatic nerve lesion in the gluteal region causes paralysis of the hamstrings and all of the muscles below the knee.

The pudendal nerve traverses the gluteal region to become the major nerve of the perineum.

TABLE 5-1. NERVES OF GLUTEAL REGION

NERVE	COURSE	STRUCTURES INNERVATED/COMMENTS
Superior gluteal nerve (L4, L5, S1)	Passes above piriformis and between gluteus medius and minimus with superior gluteal artery	Innervates gluteus medius, gluteus minimus, tensor fasciae latae, and hip joint
Inferior gluteal nerve (L5, S1, S2)	Passes below piriformis with inferior gluteal artery	Innervates gluteus maximus
Sciatic nerve (L4, L5, S1-3)	Passes through greater sciatic foramen below piriformis and descends midway between ischial tuberosity and greater trochanter of femur posterior to hip joint	Comprises tibial and common fibular nerves bound together by connective tissue; these nerves usually separate in distal thigh, but sometimes tibial nerve passes below piriformis and common fibular nerve through or above it
Posterior femoral cutaneous nerve (S1-3)	Passes below piriformis	Supplies skin of buttock, posterior thigh, and popliteal fossa; sends branch to perineum
Nerve to obturator internus (L5, S1, S2)	Enters gluteal region via greater sciatic foramen and leaves through lesser sciatic foramen	Innervates obturator internus and superior gemellus
Nerve to quadratus femoris (L4, L5, S1)	Passes below piriformis	Innervates quadratus femoris and inferior gemellus
Pudendal nerve (S2-4)	Enters gluteal region through greater sciatic foramen and leaves via lesser sciatic foramen with internal pudendal artery to reach pudendal canal	Main motor and sensory nerve of perineum

3. **Internal pudendal artery**
   a. Leaves greater sciatic foramen and enters lesser sciatic foramen with **pudendal nerve**
   b. Distributed to **perineum,** having **no branches in gluteal region**
4. **Gluteal veins**
   a. Accompany corresponding arteries as tributaries of **internal iliac vein**
   b. Communicate with tributaries of **femoral vein** and form **alternate pathway** for return of blood from lower extremity

C. **Features of Gluteal Region**
   1. **Sacrotuberous ligament**
      a. Connects **posterior iliac spines, sacrum,** and **coccyx** to **ischial tuberosity**
      b. Inferior boundary of **lesser sciatic foramen**
   2. **Sacrospinous ligament**
      a. Connects **sacrum and coccyx** to **ischial spine**
      b. Boundary between **greater** and **lesser sciatic foramina**
   3. **Greater and lesser sciatic foramina**
      a. Overview
         (1) Bony notches on posterior border of hip bone converted into foramina by **sacrotuberous** and **sacrospinous ligaments**
         (2) Transmit muscles, nerves, and vessels between pelvis and gluteal region (greater sciatic foramen) or between gluteal region and perineum (lesser sciatic foramen)
      b. **Greater sciatic foramen** transmits
         (1) Piriformis muscle
         (2) Sciatic nerve
         (3) Superior and inferior gluteal nerves and vessels
         (4) Pudendal nerve, internal pudendal artery and vein (leaving pelvis)
         (5) Posterior femoral cutaneous nerve
         (6) Nerves to obturator internus and quadratus femoris
      c. **Lesser sciatic foramen** transmits
         (1) Obturator internus muscle and its nerve
         (2) Pudendal nerve, internal pudendal artery and vein (entering perineum)
   4. **Piriformis muscle**
      a. Key **landmark** in identifying structures of gluteal region
      b. Superior gluteal nerve and vessels pass above it; sciatic nerve, inferior gluteal nerve and vessels, pudendal nerve and internal pudendal vessels, and smaller nerves and vessels pass below it.
      c. Originates inside pelvis from anterior surface of sacrum and **passes through greater sciatic foramen** to insert into greater trochanter of femur

> **Inflammation or spasm of the piriformis** may produce pain similar to that caused by sciatica ("piriformis syndrome"). Individuals with a **hypertrophied piriformis muscle** from sports that require excessive use of the gluteal muscles (e.g., cyclists, ice skaters) are more prone to this syndrome.

IV. **Thigh (Figure 5-15)**
   A. **Muscles of Thigh**

> The **pes anserinus** ("goose's foot") is a common tendinous insertion into the tibia of the semitendinosus, gracilis, and sartorius, all of which move both the hip and knee; together they form an inverted tripod that stabilizes the pelvis and extremity when standing. The associated bursa may become inflamed **(pes anserinus bursitis)** through overuse or secondary to medial knee compartment arthritis.
>
> Athletes frequently injure the **hamstring muscles,** which cross both hip and knee joints and often tear during forceful contraction while stretched to nearly maximum (e.g., when sprinting or kicking).

> The **psoas major muscle** originates on the lumbar vertebrae and passes inferiorly on the posterior abdominal wall to insert into the lesser trochanter. Infection originating in the abdomen may descend between the psoas major and its fascia to present as a **psoas abscess in the upper thigh. Spinal tuberculosis** or a **fistula related to diverticulitis** of the **sigmoid colon** is a common cause.

The gluteal veins form an alternate route of venous return in femoral vein occlusion.

Pes anserinus bursitis occurs at the common insertion of the semitendinosus, gracilis, and sartorius tendons.

The differential diagnosis of swelling in the upper thigh should include a psoas abscess.

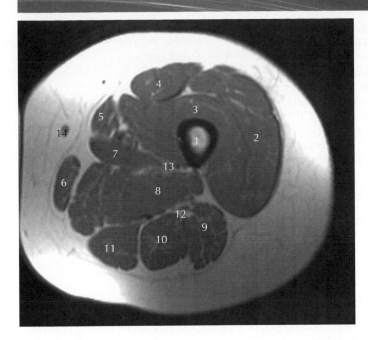

5-15: Axial MRI of upper left thigh. Femur = 1; vastus lateralis = 2; vastus intermedius = 3; rectus femoris = 4; sartorius = 5; gracilis = 6; adductor longus = 7; adductor magnus = 8; biceps femoris = 9; semitendinosus = 10; semimembranosus = 11; sciatic nerve = 12; profunda femoris artery = 13; and great saphenous vein = 14. *(From Weir, J, Abrahams, P: Imaging Atlas of Human Anatomy, 3rd ed. London, Mosby Ltd., 2003, p 197, e.)*

The quadriceps femoris muscle in the anterior thigh and the hamstrings in the posterior thigh are frequent sites of **contusion** in contact sports. Heterotopic ossification **(myositis ossficans)** may occur within the bruised muscle, usually in adolescents or young adults. The ossifying mass becomes radiopaque over time **(Figure 5-16)**. Factors contributing to myositis ossificans include vigorous massage and premature return to strenuous activity. This condition must be distinguished from **extraskeletal osteogenic sarcoma.**

Myositis ossificans is heterotopic ossification within muscles following a contusion.

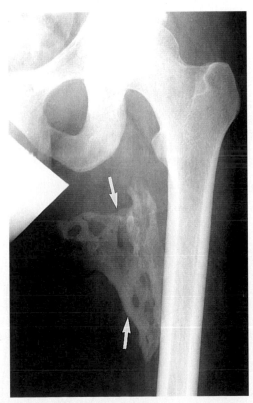

5-16: Myositis ossificans in the proximal thigh of a young soccer player. Muscles of the thigh are a common site for contusion from blunt trauma in contact sports and heterotopic ossification may occur. *(From Mettler, F A: Essentials of Radiology, 2nd ed. Philadelphia, Saunders, 2004, Figure 8-114.)*

  B. Nerves of Thigh
   1. Femoral nerve (L2-4) (Figure 5-17)
      a. Overview
         (1) Forms in **psoas major** as largest branch of **lumbar plexus**
         (2) Enters **femoral triangle** by passing deep to inguinal ligament
         (3) **Susceptible to injury** because it lies superficially just below **inguinal ligament**
      b. **Cutaneous distribution**
         • **Saphenous nerve,** only branch of femoral nerve to extend below knee, becomes cutaneous at knee and **accompanies great saphenous vein** to supply skin on medial side of leg, ankle, and foot

Hip pain is often referred to the knee joint.

> The **femoral and obturator nerves** supply both the **hip and knee joints,** providing a basis for **referred pain.** The **saphenous nerve** is at risk when the great saphenous vein is harvested as a graft for coronary bypass surgery or in a **saphenous cutdown.**

      c. **Muscular branches** supply the **anterior thigh compartment.**
   2. Obturator nerve (L2-4) (Figure 5-18)
      a. Forms from **lumbar plexus** in substance of **psoas major muscle**
      b. Enters thigh through **obturator foramen** with **obturator vessels**
      c. Splits around adductor brevis as **anterior** and **posterior branches** to supply **medial (adductor) muscles of thigh**

5-17: Muscular and cutaneous distributions of the femoral nerve.

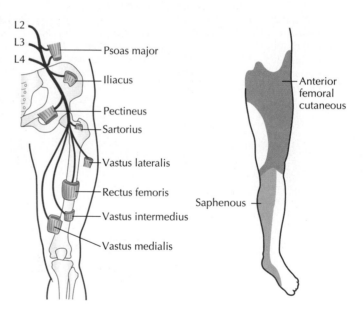

5-18: Muscular and cutaneous distributions of the obturator nerve.

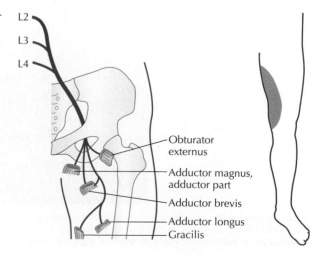

3. **Sciatic nerve** (L4, L5, S1-3) **(Figure 5-19)**
   - Usually divides in distal third of posterior thigh into **tibial nerve** and **common fibular nerve**
   a. **Tibial nerve (see Figure 5-19)**
      - Principal nerve to muscles of **posterior thigh, posterior leg,** and **sole of foot**
   b. **Common fibular nerve**
      - Supplies **lateral and anterior compartments of leg** and also **short head** of **biceps femoris in thigh**

C. **Arteries of Thigh**
   1. **Femoral artery**
      a. Overview
         (1) Begins at **inguinal ligament** as continuation of **external iliac artery** and becomes **popliteal artery** at **adductor hiatus**
         (2) **Palpable** below inguinal ligament midway between anterior superior iliac spine and pubic symphysis
         (3) Enclosed in **femoral sheath** lateral to femoral vein and descends through femoral triangle **medial to femoral nerve**
      b. **Profunda femoris artery** (deep artery of thigh)
         - Gives rise to vessels supplying thigh, gluteal region, and hip and knee joints

         > The profunda femoris artery is the chief blood supply of the thigh.

      c. **Medial femoral circumflex artery**
         (1) Usually arises from **profunda femoris** but can branch directly from **femoral artery**
         (2) Supplies **hip joint** and muscles of upper **thigh** and **gluteal region**
      d. **Lateral femoral circumflex artery**

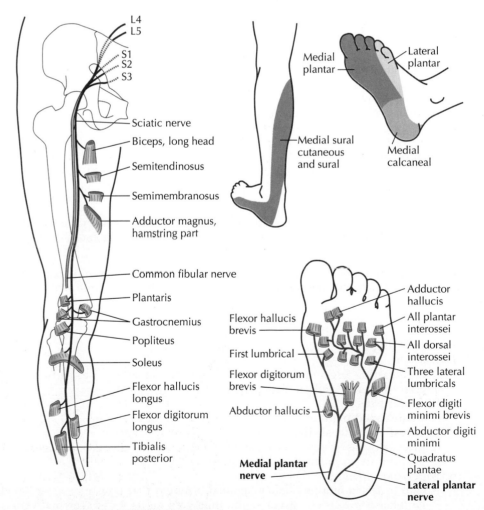

5-19: Muscular and cutaneous distributions of the tibial nerve.

(1) Usually arises as branch of **profunda femoris artery** but can branch directly from **femoral artery**

(2) Supplies **hip joint** and muscles of upper **thigh** and **gluteal region**

e. **Perforating arteries**

(1) Usually four branches of **profunda femoris**

(2) Pierce **adductor magnus** to become major supply to **posterior compartment of thigh**

f. **Descending genicular artery**

- Divides into **musculoarticular branch**, which participates in **genicular anastomosis**, and **saphenous branch**, which runs superficially with **saphenous nerve**

The femoral artery may be compressed against the superior pubic ramus or the femoral head to slow hemorrhage.

The **femoral artery** bleeds profusely when lacerated and can rapidly cause **fatal hemorrhage.** The artery may be compressed posteriorly against the superior pubic ramus or femoral head to slow bleeding. A severed artery may retract into the abdomen, making emergency access difficult.

The femoral artery is used for cardiac catheterization.

The femoral artery is used for **cardiac catheterization** to record pressure within the left ventricle or to inject contrast media to examine the coronary circulation for atherosclerosis in anticipation of coronary bypass surgery or angioplasty. Similarly, contrast media can be injected into any branch of the abdominal aorta.

Intermittent claudication: cramping pain in leg during exercise that is relieved by rest

The incidence of **occlusive arterial disease** in the lower extremity increases with age, especially in males, and often causes cramping leg pain with walking that disappears with rest **(intermittent claudication).** Quality of life is often severely compromised, and arterial bypass surgery or angioplasty may be performed to restore circulation. Bypasses usually involve the iliac, femoral, popliteal, and tibial arteries.

---

2. **Cruciate anastomosis**

a. Collateral circulation around hip joint

b. Formed by **medial femoral circumflex, lateral femoral circumflex, inferior gluteal, and first perforating arteries**

c. Can potentially extend to popliteal artery through anastomoses between **perforating arteries** and branches of **popliteal artery**

3. **Obturator artery**

- Arises from **internal iliac artery** and enters thigh through **obturator canal** with **obturator nerve** but generally does *not* accompany obturator nerve distally in thigh

Cruciate anastomosis bypasses obstruction of the external iliac or femoral artery.

In about 80% of individuals, the **artery to the head of the femur** originates from the obturator artery. It is the main blood supply to the head of the femur in children but is rarely large enough in an adult to prevent **avascular necrosis** after a **femoral neck fracture.**

The **obturator artery** may alternatively arise from the **inferior epigastric artery.** As it descends over the pelvic brim to reach the obturator foramen, this **aberrant obturator artery** is at risk in surgical repair of a **femoral hernia.**

D. **Features of Thigh**

1. **Fascia lata**

- Deep investing fascia of thigh that sends intermuscular septa to partition thigh into anterior, posterior, and medial compartments

a. **Iliotibial tract**

(1) **Thickened band** of fascia lata on lateral side of thigh between tubercle of **iliac crest** and **lateral tibial condyle** that reinforces capsule of knee joint

(2) Receives insertions from **tensor fasciae latae** and **gluteus maximus** and may contribute to **posture** and **locomotion**

The iliotibial band may cause acute inflammation by repetitive motion over the lateral femoral condyle.

b. Saphenous opening

- Gap in **fascia lata** just below inguinal ligament that transmits small blood and lymphatic vessels and **great saphenous vein** on its way to femoral vein

2. **Femoral sheath (Figure 5-20)**
   a. Overview
      (1) Funnel-shaped extension of **transversalis fascia** and **iliacus fascia** that enters thigh deep to inguinal ligament
      (2) Divided into three compartments from lateral to medial enclosing femoral artery, femoral vein, and femoral canal
   b. **Femoral canal**
      (1) **Medial compartment** of femoral sheath
      (2) Contains fat, loose connective tissue, and lymphatics
   c. **Femoral ring**
      (1) Proximal end of **femoral canal**
      (2) Bounded medially by lacunar ligament, laterally by femoral vein, anteriorly by inguinal ligament, and posteriorly by pectineus muscle over superior ramus of pubis

The femoral sheath encloses the femoral artery, vein, and canal, but not the femoral nerve.

Femoral hernia: bulge inferior and lateral to pubic tubercle

A **femoral hernia** passes through the **femoral ring** into the **femoral canal** to form a swelling in the upper thigh inferior and lateral to the pubic tubercle. The hernial sac may protrude through the **saphenous opening** into superficial fascia. A femoral hernia occurs more frequently in females and is dangerous because the hernial sac may become **strangulated.** An **aberrant obturator artery** is vulnerable during surgical repair.

An aberrant obturator artery is in danger during surgical repair of a femoral hernia.

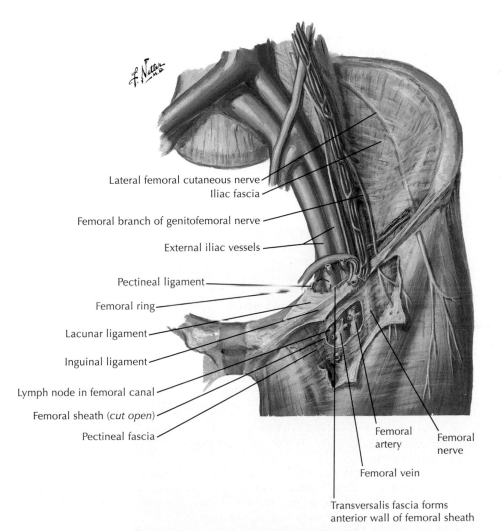

Lateral femoral cutaneous nerve
Iliac fascia
Femoral branch of genitofemoral nerve
External iliac vessels
Pectineal ligament
Femoral ring
Lacunar ligament
Inguinal ligament
Lymph node in femoral canal
Femoral sheath (*cut open*)
Pectineal fascia
Femoral artery
Femoral nerve
Femoral vein
Transversalis fascia forms anterior wall of femoral sheath

5-20: Anterior view of femoral region showing structures passing between abdominal cavity and thigh deep to the inguinal ligament. The femoral sheath is divided into three compartments, a medial femoral canal, an intermediate compartment for the femoral vein, and a lateral compartment for the femoral artery. The femoral nerve descends lateral to the femoral sheath. *(From Netter, F H: Atlas of Human Anatomy, 4th ed. Philadelphia, Saunders, 2006, Plate 262.)*

3. **Femoral triangle**
    a. Space in upper thigh bounded by **inguinal ligament, sartorius,** and medial border of **adductor longus muscle**
    b. Floor formed by **iliopsoas, pectineus, and adductor longus muscles**
    c. Contains, from lateral to medial, **femoral nerve, artery, vein,** and **canal** as they lie anterior to **hip joint**
    d. Covered only by skin and fascia, leaving its contents **vulnerable to injury**
4. **Adductor canal**
    a. Fascial tunnel from **apex** of femoral triangle to **adductor hiatus** bounded anterolaterally by **vastus medialis muscle** and posteriorly by **adductor longus and magnus muscles**
    b. Covered anteromedially by strong fascia deep to **sartorius muscle,** so consequently also called **subsartorial canal**
    c. Contains **saphenous nerve, nerve to vastus medialis,** and **femoral artery** lying anterior to **femoral vein**

V. **Popliteal Region and Leg**
    A. **Popliteal Fossa**
        1. Diamond-shaped area behind knee through which nerves and vessels pass between thigh and leg
        2. Bounded superiorly and medially by **semimembranosus and semitendinosus muscles,** superiorly and laterally by **biceps femoris muscle,** and inferiorly by medial and lateral heads of **gastrocnemius muscle**
        3. Floor formed by popliteal surface of **distal femur,** capsule of knee joint, and popliteus muscle
        4. From superficial to deep, contains **tibial nerve, popliteal vein,** and **popliteal artery; common fibular nerve** traverses fossa superolaterally

> In **fractures of the distal third of the femur,** the distal fragment may be rotated posteriorly by the **gastrocnemius muscle** and may compress or tear the **popliteal artery (see Figure 5-3, B).**
>
> The synovial lining of the knee joint can herniate through the joint capsule into the **popliteal fossa** to create a large **popliteal (Baker) cyst** that may be painful and limit joint mobility. **Rupture** of a popliteal cyst may cause sudden calf pain and swelling and be mistaken for deep venous thrombosis **(Figure 5-21).** These cysts commonly occur in rheumatoid arthritis.

Wounds to both the femoral artery and vein may cause an arteriovenous fistula.

The popliteal fossa is a diamond-shaped area behind the knee.

In a fracture of the lower femur, the distal fragment may be rotated posteriorly into the popliteal artery.

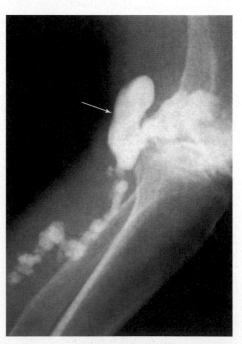

5-21: Arthrogram of rheumatoid arthritis patient showing contrast media leaking downward into calf from ruptured Baker cyst. *(From Forbes, C D, Jackson, W F: Color Atlas and Text of Clinical Medicine, 3rd ed. Mosby Ltd., 2003, Figure 3.28.)*

B. Muscles of Leg (Figure 5-22)

Rupture of the calcaneal tendon (third degree strain) greatly weakens plantar flexion, making it impossible to stand on the toes and difficult to walk. The tendon is prone to rupture after a history of **chronic tendinitis,** which often develops in runners. Paralysis of the gastrocnemius and soleus results in a **triceps surae gait,** in which the pelvis drops *on the affected side* during the stance (weight-bearing) phase of walking.

The tendon of the **plantaris** muscle, like that of the palmaris longus, is used for **tendon autografts** to the long finger flexors.

A ruptured calcaneal tendon makes standing on the toes impossible.

C. Nerves of Leg
1. **Tibial nerve (L4, L5, S1-3) (see Figure 5-19)**
   a. Branches from **sciatic nerve** to supply **muscles in posterior compartment** and **articular** branches to knee and ankle joints
   b. In **popliteal fossa,** descends superficial to **popliteal vessels**
   c. In posterior compartment, descends with **posterior tibial artery** deep to **gastrocnemius** and **soleus muscles**
   d. Ends **deep to flexor retinaculum** by dividing into **medial and lateral plantar nerves**
2. **Common fibular nerve (L4, L5, S1, S2) (Figure 5-23)**
   a. Overview
      (1) Arises from **sciatic nerve** and courses along medial margin of **biceps femoris muscle** in popliteal fossa
      (2) Passes superficially around **neck of fibula**
      (3) Divides into **superficial and deep fibular nerves**

Injury to the **common fibular nerve** is usually at the **neck of the fibula** after trauma, fracture, or pressure from a cast. Improper application of therapeutic cold (e.g., an ice pack) may also injure the nerve.

The common fibular nerve is the most frequently injured nerve in the lower extremity, usually at the neck of the fibula.

   b. **Deep fibular nerve (L4, L5, S1)**
      (1) Passes through lateral compartment of leg to descend in anterior compartment with **anterior tibial artery**
      (2) Supplies **muscles of anterior compartment**
   c. **Superficial fibular nerve (L5, S1, S2)**
      • Supplies **muscles of lateral compartment** and skin of dorsum of foot
D. Arteries of Popliteal Region and Leg (Figures 5-24 and 5-25)
   1. **Popliteal artery**

Anterior compartment leg muscles: deep fibular nerve. Lateral compartment muscles: superficial fibular nerve

5-22: Axial MRI of left leg. Tibia = 1; interosseous membrane — 2; fibula = 3; fibularis longus = 4; fibularis brevis = 5; extensor digitorum longus = 6; extensor hallucis longus = 7; tibialis anterior = 8; tibialis posterior = 9; flexor hallucis longus = 10; flexor digitorum longus 11; soleus = 12; lateral head of gastrocnemius = 13; medial head of gastrocnemius = 14; aponeurosis of gastrocnemius = 15; anterior tibial artery = 16; posterior tibial artery = 17; and small saphenous vein = 18. (*From Weir, J, Abrahams, P: Imaging Atlas of Human Anatomy, 3rd ed. London, Mosby Ltd., 2003, p 205, e.*)

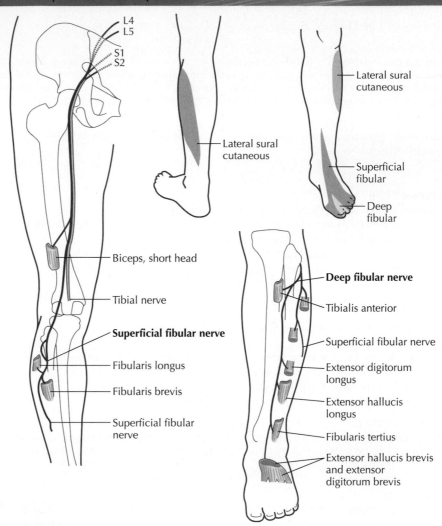

L4
L5
S1
S2

Lateral sural
cutaneous

Lateral sural
cutaneous

Superficial
fibular

Deep
fibular

Biceps, short head

Tibial nerve

Deep fibular nerve

Tibialis anterior

Superficial fibular nerve

Superficial fibular nerve

Fibularis longus

Extensor digitorum
longus

Fibularis brevis

Extensor hallucis
longus

Superficial fibular
nerve

Fibularis tertius

Extensor hallucis brevis
and extensor
digitorum brevis

5-23: Muscular and cutaneous distributions of deep fibular and superficial fibular nerves.

5-24: Arteries of the popliteal region, including genicular anastomosis, anterior view.

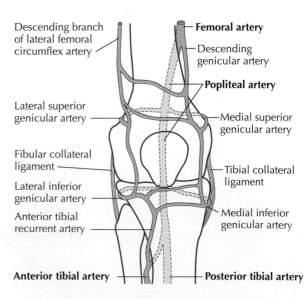

Descending branch
of lateral femoral
circumflex artery

Femoral artery

Descending
genicular artery

Popliteal artery

Lateral superior
genicular artery

Medial superior
genicular artery

Fibular collateral
ligament

Tibial collateral
ligament

Lateral inferior
genicular artery

Anterior tibial
recurrent artery

Medial inferior
genicular artery

Anterior tibial artery

Posterior tibial artery

Femoral artery →
popliteal artery →
anterior and posterior
tibial arteries

a. Continuation of **femoral artery** at adductor hiatus
b. Ends at inferior border of popliteus muscle by dividing into **anterior and posterior tibial arteries**
c. Most anterior structure in **popliteal fossa,** lying against popliteal surface of **femur,** capsule of **knee joint,** and **popliteus muscle**

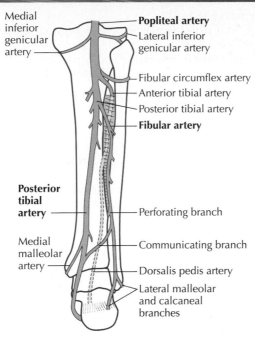

Medial inferior genicular artery

Popliteal artery

Lateral inferior genicular artery

Fibular circumflex artery

Anterior tibial artery

Posterior tibial artery

Fibular artery

Posterior tibial artery

Medial malleolar artery

Perforating branch

Communicating branch

Dorsalis pedis artery

Lateral malleolar and calcaneal branches

5-25: Arteries of the leg, posterior view.

A **dislocated knee** or **fractured distal femur** can injure the **popliteal artery** because of its deep position adjacent to the femur and capsule of the knee joint **(see Figure 5-3, B).** An **arterial embolus** at the bifurcation of the popliteal artery may block blood flow to the leg.

2. **Genicular anastomosis**
   • Allows blood to flow to leg and foot when popliteal artery is blocked (e.g., when knee is fully flexed)
3. **Posterior tibial artery**
   a. Descends with **tibial nerve** in **posterior compartment**
   b. Terminates deep to **flexor retinaculum** behind **medial malleolus** by dividing into **medial and lateral plantar arteries**
4. **Fibular artery**
   a. Largest branch of posterior tibial artery, which it sometimes replaces in lower leg
   b. Descends close to fibula to supply lateral side of **posterior compartment** and muscles of **lateral compartment**

> Posterior tibial artery pulse: palpable between medial malleolus and calcaneus

The **dorsalis pedis pulse** may not be palpable if the artery arises from the **perforating branch of the fibular artery,** which pierces the interosseous membrane to reach the anterior compartment.

> The dorsalis pedis artery occasionally arises from the perforating branch of the fibular artery.

5. **Anterior tibial artery**
   a. Descends in **anterior compartment** on interosseous membrane with **deep fibular nerve**
   b. Becomes **dorsalis pedis artery** as it crosses ankle joint

VI. **Foot**
   A. **Nerves of Foot (see Figures 5-19 and 5-23)**
      1. **Deep fibular nerve** (L4, L5, S1)
         a. Passes onto **dorsum of foot** to supply **extensor digitorum brevis** and **extensor hallucis brevis muscles**
         b. Supplies adjacent sides of **toes 1 and 2** and web of skin between
      2. **Medial plantar nerve** (L4, L5)
         • Terminal branch of **tibial nerve** analogous to median nerve in hand

3. **Lateral plantar nerve** (S1, S2)
   • Terminal branch of **tibial nerve** analogous to ulnar nerve in hand

B. **Arteries of Foot (Figure 5-26)**
   1. **Medial and lateral plantar arteries** accompany nerves of the same name.
   2. **Plantar arch** is formed by anastomosis of **lateral plantar artery** with **deep plantar** branch of dorsalis pedis
   3. **Dorsalis pedis artery** (dorsal artery of foot)

C. **Features of Leg and Foot**
   1. **Crural fascia (Figure 5-27)**
      a. **Deep investing fascia of leg** continuous proximally with fascia lata
      b. Closely binds muscles of **anterior and lateral compartments,** providing attachment for some muscles
      c. Sends **anterior and posterior intermuscular septa** to fibula, enclosing **lateral compartment,** and sends **transverse intermuscular septum** between superficial and deep posterior leg muscles

Dorsalis pedis pulse: palpable on the dorsum of the foot lateral to the tendon of extensor hallucis longus

---

Osseofibrous compartments of the extremities have unyielding walls; therefore **bleeding** or **edema** in a compartment may cause **compartment syndrome,** which most commonly affects the **anterior compartment.** The syndrome is characterized by **"five P's": pain, pallor, puffiness, paresthesia, and paralysis.** A distal pulse may not be palpable. Without a reduction of compartment pressure by **fasciotomy,** muscles of the compartment undergo necrosis and are replaced by dense fibrous scar tissue that shortens in **Volkmann ischemic contracture.**

Compartment syndrome is indicated by pain, pallor, puffiness, paresthesia, and paralysis.

---

2. **Flexor retinaculum**
   a. Localized thickening of deep fascia extending from medial malleolus to calcaneus as superficial boundary of **tarsal tunnel**
   b. Covers, from anterior to posterior, tendons of **tibialis posterior and flexor digitorum longus,** posterior tibial artery, tibial nerve, and tendon of **flexor hallucis longus**
3. **Superior and inferior extensor retinacula**
   • Localized thickenings of **anterior crural fascia** at ankle that bind tendons of anterior compartment
4. **Superior and inferior fibular retinacula**
   • Bind tendons of **fibularis longus** and **fibularis brevis muscles**

Tarsal tunnel structures: "Tom, Dick an' Harry" for Tibialis posterior, flexor Digitorum longus, posterior tibial Artery, tibial Nerve, and flexor Hallucis longus.

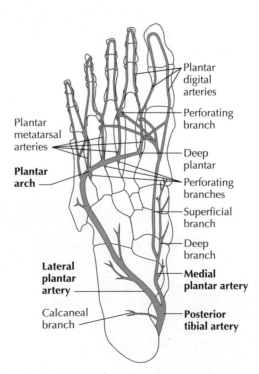

5-26: Arteries of the plantar foot.

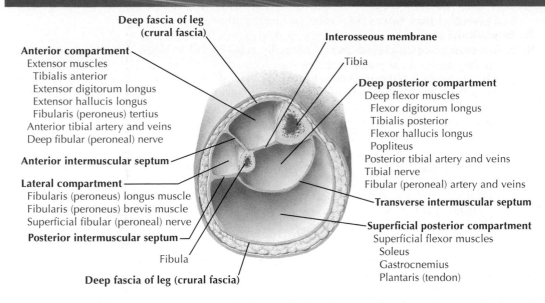

Deep fascia of leg (crural fascia)

Interosseous membrane

Anterior compartment
Extensor muscles
Tibialis anterior
Extensor digitorum longus
Extensor hallucis longus
Fibularis (peroneus) tertius
Anterior tibial artery and veins
Deep fibular (peroneal) nerve

Tibia

Deep posterior compartment
Deep flexor muscles
Flexor digitorum longus
Tibialis posterior
Flexor hallucis longus
Popliteus
Posterior tibial artery and veins
Tibial nerve
Fibular (peroneal) artery and veins

Anterior intermuscular septum

Transverse intermuscular septum

Lateral compartment
Fibularis (peroneus) longus muscle
Fibularis (peroneus) brevis muscle
Superficial fibular (peroneal) nerve

Superficial posterior compartment
Superficial flexor muscles
Soleus
Gastrocnemius
Plantaris (tendon)

Posterior intermuscular septum

Fibula

Deep fascia of leg (crural fascia)

Cross section just above middle of leg

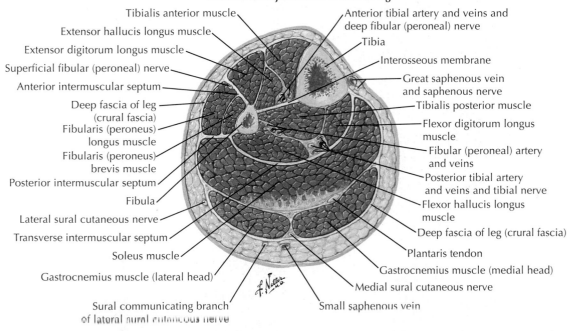

Tibialis anterior muscle

Anterior tibial artery and veins and deep fibular (peroneal) nerve

Extensor hallucis longus muscle

Tibia

Extensor digitorum longus muscle

Interosseous membrane

Superficial fibular (peroneal) nerve

Great saphenous vein and saphenous nerve

Anterior intermuscular septum

Deep fascia of leg (crural fascia)

Tibialis posterior muscle

Fibularis (peroneus) longus muscle

Flexor digitorum longus muscle

Fibularis (peroneus) brevis muscle

Fibular (peroneal) artery and veins

Posterior intermuscular septum

Posterior tibial artery and veins and tibial nerve

Fibula

Flexor hallucis longus muscle

Lateral sural cutaneous nerve

Deep fascia of leg (crural fascia)

Transverse intermuscular septum

Plantaris tendon

Soleus muscle

Gastrocnemius muscle (medial head)

Gastrocnemius muscle (lateral head)

Medial sural cutaneous nerve

Sural communicating branch of lateral sural cutaneous nerve

Small saphenous vein

5-27: Deep fascia and cross-section of the right leg viewed from below. Bones and deep fascia divide the leg into anterior, lateral, and posterior compartments. Each compartment has an associated nerve and artery, except the lateral compartment, which receives blood from the fibular artery of the posterior compartment. *(From Netter, F H: Atlas of Human Anatomy, 4th ed. Philadelphia, Saunders, 2006, Plate 522.)*

5. **Plantar aponeurosis**
   a. Central thickening of **deep fascia** on sole of foot attaching proximally to **calcaneal tuberosity** and distally ending in slips to five **digital tendon sheaths**
   b. Gives origin proximally to **flexor digitorum brevis** muscle fibers
   c. Functions as **ligament** to support longitudinal arches of foot

Plantar fasciitis produces pain and tenderness of the sole of the foot from overuse (e.g., running). Recurrent episodes may induce formation of a **calcaneal bone spur.**

VII. **Veins of Lower Extremity**
   A. **Overview**
      1. Divided into **superficial and deep veins** connected by **perforating veins**

Blood passes from the superficial to the deep veins of the extremities via perforating veins.

2. Contain **more valves** than veins of upper extremity
B. **Superficial Veins**
  • Located in superficial fascia and normally **send blood to deep veins** via perforating veins
1. **Great (long) saphenous vein (Figure 5-28)**
  • Arises from **medial side** of **dorsal venous arch** of foot, passes **anterior** to **medial malleolus,** and ascends on medial side of leg adjacent to **saphenous nerve**

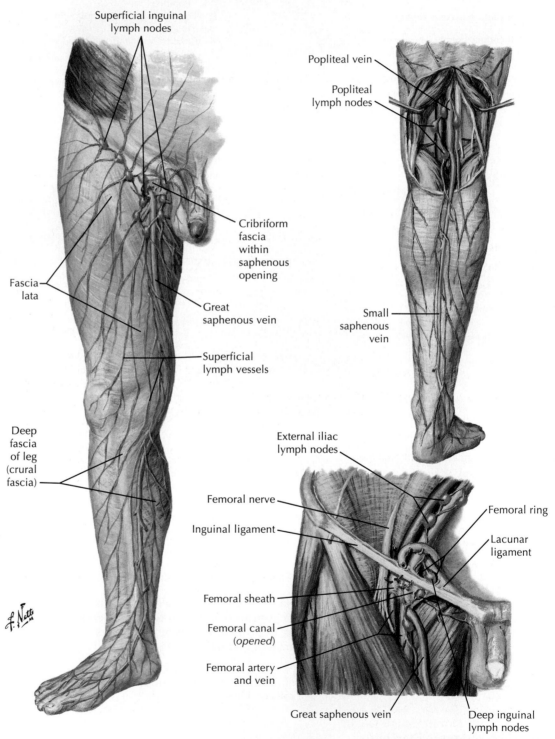

5-28: Superficial veins and lymphatics of the lower extremity. The great and small saphenous veins are the major superficial veins. Superficial lymphatic vessels accompany the saphenous veins and deep lymphatic vessels accompany the deep veins of the extremity. *(From Netter, F H: Atlas of Human Anatomy, 4th ed. Philadelphia, Saunders, 2006, Plate 546.)*

Even when collapsed (e.g., patient in shock), the **great saphenous vein** can be located anterior to the medial malleolus by a **saphenous cutdown.** The **saphenous nerve** may be damaged during a cutdown, producing pain or numbness along the medial border of the foot.

The great saphenous vein may be removed and used for **coronary artery bypass surgery.** The vein is **reversed** so its valves don't obstruct blood flow in the graft.

In **obstruction** of either the **inferior or superior vena cava,** communications between the superficial epigastric veins, which are great saphenous tributaries, and the lateral thoracic veins **(thoracoepigastric veins)** enlarge and provide a **caval-caval shunt** to return venous blood to the heart.

The terminal part of the great saphenous vein may be locally dilated in a **saphenous varix,** which can be confused with a femoral hernia or psoas abscess.

> Saphenous cutdown: the great saphenous vein can be accessed by incision anterior to the medial malleolus.

> 2. **Small** (short) **saphenous vein** (see Figure 5-28)
>   a. Arises from **lateral side** of **dorsal venous arch,** passes **posterior to lateral malleolus,** and ascends the posterior leg adjacent to **sural nerve**
>   b. Pierces popliteal fascia to end in **popliteal vein**

Varicose veins are abnormally dilated, tortuous superficial veins often developing in the lower extremity where elasticity is reduced and valves in the superficial or perforating veins are incompetent. Additional causes are **increased intraabdominal pressure from pregnancy** or an **abdominal tumor,** obesity, prolonged standing, and **thrombophlebitis** of the deep lower extremity veins.

> Varicose veins are dilated, tortuous superficial veins often developing in the lower extremity.

> C. **Deep Veins**
>   1. Accompanying veins **(venae comitantes)** for deep arteries
>   2. Normally receive blood from superficial veins via perforating veins
>   3. Compressed by contraction of surrounding muscles (musculovenous pump), pushing blood toward heart
>   4. Include **femoral vein,** which receives **great saphenous vein** at **saphenous opening** in fascia lata

The **femoral vein** is a deep vein and is sometimes mistakenly called the "superficial femoral vein." Unfortunately, this careless naming can contribute to overlooking a source of emboli because **deep veins of the lower extremity** are the most common source of **pulmonary thromboemboli,** which may be rapidly fatal **(Figure 5-29).** Risk factors for **pulmonary thromboembolism** include **prolonged immobilization,** malignancy, aging, obesity, and oral contraceptives. Approximately half of pulmonary emboli result from **undetected (silent) thrombi.**

The femoral vein provides rapid access to a large vein for **catheterization** and is easily located medial to the femoral artery just below the inguinal ligament.

> Most pulmonary emboli originate in the deep veins of the lower extremity.

VIII. **Innervation of Lower Extremity**
    A. **Motor Innervation (Table 5-2)**
    B. **Muscle Function and Related Segmental Innervation**
      • Generally, lumbar segmental nerves supply anterior limb, and sacral segmental nerves supply posterior limb
      1. **Hip**
        a. **Extension:** L4, L5
        b. **Flexion:** L2, L3
      2. **Knee**
        a. **Extension:** L3, L4
        b. **Flexion:** L5, S1
      3. **Ankle**
        a. **Plantar flexion:** S1, S2
        b. **Dorsiflexion:** L4, L5
      4. **Foot**
        a. **Inversion:** L4, L5
        b. **Eversion:** L5, S1

> Anterior thigh muscles: femoral nerve. Medial thigh: obturator nerve. Posterior thigh: tibial division of sciatic nerve

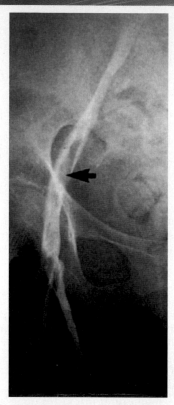

5-29: Venogram showing deep vein thrombosis *(arrow)* in the external iliac vein just above its junction with the femoral vein. Venography is still the "gold standard" when a diagnosis of deep venous thrombosis is uncertain. *(From Forbes, C D, Jackson, W F: Color Atlas and Text of Clinical Medicine, 3rd ed. Mosby Ltd., 2003, Figure 5.194.)*

TABLE 5-2. MOTOR INNERVATION OF LOWER EXTREMITY

NERVE	MUSCLES INNERVATED	COMMENTS
Femoral nerve	Iliacus muscle, anterior compartment muscles of thigh	Supplies muscles that flex hip and extend knee
Obturator nerve	Medial (adductor) compartment muscles of thigh (except hamstring part of adductor magnus)	Supplies muscles that adduct thigh; may help innervate pectineus
Tibial nerve	Posterior compartment muscles of thigh (except short head of biceps femoris) and hamstring part of adductor magnus; posterior compartment muscles of leg	Division of sciatic nerve Supplies muscles that extend thigh and flex knee and muscles that plantar flex foot and toes
Medial plantar nerve	Abductor hallucis, flexor hallucis brevis, flexor digitorum brevis, and first lumbrical muscle	Terminal branch of tibial nerve deep to flexor retinaculum
Lateral plantar nerve	Intrinsic plantar muscles of foot not innervated by medial plantar nerve	Terminal branch of tibial nerve deep to flexor retinaculum
Common fibular nerve	Short head of biceps femoris	Division of sciatic nerve
Deep fibular nerve	Anterior compartment muscles of leg; extensor digitorum brevis and extensor hallucis brevis	Terminal branch of common fibular nerve
Superficial fibular nerve	Lateral compartment muscles of leg	Terminal branch of common fibular nerve

  C. **Dermatomes of Lower Extremity (Figure 5-30)**

IX. **Nerve Injuries of Lower Extremity**
  A. **Overview**
    1. Much less common than nerve injuries to upper extremity
    2. Frequently caused by **neoplasms, pelvic surgery, psoas major hematoma,** or **diabetes**
    3. Rarely caused by direct trauma to **lumbosacral plexus**
  B. **Injury to Femoral Nerve (see Figure 5-17)**

Femoral nerve lesion: loss of knee extension

    1. At lumbar plexus: **weakness of hip flexion** (iliopsoas, rectus femoris, and sartorius muscles) in addition to loss of **knee extension** (quadriceps femoris muscle)

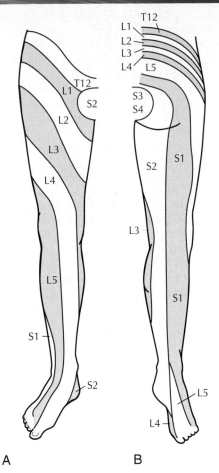

5-30: Dermatomes of the lower extremity. **A,** Anterior view. **B,** posterior view.

2. At inguinal ligament: **loss of knee extension** (quadriceps femoris muscle)
3. **Loss of sensation** over anterior thigh and medial leg and foot
4. May occur during **catheterization of femoral artery**

C. **Injury to Obturator Nerve (see Figure 5-18)**
1. Difficulty adducting thigh (e.g., crossing legs while sitting)
2. **Decreased sensation** over upper medial thigh
3. May occur from compression by uterus during pregnancy, obstetric procedures, or pelvic disease

D. **Injury to Superior Gluteal Nerve**
1. **Loss of thigh abduction** and **medial rotation** (gluteus medius, gluteus minimus, tensor fasciae latae muscles)
2. Causes positive **Trendelenburg sign (see Figure 5-8)**
3. **Gluteus medius gait:** trunk leans toward affected side during stance phase to compensate for loss of hip abduction

E. **Injury to Inferior Gluteal Nerve**
1. Weakened hip extension (gluteus maximus), most noticeable when **climbing stairs** or **standing from a seated position**
2. **Gluteus maximus gait:** trunk leans backward on affected side when walking to compensate for loss of hip extension

F. **Injury to Sciatic Nerve**
1. Overview
   a. Weakened hip extension and knee flexion
   b. Inability to dorsiflex, plantar flex, evert, or invert foot
   c. **Loss of cutaneous sensation** over leg and foot except medial area supplied by saphenous nerve
   d. **Footdrop** (lack of dorsiflexion) and **flail foot** (lack of both dorsiflexion and plantar flexion)

Positive Trendelenburg sign: unsupported side of pelvis drops when bearing weight on the affected extremity

Superior gluteal nerve lesion: positive Trendelenburg sign and gluteus medius gait

Inferior gluteal nerve lesion: difficultly climbing stairs or standing from a seated position

Tibial nerve injury: loss of plantar flexion

        e. Most often caused by **improperly placed gluteal injections** but may result from **posterior hip dislocation**

  2. **Injury to tibial nerve (see Figure 5-19)**

      a. In popliteal fossa: **loss of plantar flexion** of foot (mainly gastrocnemius and soleus muscles) and weakened **inversion** (tibialis posterior muscle), causing **calcaneovalgus.** Pelvis drops on **affected weight-bearing side** during walking **(triceps surae gait)** instead of on nonaffected side as in gluteus medius gait.

      b. At medial malleolus **(tarsal tunnel syndrome)** or in foot affects intrinsic foot muscles but spares plantar flexion and inversion of foot

  3. **Injury to common fibular nerve (see Figure 5-23)**

      a. Overview

         (1) Often results from direct trauma as nerve passes superficially around **neck of fibula**

         (2) **Footdrop** and **loss of eversion,** causing **equinovarus**

         (3) May result from **fractured fibula, blow to fibula,** or **compression**

         (4) May cause **sensory loss** over lateral leg and dorsum of foot

Deep fibular nerve injury: footdrop. Superficial fibular nerve injury: loss of eversion

      b. **Injury to deep fibular nerve**

         (1) **Footdrop** (tibialis anterior, extensor digitorum longus, and extensor hallucis longus muscles), **loss of toe extension** (extensor digitorum longus and brevis, extensor hallucis longus and brevis muscles), and weakened inversion (tibialis anterior muscle)

         (2) **Sensory loss** from **skin** between toes 1 and 2

      c. **Injury to superficial fibular nerve**

         (1) **Loss of eversion** (fibularis longus and brevis muscles)

         (2) **Sensory loss** over distal lateral portion of leg and dorsum of foot

X. Lymphatics of Lower Extremity

    • Lymph passes through superficial or deep inguinal lymph nodes en route to **external iliac nodes.**

  A. Superficial Inguinal Lymph Nodes (Figure 5-31)

    • Lie in superficial fascia just inferior to inguinal ligament and receive lymph vessels that parallel great saphenous vein and its tributaries

Enlarged superficial inguinal lymph nodes may be the first sign of uterine cancer.

> Because of the length of the lower extremity, **painful, enlarged superficial inguinal lymph nodes** can occur three feet or farther away from the point of infection. Enlarged nodes can also suggest involvement of the perineal, gluteal, pelvic, and lower abdominal wall regions. In female patients an occasional cause of inguinal lymphadenopathy is **uterine cancer** that has metastasized along the round ligament to the labium majus. Lymph drainage from the **testis** parallels its blood supply to reach the aortic nodes in the abdominal cavity and so does *not* metastasize to inguinal lymph nodes.

  B. Deep Inguinal Lymph Nodes

    • Lie deep to fascia lata along femoral vein and receive lymph from deep structures and **popliteal nodes**

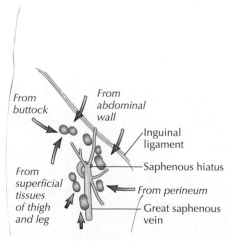

5-31: Lymph drainage (*arrows*) to superficial inguinal lymph nodes.

C. **Popliteal Lymph Nodes**
- Receive deep lymph vessels and superficial lymph vessels that parallel small saphenous vein

XI. **Limb Development**

A. **Development of Upper and Lower Extremities**
- Similar, except lower extremity development lags behind that of upper **(see Chapter 6, VIII).**

B. **Rotation of Lower Extremity**
- Is **90° medial rotation** instead of 90° lateral rotation as in upper extremity; therefore, flexion at knee is posterior movement of leg

Lymph from the perineum drains to the superficial inguinal nodes, but lymph from the testis does not.

I. Skeleton of Upper Extremity
   A. Pectoral Girdle and Proximal Humerus (Figure 6-1)
      - Bones of shoulder with **pectoral girdle** consisting of **clavicle** and **scapula**
      1. **Clavicle**
         a. Articulates medially with **sternum** at **sternoclavicular joint** and laterally with **acromion** at **acromioclavicular joint**
         b. **Coracoclavicular ligament** attaches laterally, and **costoclavicular ligament** attaches medially on its inferior surface.

> The clavicle is the most frequently fractured bone in the body.

Clavicle fractures occur most frequently at the junction of the middle and lateral thirds of the clavicle **(Figure 6-2).** The patient characteristically supports the sagging limb with the opposite hand. Subclavian vessels and trunks of the brachial plexus are at risk in fractures of the middle third because they lie behind only the thin **subclavius muscle.** As the fractured clavicle heals, **supraclavicular nerves** may be trapped by callous formation, causing **chronic neck pain.**

      2. **Scapula**
         a. Overview
            (1) Articulates laterally with **humerus** at **glenohumeral joint**
            (2) Overlies posterior thoracic wall at **ribs 2-7** with **spine** typically lying at level of spinous process of vertebra T3
         b. **Acromion**
            - Articulates with **clavicle** and overhangs head of humerus as **bony point of shoulder**
         c. **Coracoid process**
            (1) Palpable below clavicle under anterior margin of deltoid
            (2) Provides attachment for coracoclavicular, coracoacromial, and coracohumeral ligaments and costocoracoid membrane in addition to muscles
         d. **Glenoid cavity**
            - Shallow, deepened slightly by fibrocartilaginous **glenoid labrum,** for articulation with **head of humerus**
         e. **Suprascapular notch** on superior border converted by **superior transverse scapular ligament** into **suprascapular foramen** that transmits **suprascapular nerve**

> Suprascapular nerve entrapment at the suprascapular notch weakens the supraspinatus and infraspinatus muscles.

The **suprascapular nerve** may be **trapped and compressed** as it passes through the suprascapular foramen, which affects functions of the **supraspinatus and infraspinatus muscles.** The patient has difficulty initiating abduction and weak lateral rotation of the arm.

      3. **Proximal humerus**
         a. **Head**
            - Articulates with glenoid cavity at glenohumeral joint
         b. **Anatomical neck**
            - Provides attachment for fibrous joint capsule
         c. **Greater tubercle**
            - Provides insertion for supraspinatus, infraspinatus, and teres minor muscles

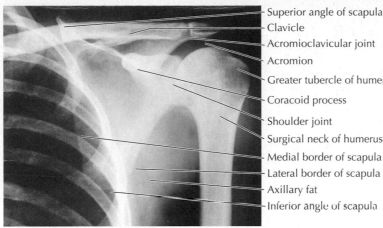

Superior angle of scapula
Clavicle
Acromioclavicular joint
Acromion
Greater tubercle of humerus
Coracoid process
Shoulder joint
Surgical neck of humerus
Medial border of scapula
Lateral border of scapula
Axillary fat
Inferior angle of scapula

6-1: Radiograph of the left shoulder, anteroposterior view.

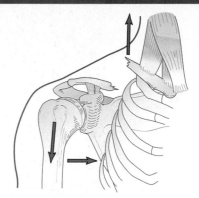

6-2: Clavicle fracture, anterior view. *Arrows*, direction of force. Lateral fragment is depressed by weight of the limb and pulled anteromedially by the pectoralis major muscle, with the medial fragment pulled upward by the sternocleidomastoid muscle.

    d. **Lesser tubercle**
      • Provides insertion for subscapularis muscle

Avulsion fractures of the **greater tubercle** are relatively common, often in association with anterior dislocation of the shoulder joint. The attachments of the **supraspinatus, infraspinatus, and teres minor muscles** hold the tubercle posteriorly, while the subscapularis and other muscles rotate the rest of the humerus medially.

Greater or lesser tubercle of humerus may be avulsed by attached rotator cuff muscles.

The **lesser tubercle,** which receives the insertion of the **subscapularis muscle,** may be avulsed in violent lateral rotation of the abducted arm (e.g., a football player attempting to tackle a ball carrier running by) or in a rare **posterior dislocation of the shoulder joint.**

    e. **Intertubercular sulcus (bicipital groove)**
      (1) Transmits **tendon of long head of biceps brachii muscle**
      (2) Bridged by **transverse humeral ligament**
    f. **Surgical neck**
      • Proximal end of **shaft** named for its frequency of fracture

Surgical neck fracture injures the axillary nerve and the posterior humeral circumflex artery.

Surgical neck fractures, which are common, may damage the **axillary nerve** and the **posterior humeral circumflex artery** as they pass through the **quadrangular space (Figure 6-3).**

  B. **Shaft**
    1. **Radial groove** (spiral groove)
      • Separates origins of **lateral and medial heads** of triceps brachii muscle and contains **radial nerve** and **profunda brachii artery**
    2. **Deltoid tuberosity**
      • Marks insertion of **deltoid muscle** about halfway down lateral border

Humeral shaft fracture injures the radial nerve and the profunda brachii artery.

Fractures of the humeral shaft may damage the **radial nerve** and **profunda brachii artery** in the **radial groove.** Fractures proximal to the deltoid insertion will cause **adduction of the proximal fragment** by the pectoralis major with the distal fragment pulled proximally by the deltoid. In contrast, **fracture distal to the deltoid insertion** will cause **abduction of the proximal fragment** by the deltoid, with the distal fragment pulled proximally by the biceps and triceps.

  C. **Elbow (Figure 6-4)**
    1. **Distal humerus**
    a. **Medial epicondyle**
      (1) Gives **origin** to **superficial flexor muscles** of forearm
      (2) **Grooved posteriorly** by **ulnar nerve**

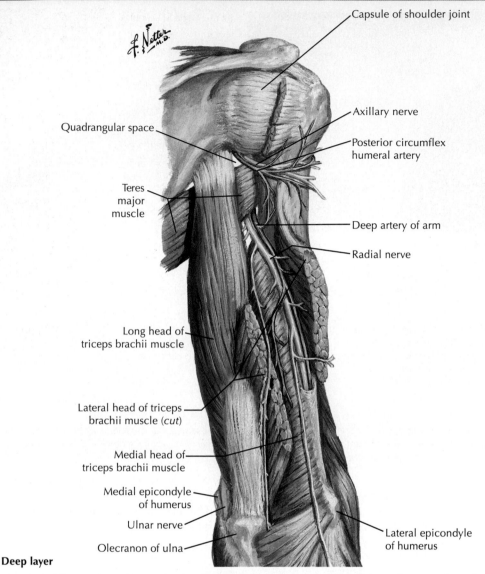

Capsule of shoulder joint

Axillary nerve

Posterior circumflex humeral artery

Quadrangular space

Teres major muscle

Deep artery of arm

Radial nerve

Long head of triceps brachii muscle

Lateral head of triceps brachii muscle (*cut*)

Medial head of triceps brachii muscle

Medial epicondyle of humerus

Ulnar nerve

Olecranon of ulna

Lateral epicondyle of humerus

Deep layer

6-3: Posterior view of dissected arm. Nerves closely related to the humerus may be injured during fractures: the axillary nerve at the surgical neck, the radial nerve in the radial groove at midshaft, and the ulnar nerve behind the medial epicondyle. Not seen in a posterior view is the median nerve, which may be injured in a supracondylar fracture of the humerus. *(From Greene, W B: Netter's Orthopaedics. Philadelphia, Saunders, 2006, Figure 14-5.)*

    b. **Lateral epicondyle**
- Gives **origin** to **superficial extensor muscles** of forearm

Supracondylar humeral fracture may cause forearm compartment syndrome.	**Supracondylar fractures** may injure the **brachial artery** and **median nerve** and are common in children and in arm wrestlers. Damage to the brachial artery may compromise the blood supply of the forearm, resulting in **compartment syndrome** with **Volkmann ischemic contracture,** usually involving the flexor compartment. Anterior displacement of the jagged proximal fragment damages the attached **brachialis,** possibly causing heterotopic ossification **(posttraumatic myositis ossificans).**
Medial epicondyle may be avulsed before skeletal maturity by the forceful abduction of the extended elbow.	Forceful abduction of the extended elbow may produce **avulsion of the medial epicondyle** in children because the **ulnar collateral ligament** is stronger than the epiphysis for the medial epicondyle. The common flexor tendon of the superficial forearm muscles will pull the avulsed fragment distally. The **ulnar nerve may be damaged.**

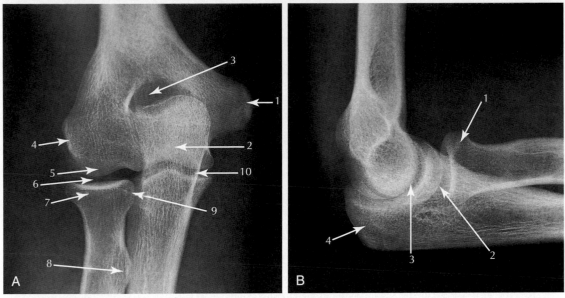

6-4: Anteroposterior **(A)** and lateral **(B)** radiographs of adult elbow joint. Elbow joint is flexed in **B**. *(From Standring, S: Gray's Anatomy: The Anatomical Basis of Clinical Practice, 39th ed. London, Churchill Livingstone, 2005, Figure 51.3.)* A: 1. Medial humeral epicondyle. 2. Shadow of olecranon superimposed on trochlea. 3. Olecranon fossa. 4. Lateral epicondyle. 5. Capitulum. 6. Humero-radial joint. 7. Head of radius. 8. Radial tuberosity. 9. Radial head articulating with radial notch of ulna. 10. Humero-ulnar joint. B: 1. Head of radius. 2. Profile of capitulum. 3. Profile of trochlea. 4. Olecranon.

The **ulnar nerve** behind the **medial epicondyle** can be bumped or compressed, causing "funny bone" paresthesia or numbness.

---

2. **Proximal radius**
   a. **Head**
      (1) **Articulates proximally** with **capitulum** and **medially** with **radial notch of ulna at proximal radioulnar joint**
      (2) Encircled by strong **anular ligament** except at radial notch of ulna
   b. **Neck**
      • Related to **deep radial nerve** as it pierces supinator muscle
   c. **Tuberosity**
      • Insertion of **biceps brachii tendon,** just lateral to brachial artery

---

The **brachial artery** lies just medial to the **biceps brachii tendon** in the cubital fossa, where the stethoscope is placed when **taking blood pressure.** The **deep branch of the radial nerve** may be injured in a **fracture of the neck of the radius.** See **Figure 6-5** for **fractures of the radial shaft.**

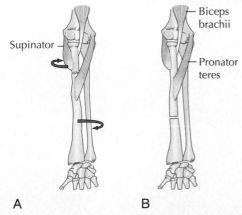

Supinator

Biceps brachii

Pronator teres

A   B

6-5: Effect of the pronator teres and biceps brachii on proximal and distal fragments of the fractured radius. **A,** If fracture is proximal to the insertion of the pronator teres, the distal fragment will be pronated. Fragments must be aligned before setting the fracture. **B,** If fracture is distal to the insertion of the pronator teres, fragments approximate the normal "at rest" position. *Arrows,* direction of force.

3. **Proximal ulna**
   a. **Olecranon**
      - Separated from skin by **olecranon bursa**

The olecranon may be avulsed by forcible triceps brachii contraction or a direct blow.

The **olecranon** may be avulsed by forcible contraction of the **triceps brachii** during a fall or by a direct blow. The pull of the triceps may displace the olecranon fragment proximally. "Student's elbow" is **olecranon bursitis** caused by repeated friction against the **olecranon bursa**.

   b. **Coronoid process** is distal attachment of brachialis muscle
   c. **Radial notch** is lateral facet for **head of radius** at **proximal radioulnar joint**
D. **Wrist and Hand (Figure 6-6)**
   1. **Distal radius**
      - Concave for articulation with carpal bones at **radiocarpal joint**
      a. **Ulnar notch**
         - Medial facet for **head of ulna** at **distal radioulnar joint**
      b. **Styloid process**
         - Lateral prolongation of radius **palpable in anatomical snuffbox**

Transverse fractures of the **distal radius** are often characterized by shortening of the radius, with the **radial styloid process repositioned proximal to the ulnar styloid process**. As a result of the fracture, the roughened **dorsal tubercle of the radius** may **rupture the extensor pollicis longus tendon**.

Colles fracture: "dinner fork deformity"

Colles fracture, in which the distal radial fragment is displaced posteriorly ("dinner fork deformity"), is common after age 50 and most often occurs when an individual breaks a fall with an outstretched hand. It is the second most common fracture in women with osteoporosis.

The distal fragment of the radius is *anteriorly* displaced in **Smith fracture**.

   2. **Distal ulna**
      - Separated from carpal bones by **articular disc** (triangular ligament) of radiocarpal joint
   3. **Carpal bones**
      a. **Proximal row**
         (1) Lateral to medial: **scaphoid, lunate, triquetrum,** and **pisiform**
         (2) Articulates at **radiocarpal joint** except for pisiform

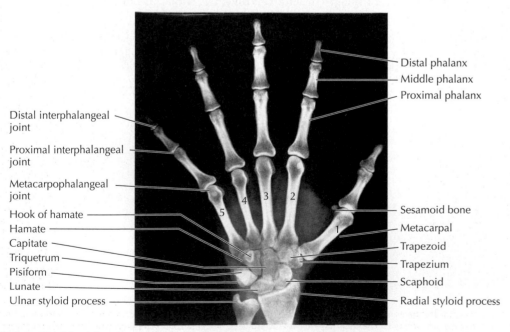

6-6: Radiograph of the right wrist and hand, anteroposterior view.

b. **Distal row**
  (1) Lateral to medial: **trapezium, trapezoid, capitate,** and **hamate**
  (2) Articulates with **proximal row of carpal bones** at **midcarpal joint** and with **metacarpal bones** at **metacarpophalangeal joints**
c. **Scaphoid** (navicular)
  • Lies in floor of **anatomical snuffbox**
d. **Lunate**

Scaphoid fractures may not show on radiographs for 10 days to 2 weeks, but deep tenderness will be present in the **anatomical snuffbox.** The proximal fragment may undergo **avascular necrosis** because the blood supply is interrupted **(Figure 6-7),** or **nonunion** of the fracture may occur.

The scaphoid is the most frequently fractured carpal bone, with a risk of avascular necrosis.

Forced hyperextension of the wrist may cause **anterior dislocation of the lunate, compressing the median nerve.**

Deep tenderness in anatomical snuffbox: scaphoid fracture

e. **Pisiform**
  • Palpable **sesamoid bone** in tendon of flexor carpi ulnaris muscle
f. **Trapezium**
  • Forms a saddle joint with **first metacarpal bone**
g. **Hamate**
  • On its palmar surface has prominent **hook of hamate**

The **hook of the hamate bone** frequently is **fractured** in racket sports and golf. Dense connective tissue converts the depression between the **hook of hamate** and the **pisiform** into **Guyon canal (ulnar tunnel),** where the **ulnar nerve may be compressed** (e.g., by a ganglion cyst).

The ulnar nerve may be compressed in Guyon canal between the pisiform and hamate bones.

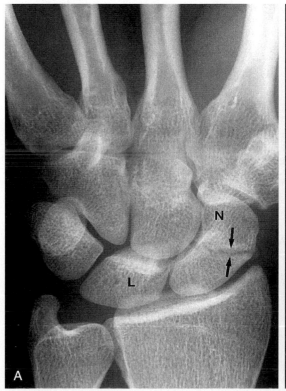
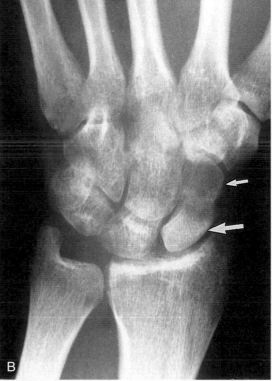

6-7: Scaphoid fracture. **A,** PA radiograph of wrist showing radiolucent fracture line through midportion of scaphoid (N). Fracture line may not become apparent for 10-14 days. **B,** Avascular necrosis of proximal fragment due to interrupted blood supply (*large arrow*) is shown by relative radiodensity while distal portion (*small arrow*) demonstrates mineral loss from disuse osteoporosis after fracture. (*From Mettler, F A: Essentials of Radiology, 2nd ed. Philadelphia, Saunders, 2004, Figure 8-70.*)

4. **Metacarpal bones**
   • Articulate proximally with **carpal bones** and distally with **proximal phalanges**

The **necks of metacarpal bones** are **frequently fractured** during fistfights. Typically, fractured fifth metacarpals are seen in unskilled fighters **(boxer's fracture).** Professional boxers punch mainly with the second and third metacarpals and rarely suffer these fractures.

5. **Phalanges**
   • Two in thumb; three each in fingers 2-5

II. Joints of Upper Extremity
A. Sternoclavicular Joint
   1. Formed between **clavicle** laterally and **manubrium and first costal cartilage** medially as only true joint between **upper extremity** and **axial skeletons**
   2. Contains two joint cavities separated by **articular disc**
   3. Fibrous **capsule** reinforced by **anterior and posterior sternoclavicular ligaments** and superiorly by **interclavicular ligament**
   4. Stabilized mainly by strong **costoclavicular ligament,** which anchors medial end of clavicle to rib 1 and its costal cartilage

Sternoclavicular joint only bony union between axial and upper extremity skeletons

A posterior dislocation of the sternoclavicular joint may compress the trachea or great vessels.

The **sternoclavicular joint** is so stable that the clavicle usually will fracture before the joint dislocates. If the joint dislocates, it is usually anteriorly. In a rare **posterior dislocation,** however, the medial end of the clavicle may **compress the trachea** or **major blood vessels.**

B. Functional Scapulothoracic Joint
   1. Movements of scapula on thoracic wall function like a joint
   2. **Elevation:** trapezius (upper fibers) and levator scapulae muscles
   3. **Depression:** gravity, trapezius (lower fibers), and serratus anterior (lower fibers) muscles

The **latissimus dorsi muscle,** and to a lesser extent the **pectoralis major muscle,** acts through attachments on the humerus to **depress the shoulder girdle. Without functioning** of these muscles, an individual **cannot walk with axillary crutches** or **negotiate wheelchair transfers.**

   4. **Superior rotation:** serratus anterior and trapezius muscles (upper and lower fibers together)
   5. **Inferior rotation:** levator scapulae, rhomboid major and minor muscles
   6. **Protraction:** serratus anterior and pectoralis minor muscles
   7. **Retraction:** trapezius (middle fibers), rhomboid major and minor muscles
C. Acromioclavicular Joint (Figure 6-8)
   1. Formed between **acromion** and **lateral end of clavicle**
   2. Stabilized by **coracoclavicular ligament** between coracoid process of scapula and clavicle

Shoulder separation: acromioclavicular joint dislocates with tearing of the coracoclavicular ligament

Falling on an outstretched hand or a point of the shoulder often **dislocates the acromioclavicular joint (shoulder separation).** The **coracoclavicular ligament** tears when the lateral end of the clavicle rides up over the acromion. The weight of the shoulder causes it to drop away, or separate, from the clavicle **(see Figure 6-8).**

D. Glenohumeral (Shoulder) Joint (see Figure 6-1)
   1. Overview

The shoulder joint accounts for 120° of shoulder abduction, and scapular rotation for 60°.

   a. Synovial **ball-and-socket joint** between **head of humerus** and **glenoid cavity** of scapula
   b. Has fibrocartilaginous **glenoid labrum** that slightly deepens glenoid cavity
   c. Responsible for two-thirds (120°) of possible shoulder flexion and abduction; upward rotation of scapula by serratus anterior and trapezius responsible for other 60°
   d. Surrounded and stabilized by **rotator cuff muscles**

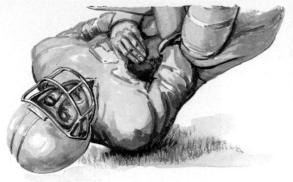

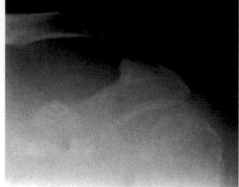

Injury to acromioclavicular joint. Usually caused by fall on tip of shoulder, depressing acromion (shoulder separation).

Stress radiograph. Taken with patient holding 10-lb weight, accentuating separation of acromioclavicular joint.

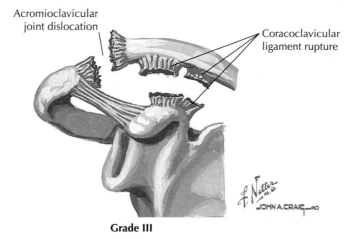

Acromioclavicular joint dislocation

Coracoclavicular ligament rupture

Grade III

6-8: Shoulder separation (acromioclavicular dislocation) with rupture of coracoclavicular ligament. *(From Greene, W B: Netter's Orthopaedics. Philadelphia, Saunders, 2006, Figure 14-19.)*

2. **Fibrous capsule**
   a. Attaches to **glenoid labrum** and **anatomical neck** of humerus
   b. Reinforced by **glenohumeral ligaments** anteriorly, **coracohumeral ligament** superiorly, and by **rotator cuff muscles** except inferiorly
   c. Separated from acromion and deltoid by **subacromial bursa**
   d. Bridges intertubercular groove as the **transverse humeral ligament**
3. **Movements of glenohumeral joint (Table 6-1)**

The **glenohumeral** joint is the **most frequently dislocated large joint (shoulder dislocation).** In the usual **anterior-inferior dislocation,** muscle traction pulls the dislocated humeral head into a subcoracoid position **(Figure 6-9).** The **axillary nerve** may be injured. **Posterior dislocations** comprise only 5% but are seen following **convulsions** or **electric shock.** A posterior dislocation may not be apparent on standard AP radiographs.

The supraspinatus initiates arm abduction, and the deltoid continues it after the first 15°.

The shoulder joint is the most frequently dislocated large joint.

TABLE 6-1. MUSCLES PRODUCING MOVEMENTS OF GLENOHUMERAL JOINT

MOVEMENT	MUSCLES INVOLVED
Flexion	Deltoid (anterior fibers), coracobrachialis, biceps, and pectoralis major
Extension	Latissimus dorsi, deltoid (posterior fibers), teres major, and long head of triceps
Abduction	Supraspinatus (initiation) and deltoid
Adduction	Pectoralis major, latissimus dorsi, and teres major
Medial rotation	Subscapularis, pectoralis major, deltoid (anterior fibers), latissimus dorsi, and teres major
Lateral rotation	Infraspinatus, teres minor, and deltoid (posterior fibers)

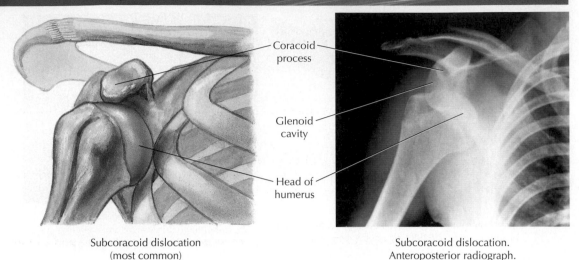

Subcoracoid dislocation
(most common)

Subcoracoid dislocation.
Anteroposterior radiograph.

6-9: Dislocation of glenohumeral joint in usual anteroinferior direction (subcoracoid dislocaton). *(From Greene, W B: Netter's Orthopaedics. Philadelphia, Saunders, 2006, Figure 14-17.)*

Abduction of the arm is initiated (first 15°) by the **supraspinatus muscle** (suprascapular nerve). Further abduction to the horizontal position is a function of the **deltoid muscle** (axillary nerve). Raising the extremity above the horizontal position requires upward scapular rotation by action of the **trapezius** (accessory nerve) and **serratus anterior** (long thoracic nerve). **Injury** to these muscles or nerves **compromises abduction.**

Subcromial bursitis is often due to deposition of calcium within the supraspinatus tendon **(calcific supraspinatus tendinitis)** in middle-aged males. The patient typically experiences a **painful arc of movement** from 50 to 130° of abduction.

Osteoarthritic changes in the glenohumeral joint or **chronic tendinitis** may cause a **rupture of the long head of the biceps tendon.** Alternatively, the tendon may be **avulsed** from the supraglenoid tubercle of the scapula. The detached muscle belly contracts into a ball in the anterior arm on attempted elbow flexion (Popeye deformity).

Ruptured long head of biceps tendon: Popeye deformity

Disorders such as bicipital tendinitis and cervical disc herniation that produce shoulder pain or **prolonged immobilization** in a cast or sling may cause **adhesive capsulitis** ("frozen shoulder"), significantly restricting movement.

Pain may be referred to the shoulder in various disorders, such as cervical disc herniation, angina pectoris, pleuritis, cholecystitis, or ruptured spleen.

The **trapezius** is the only muscle that can elevate the shoulder. Its paralysis from a **lesion of the spinal accessory nerve** or a **stroke** causes a drooping shoulder and an **inability to shrug. Inferior subluxation** of the head of the humerus is common following paralysis of the trapezius due to the drooping shoulder.

The shoulder joint usually dislocates in an anteroinferior direction.

E. **Elbow Joint (see Figure 6-4)**
   1. **Hinge joint** consisting of **humeroradial and humeroulnar joints**
   2. Fibrous **capsule** that is strengthened medially and laterally by strong **ulnar and radial collateral ligaments**
   3. **Flexion:** brachialis, biceps brachii, and brachioradialis muscles
   4. **Extension:** triceps brachii and anconeus muscles

Brachioradialis provides weak elbow flexion if the brachialis and biceps are paralyzed.

The **brachialis muscle** is the main flexor of the elbow; the **biceps brachii muscle** flexes and assists in supination. Both are innervated by the **musculocutaneous nerve.** When these primary elbow flexors are paralyzed, the **brachioradialis muscle** (radial nerve) provides some ability to flex the elbow.

In a **supracondylar fracture** of the humerus, the medial and lateral epicondyles and olecranon process maintain their triangular relationship. In **elbow dislocation,** the olecranon aligns with the epicondyles. **Posterior dislocations** of the elbow are frequent in children.

F. Radioulnar Joints
- Necessary for **pronation** and **supination** of forearm, compensating for lack of rotation at wrist

A **lesion of the median nerve** at or above the elbow **paralyzes the pronator quadratus and pronator teres muscles,** with loss of ability to pronate the forearm. When the **supinator muscle** is paralyzed from a **radial nerve lesion,** the **biceps brachii muscle** can still supinate the forearm.

Median nerve lesion at elbow: loss of forearm pronation

1. **Proximal radioulnar joint (see Figure 6-4)**
   a. Allows **head of radius to rotate** in ring formed by **radial notch of ulna** and **anular ligament,** its main stabilizer
   b. Shares **articular cavity** with elbow joint

In adults, the **head of the radius** is not dislocated without **tearing the anular ligament.** Young children are prone to dislocation of the immature head of the radius from the encircling anular ligament, a **"pulled elbow"** or **"nursemaid's elbow,"** caused by sudden traction on an extended forearm.

Infections of the elbow joint always involve the **proximal radioulnar joint** because of their shared joint cavity.

Lifting a preschool child by the forearm or hand may dislocate the head of the radius from the anular ligament.

2. **Distal radioulnar joint (see Figure 6-6)**
   a. **Pivot joint** between **head of ulna** and **ulnar notch of radius**
   b. Fibrocartilaginous **articular disc** (triangular ligament) separating it from radiocarpal joint
3. **Movements of proximal and distal radioulnar joints**
   a. **Pronation:** pronator quadratus and pronator teres muscles
   b. **Supination:** supinator and biceps brachii muscles
4. **Interosseous membrane**
   a. Connects radius and ulna and provides for muscle attachments
   b. Allows much of the force applied at the wrist to be transferred from the radius to the ulna, which has more stable articulation with humerus

Force transmission: hand → radius → interosseous membrane → ulna → humerus

G. Joints of Wrist and Hand (see Figure 6-6)
1. **Radiocarpal (wrist) joint**
   a. Formed between **radius and articular disc** proximally and **scaphoid, lunate, and triquetrum** distally
   b. Capsule strengthened mainly by **radial and ulnar collateral ligaments**
   c. Movements (Table 6-2)
2. **Carpometacarpal (CM) joints of fingers**
   - Allow limited movement at fourth and fifth fingers to facilitate gripping
3. **Carpometacarpal (CM) joint of thumb**
   - **Saddle joint between first metacarpal and trapezium allowing thumb opposition, adduction, abduction, flexion, and extension**
   a. **Flexion:** flexor pollicis brevis and flexor pollicis longus muscles
   b. **Extension:** abductor pollicis longus, extensor pollicis brevis, and extensor pollicis longus muscles
   c. **Abduction:** abductor pollicis longus and abductor pollicis brevis muscles
   d. **Adduction:** adductor pollicis muscle
   e. **Opposition:** opponens pollicis muscle

Wrist extension is necessary for effective finger flexion.

TABLE 6-2. MUSCLES PRODUCING MOVEMENTS OF RADIOCARPAL (WRIST) JOINT

MOVEMENT	MUSCLES INVOLVED
Flexion	Flexor carpi ulnaris, flexor carpi radialis, palmaris longus, long finger flexors
Extension	Extensor carpi ulnaris, extensor carpi radialis longus and brevis
Abduction	Flexor carpi radialis, extensor carpi radialis longus and brevis
Adduction	Flexor carpi ulnaris and extensor carpi ulnaris

4. **Metacarpophalangeal (MP) joints of fingers**
   a. Allow **flexion, extension, abduction, adduction,** and **circumduction**
   b. **Flexion:** lumbricals, interossei, flexor digitorum superficialis and profundus muscles; (Note: wrist extensors are synergist muscles necessary for effective finger flexion)
   c. **Extension:** extensor digitorum, extensor indicis (finger 2), and extensor digiti minimi (finger 5) muscles
   d. **Abduction:** dorsal interosseous muscles
   e. **Adduction:** palmar interosseous muscles

5. **Metacarpophalangeal (MP) joint of thumb**
   a. **Acts with first (CM) joint** in many movements
   b. **Flexion:** flexor pollicis brevis and flexor pollicis longus muscles
   c. **Extension:** extensor pollicis brevis and extensor pollicis longus muscles

6. **Interphalangeal (IP) joints of fingers**
   a. **Proximal (PIP)** and **distal (DIP) interphalangeal joints** except in thumb
   b. Synovial **hinge joints** allowing only **flexion** and **extension** because of strong **collateral ligaments** that prevent abduction and adduction
   c. **Flexion:** flexor digitorum superficialis (PIP) and flexor digitorum profundus (DIP) muscles
   d. **Extension:** extensor digitorum, lumbricals, interossei, extensor indicis (finger 2), and extensor digiti minimi (finger 5) muscles

III. **Pectoral Region, Shoulder, and Axilla**
   A. **Pectoral and Axillary Fasciae**
      1. **Pectoral fascia**
         • Invests pectoralis major and is continuous posteriorly with axillary fascia
      2. **Axillary fascia**
         • Forms base (floor) of axilla
   B. **Rotator (Musculotendinous) Cuff**
      1. **Stabilizes shoulder joint,** holding head of humerus in glenoid fossa
      2. **Reinforces joint** on all sides except inferiorly, where dislocation usually occurs initially (before muscular traction pulls humeral head into subcoracoid position)

> The **subacromial bursa** separates the tendon of the supraspinatus from the acromion and coracoacromial ligament. **Subacromial bursitis** and **supraspinatus tendinitis** are common conditions and cause painful abduction of the arm. **Supraspinatus tendon rupture** is common after middle age, resulting in **inability to initiate abduction** of the arm. However, if the arm can be passively abducted to 90°, that position can often be maintained by the **deltoid** muscle.
>
> **Rotator cuff muscles** may be **injured traumatically** or tear by **attrition** without significant injury or awareness other than shoulder pain that may be severe at night.

   C. **Axilla**
      1. **Boundaries of axilla**
         a. **Base** consists of axillary fascia and skin of armpit
         b. **Apex** is bounded by clavicle, rib 1, and superior border of scapula
         c. **Medial wall** is the upper rib cage covered by serratus anterior muscle.
         d. **Lateral wall** is formed by the intertubercular groove of humerus.
         e. **Anterior wall** consists of pectoralis major and minor muscles.
         f. **Posterior wall** is formed by the subscapularis, teres major, and latissimus dorsi muscles.
      2. **Contents of axilla**
         a. **Axillary artery** and **axillary vein**
         b. Parts of **brachial plexus** and its branches
         c. **Axillary sheath,** an extension of prevertebral layer of deep cervical fascia enclosing **axillary vessels** and **brachial plexus**
         d. **Axillary lymph nodes,** which are often the first involved in breast cancer
   D. **Axillary Artery (Figure 6-10)**
      1. Overview
         a. Continuous with **subclavian artery** at lateral border of rib 1 and becomes **brachial artery** at inferior border of teres major
         b. Crossed anteriorly by **pectoralis minor muscle,** which divides artery into three parts; second part is related medially, laterally, and posteriorly to **cords of brachial plexus**

MP joints allow abduction-adduction only in extension due to collateral ligaments.

Dorsal interossei **abduct** = **DAB.** Palmar interossei **adduct** = **PAD**

Rotator cuff muscles are **S**upraspinatus, **I**nfraspinatus, **T**eres minor, **S**ubscapularis: **SITS.**

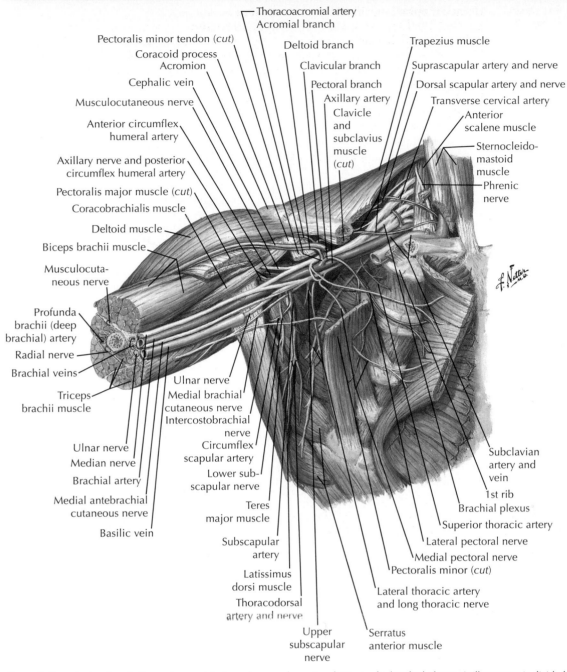

Thoracoacromial artery
Acromial branch
Pectoralis minor tendon (cut)
Coracoid process
Acromion
Cephalic vein
Musculocutaneous nerve
Anterior circumflex humeral artery
Axillary nerve and posterior circumflex humeral artery
Pectoralis major muscle (cut)
Coracobrachialis muscle
Deltoid muscle
Biceps brachii muscle
Musculocutaneous nerve
Profunda brachii (deep brachial) artery
Radial nerve
Brachial veins
Triceps brachii muscle
Ulnar nerve
Median nerve
Brachial artery
Medial antebrachial cutaneous nerve
Basilic vein
Ulnar nerve
Medial brachial cutaneous nerve
Intercostobrachial nerve
Circumflex scapular artery
Lower subscapular nerve
Teres major muscle
Subscapular artery
Latissimus dorsi muscle
Thoracodorsal artery and nerve
Upper subscapular nerve
Serratus anterior muscle
Deltoid branch
Clavicular branch
Pectoral branch
Axillary artery
Clavicle and subclavius muscle (cut)
Trapezius muscle
Suprascapular artery and nerve
Dorsal scapular artery and nerve
Transverse cervical artery
Anterior scalene muscle
Sternocleidomastoid muscle
Phrenic nerve
Subclavian artery and vein
1st rib
Brachial plexus
Superior thoracic artery
Lateral pectoral nerve
Medial pectoral nerve
Pectoralis minor (cut)
Lateral thoracic artery and long thoracic nerve

6-10: Axilla, anterior view. Axillary artery and its branches are shown in relation to the brachial plexus. Axillary artery is divided into three parts: medial, deep, and lateral to the pectoralis minor muscle. (From Netter, F H: Atlas of Human Anatomy, 4th ed. Philadelphia, Saunders, 2006, Plate 429.)

2. **First part** has one branch:
   - **Superior thoracic artery,** which supplies area over upper two intercostal spaces and pectoral muscles
3. **Second part** has two branches:
   a. **Thoracoacromial artery**
      - Multiple branches piercing clavipectoral fascia to supply pectoral and shoulder regions
   b. **Lateral thoracic artery**
      - Descends along lateral chest wall to supply serratus anterior and breast
4. **Third part** has three branches:
   a. **Subscapular artery**
      - Divides into **scapular circumflex artery,** which passes through **triangular space,** and **thoracodorsal artery,** which accompanies thoracodorsal nerve to **latissimus dorsi**

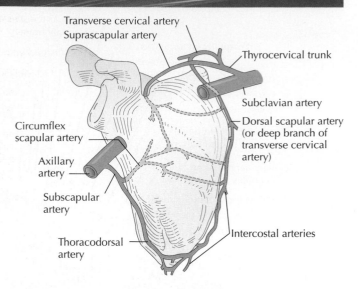

6-11: Arterial anastomoses around the right scapula.

Labels on figure: Transverse cervical artery, Suprascapular artery, Thyrocervical trunk, Subclavian artery, Dorsal scapular artery (or deep branch of transverse cervical artery), Circumflex scapular artery, Axillary artery, Subscapular artery, Intercostal arteries, Thoracodorsal artery

---

Collateral circulation around the scapula bypasses axillary artery obstruction proximal to the subscapular artery.

Blockage of the axillary artery (e.g., by atherosclerosis) can be bypassed by anastomoses between branches of the thyrocervical and subscapular arteries, forming **collateral circulation around the scapula.** The collateral circulation also often allows ligation of the axillary artery proximal to the **subscapular artery (Figure 6-11).** Ligation between the subscapular and profunda brachii arteries would cut off the blood supply and result in loss of the limb.

b. **Anterior humeral circumflex artery**
c. **Posterior humeral circumflex artery**
 (1) Passes with **axillary** nerve through **quadrangular space**
 (2) **Anastomoses** with anterior humeral circumflex artery and ascending branch of profunda brachii artery

To control bleeding, compress the subclavian artery against rib 1 or the axillary artery against the proximal humerus.

Aneurysms sometimes develop on the **axillary artery** (e.g., from trauma, as in baseball pitchers, or from atherosclerosis). If the first part is involved, the aneurysm can **compress the trunks of the brachial plexus.** Chronic improper crutch use may cause aneurysms more distally. **Thromboemboli** can travel to the hands from aneurysms, resulting in ischemic necrosis of involved digits.

E. **Axillary Vein**
 • Continuous with basilic vein and receives brachial and cephalic veins before becoming subclavian vein

An injured **axillary vein** may bleed profusely and allow **air emboli** to pass to the right side of the heart. The axillary vein may undergo **spontaneous thrombosis** after excessive movements of the shoulder **(effort thrombosis)**—for example, in baseball pitchers and weightlifters.

Upper extremity deep venous thrombosis is an occasional source of pulmonary emboli.

The brachial plexus is formed by the anterior rami of spinal nerves C5-T1.

A **central venous catheter** is placed in the **axillary vein** (subclavian vein puncture) to administer parenteral fluids and medications and to measure central venous pressure. An indwelling venous catheter may cause secondary **venous thrombosis.** Other causes include cancer and coagulation defects. Potential complications of axillary vein thrombosis include **pulmonary thromboemboli** and **superior vena cava syndrome.**

Prefixed or postfixed brachial plexus complicates the interpretation of nerve lesions.

F. **Brachial Plexus (Figure 6-12)**
 1. Overview
  a. Formed from **anterior rami** of spinal nerves **C5-T1** to supply upper extremity
  b. **Prefixed** if formed by anterior rami of C4-C8 and **postfixed** if formed by C6-T2

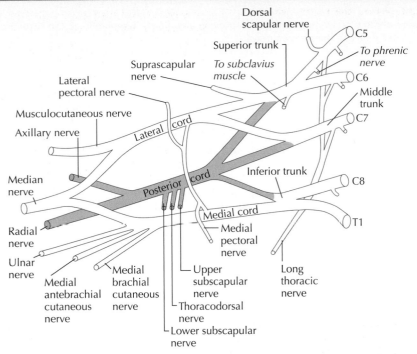

6-12: Brachial plexus and its branches. *Red,* posterior divisions of the trunks, which are nerve fibers destined for extensor regions of the upper extremity.

> As an alternative to general anesthesia, the **brachial plexus** may be blocked to anesthetize the deep structures of the upper extremity and skin distal to the middle of the arm. The block is made easier by the **axillary sheath** of fascia, which encloses the axillary vessels and brachial plexus.

    c. Comprised of **roots, trunks, divisions, cords, and branches**
  2. **Roots**
     • **Anterior rami** of five spinal nerves emerging from neck between anterior and middle scalene muscles
     a. **Dorsal scapular nerve** (C5)
        • Pierces middle scalene to supply levator scapulae and rhomboid muscles
     b. **Long thoracic nerve** (C5-7)
        • Pierces middle scalene to supply serratus anterior muscle

Roots, trunks, divisions, cords, branches = Robert Taylor drinks cold beer

> During a **radical mastectomy** or **traumatic injury**, the **long thoracic nerve** is vulnerable because it lies on the **superficial surface of the serratus anterior.** Injury produces a "winged scapula." The **thoracodorsal nerve** also may be damaged during axillary lymph node dissection.

  3. **Trunks**
     a. Overview
        (1) **Upper trunk** from union of C5 and C6, **middle trunk** from C7, and **lower trunk** from union of C8 and T1
        (2) Pass behind middle third of clavicle, forming **supraclavicular** and **infraclavicular** portions of plexus
     b. **Suprascapular nerve** (C5-6)
        • Passes through suprascapular foramen to supply **supraspinatus and infraspinatus muscles**
     c. **Nerve to subclavius** (C5)
        • May give **accessory phrenic nerve** that joins phrenic nerve at variable level

An **accessory phrenic nerve** may continue to provide significant innervation to the respiratory diaphragm after injury to the **phrenic nerve.**

4. Divisions
   a. Arise from each trunk as **anterior and posterior divisions** at apex of axilla
   b. **Separate nerve fibers destined for flexor and extensor compartments** of upper extremity
5. Cords
   • Designated **medial, lateral, and posterior** according to relationship to **second part of axillary artery**
   a. Posterior cord
      • Formed by **posterior divisions** of all three trunks
      (1) **Upper subscapular nerve (C5-6)** supplies **subscapularis muscle**
      (2) **Middle subscapular nerve** (thoracodorsal nerve) **(C6-8)** supplies **latissimus dorsi muscle**
      (3) **Lower subscapular nerve (C5-6)** innervates **subscapularis and teres major muscles.**
      (4) **Axillary nerve (C5-6)** innervates **deltoid and teres minor muscles.**
      (5) **Radial nerve (C5-T1)** supplies **extensor compartments of arm and forearm**
   b. Lateral cord
      • Formed by **anterior divisions** of upper and middle trunks
      (1) **Lateral pectoral nerve (C5-7)** pierces costocoracoid membrane to supply **pectoralis major muscle**
      (2) **Lateral root of median nerve (C5-7)** joins medial root from medial cord to form **median nerve**
      (3) **Musculocutaneous nerve (C5-7)** pierces coracobrachialis muscle to supply **flexor muscles of arm** and then continues as **lateral antebrachial cutaneous nerve**
   c. Medial cord
      • Formed by **anterior division** of lower trunk
      (1) **Medial pectoral nerve (C8-T1)** pierces **pectoralis minor** to supply it and **pectoralis major muscle**
      (2) **Medial brachial cutaneous nerve (C8-T1)** supplies medial side of arm and communicates with **intercostobrachial nerve** (T2), providing basis for referral of **cardiac pain** at spinal cord segments T1-2
      (3) **Medial antebrachial cutaneous nerve (C8-T1)** supplies skin of medial forearm along course of basilic vein.
      (4) **Ulnar nerve (C8-T1)** supplies two muscles of forearm and most intrinsic muscles of hand and is sensory to skin of medial hand and medial 1½ fingers
      (5) **Medial root of median nerve (C8-T1)** joins lateral root to form **median nerve**
      (6) **Median nerve (C5-T1)** is formed by lateral root from lateral cord and medial root from medial cord and supplies most of forearm flexor, thenar compartment, and lateral two lumbrical muscles

G. **Quadrangular Space**
   1. Bounded by **surgical neck of humerus, long head of triceps brachii muscle, subscapularis muscle,** and overlying **teres minor and teres major muscles**
   2. Transmits **axillary nerve** and **posterior humeral circumflex artery,** which are in jeopardy in fractured surgical neck of humerus or dislocated shoulder

H. **Axillary Lymph Nodes**
   1. Drain **upper extremity** and **upper trunk** along branches of axillary vessels
   2. Receive about 75% of lymph from **breast**
   3. Five groups that ultimately drain to **subclavian lymph trunk:** pectoral, subscapular, humeral, central, and apical nodes

The pectoral nodes lie along the **lateral thoracic vessels** and drain the lateral quadrants of the breast and anterior thoracic wall. **Breast cancer** that metastasizes from the lateral quadrants usually involves the **axillary lymph nodes** first.

Anterior divisions of brachial plexus: flexor compartments. Posterior divisions of brachial plexus: extensor compartments

The cords of the brachial plexus are named for their relationship to the second part of the axillary artery.

Cardiac pain is referred to the medial arm via the intercostobrachial and medial brachial cutaneous nerves.

The axillary nerve and the posterior humeral circumflex artery traverse the quadrangular space.

Lateral quadrant breast cancer metastasizes first to the axillary lymph nodes.

IV. Arm and Forearm
A. Muscles of Arm and Forearm
- **Flexor and extensor compartments** enclosed by deep fascia, but separated from each other by bone and dense fascia

Because the walls of the osseofibrous compartments of the extremities are unyielding, **bleeding** into or **edema** in a compartment may cause **compartment syndrome.** In the flexor forearm, symptoms include compartment pain and impaired cutaneous sensation along ulnar and median nerve distribution in the hand. If untreated, muscles of the flexor compartment may undergo ischemic necrosis, with the resulting flexion deformity of **Volkmann ischemic contracture.** A cast that fits too tightly and compresses the brachial artery may have the same result.

1. **Muscles of arm (Figure 6-13)**
   - Enclosed by **brachial fascia** and innervated by **musculocutaneous nerve** (flexor compartment) or **radial nerve** (extensor compartment)

The **biceps reflex** is commonly tested as part of routine physical examinations. The tendon of insertion (or the examiner's thumb placed over it) is tapped with a reflex hammer, momentarily jerking the elbow into flexion. The reflex tests spinal cord segments **C5-6** with both afferent and efferent limbs of the reflex arc in the **musculocutaneous nerve (C5-7).**

> Biceps reflex tests spinal nerves C5-6.

Chronic inflammation of the **tendon of the long head of the biceps (bicipital tendinitis)** in the bicipital groove may cause shoulder pain. **Degenerative changes** may cause the tendon to **rupture** during elbow flexion against resistance, with the muscle belly of the long head contracting into a ball (Popeye deformity).

> Chronic tendinitis predisposes to tendon rupture.

2. **Muscles of forearm: flexor compartment (Figure 6-14)**
   - Enclosed by **antebrachial fascia** and innervated by **median nerve** except for flexor carpi ulnaris and medial half of flexor digitorum profundus, which are innervated by **ulnar nerve**
3. **Muscles of forearm: extensor compartment**
   - Receive innervation from **radial nerve** or its **deep radial/posterior interosseous branch**

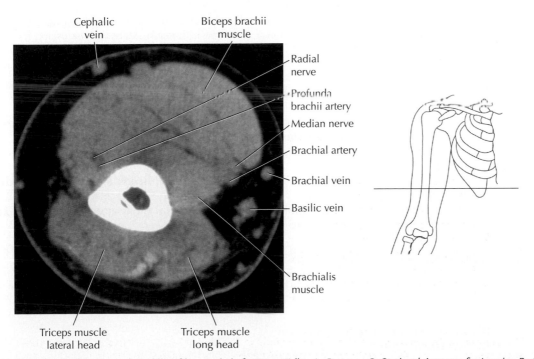

6-13: Axial CT of right arm near middle of humeral shaft. *(From Kelley, L, Petersen, C: Sectional Anatomy for Imaging Professionals, 2nd ed. Mosby, 2007, Figure 9.64.)*

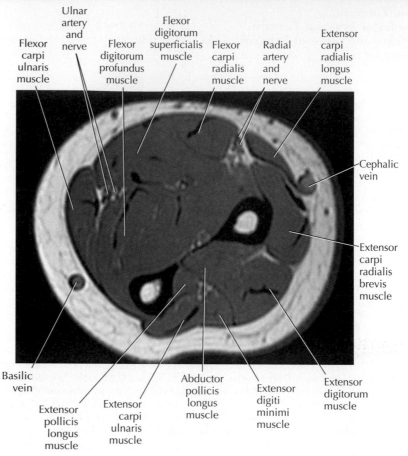

Flexor
carpi
ulnaris
muscle

Ulnar
artery
and
nerve

Flexor
digitorum
profundus
muscle

Flexor
digitorum
superficialis
muscle

Flexor
carpi
radialis
muscle

Radial
artery
and
nerve

Extensor
carpi
radialis
longus
muscle

Cephalic
vein

Extensor
carpi
radialis
brevis
muscle

Basilic
vein

Extensor
pollicis
longus
muscle

Extensor
carpi
ulnaris
muscle

Abductor
pollicis
longus
muscle

Extensor
digiti
minimi
muscle

Extensor
digitorum
muscle

6-14: Axial, T1-weighted MR scan of left forearm muscles. *(From Kelley, L, Petersen, C: Sectional Anatomy for Imaging Professionals, 2nd ed. Mosby, 2007, Figure 9.91.)*

Lateral epicondylitis is tennis elbow. Medial epicondylitis is golfer's elbow.

Local injury or **repetitive overuse** can cause pain and tenderness over the humeral epicondyles. In **lateral epicondylitis** ("tennis elbow"), pain is felt over the origin of **forearm extensor muscles** and may radiate down the forearm. **Medial epicondylits** ("golfer's elbow") is a frequent complaint in golfers and arm wrestlers with pain over the origin of **forearm flexor muscles.**

B. Cubital Fossa
1. Triangular interval anterior to elbow bounded by **brachioradialis, pronator teres,** and **line connecting epicondyles** of humerus
2. Floor formed by **brachialis** and **supinator** muscles and roof formed by **skin, fascia,** and **bicipital aponeurosis**
3. Contents from lateral to medial: **biceps brachii tendon, brachial artery,** and **median nerve**
4. Contains **bifurcation of brachial artery** into radial and ulnar arteries **(Figure 6-15)**
5. Crossed superficially by **median cubital vein**

Cubital fossa contents from lateral to medial are **TAN**: biceps brachii **T**endon, brachial **A**rtery, median **N**erve.

The bicipital aponeurosis separates the median cubital vein from the brachial artery in the cubital fossa.

The **median cubital vein** is separated from the underlying **brachial artery** by the **bicipital aponeurosis,** which **protects the artery** from **errant phlebotomy** or **injection of drugs** intended for the venous system. The **median nerve** on the medial side of the artery is also vulnerable to an incorrectly placed needle.

C. Blood Vessels of Arm and Forearm
1. **Superficial veins**
   a. Begin in **dorsal venous arch** of hand
   b. **Cephalic vein** laterally and **basilic vein** medially joined by **median cubital vein** over cubital fossa

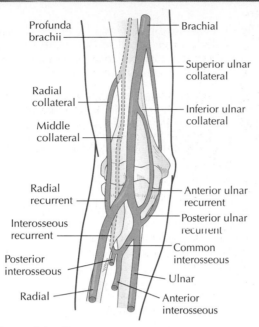

6-15: Arteries and collateral circulation of the elbow.

Cutdown in a patient with **collapsed superficial veins** can be performed over the beginning of the **cephalic vein,** which occupies a relatively constant position crossing the **anatomical snuffbox** just posterior to the radial styloid process. More commonly, however, the **basilic vein** is entered near the cubital fossa if an upper extremity vein is used.

---

    2. **Deep veins**
        a. **Venae comitantes,** usually paired, accompanying arteries
        b. Include **basilic vein,** which becomes **axillary vein** at lower border of teres major
    3. **Arteries (see Figure 6-15 and Figure 6-18)**
       • **Brachial artery** in arm, its **radial and ulnar branches** in forearm, and **interosseous branches** of ulnar artery
        a. **Brachial artery**
          (1) Continuous with **axillary artery** at lower border of teres major
          (2) Gives off **profunda brachii artery** (deep artery of the arm)
          (3) Divides into **radial** and **ulnar** arteries in cubital fossa

---

Occasionally the **brachial artery divides proximally,** with the radial or ulnar artery coursing superficially through the arm and forearm. **Injection of some drugs** into a **superficial radial or ulnar artery** can cause **necrosis of hand tissues.** These vessels are also more prone to injury by a relatively **superficial laceration.**

Asymmetry of brachial blood pressure of at least 20 mm Hg is a classic sign of **subclavian steal syndrome,** which is retrograde blood flow through a **vertebral artery** from ipsilateral arm exertion due to proximal **subclavian artery stenosis.** It produces transient upper-extremity and cerebral ischemic symptoms.

Subclavian steal syndrome is retrograde vertebral artery flow into the subclavian with brainstem hypoperfusion.

In a **humeral fracture,** the **profunda brachii artery** may be injured in the radial groove with the radial nerve.

Superficial palmar arterial arch: ulnar artery. Deep palmar arch: radial artery

---

        b. **Radial artery**
          (1) Courses under brachioradialis to distal forearm
          (2) Lies between flexor carpi radialis and brachioradialis tendons near wrist (where pulse is taken)
          (3) Winds dorsally through **anatomical snuffbox** to reach dorsum of hand

c. **Ulnar artery**
   (1) In middle third of forearm is joined by ulnar nerve deep to flexor carpi ulnaris and then distally courses lateral to flexor carpi ulnaris tendon
   (2) Passes with ulnar nerve **lateral to pisiform** and **superficial to flexor retinaculum** in Guyon canal to reach hand

> In **wrist wounds,** the **ulnar artery** is often **lacerated** lateral to the pisiform bone. In the **Allen test, patency and collateral circulation between the ulnar and radial arteries** is determined by observing the return of color to the palm after compressing both vessels and then releasing one while the patient tightly clenches and then opens the fist. It is performed before a radial artery puncture.

d. **Common interosseous artery**
   - Short branch from ulnar artery that divides into anterior and posterior interosseous arteries
   (1) **Anterior interosseous artery** descends with anterior interosseous nerve to supply forearm flexor muscles.
   (2) **Posterior interosseous artery** enters posterior compartment and descends with posterior interosseous nerve to supply forearm extensor muscles.
e. **Collateral circulation around elbow (see Figure 6-15)**

V. **Wrist and Hand**
   A. **Muscles of Hand**
      1. **Thenar muscles**
         a. Located in **thenar compartment** at base of thumb
         b. Include **flexor pollicis brevis, abductor pollicis brevis,** and **opponens pollicis muscles,** all innervated by **median nerve**
      2. **Hypothenar muscles**
         a. Located in **hypothenar compartment** at base of finger 5
         b. Include **flexor digiti minimi brevis, abductor digiti minimi,** and **opponens digiti minimi muscles,** all innervated by **ulnar nerve**

> Trauma to the distal ulnar artery by using the palm as a tool to pound may result in aneurysm formation with thromboembolization to the fingers **(hypothenar hammer syndrome).**

      3. **Interosseous and lumbrical muscles**
         a. Four **dorsal** and three **palmar interosseous muscles,** all innervated by **ulnar nerve**
         b. Four **lumbrical muscles** originate from tendons of flexor digitorum profundus muscle. **Medial two: ulnar nerve; lateral two: median nerve**
   B. **Nerves of Hand**
      1. Overview
         a. **Motor innervation** to intrinsic muscles of hand is derived mostly from **T1** spinal cord segment via **median and ulnar nerves**
         b. **Cutaneous innervation** of the hand is from **median, ulnar,** and **radial nerves.**

      2. **Median nerve (Figure 6-16; see Figure 6-19)**
         a. At wrist lies deep to tendon of **palmaris longus** when present
         b. Enters hand through **carpal tunnel** anterior to long flexor tendons and gives rise to superficial **recurrent branch** to supply thenar compartment muscles
         c. Gives **digital nerves** supplying palmar skin of lateral 3½ digits
         d. Supplies first and second **lumbrical muscles**
         e. Supplies dorsal skin over distal phalanges of lateral 3½ digits
      3. **Ulnar nerve (Figure 6-17)**
         a. Overview
            (1) Enters hand by passing **superficial to flexor retinaculum** in Guyon canal (ulnar tunnel)
            (2) Terminates by dividing into **superficial and deep branches**
         b. Superficial branch of ulnar nerve
            - Supplies **palmaris brevis muscle** and sends **palmar digital cutaneous nerves** to medial 1½ digits

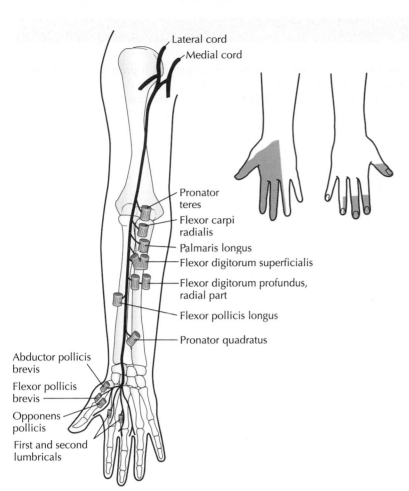

Lateral cord
Medial cord

6-16: Muscular and cutaneous distributions of the median nerve.

Pronator teres
Flexor carpi radialis
Palmaris longus
Flexor digitorum superficialis
Flexor digitorum profundus, radial part
Flexor pollicis longus
Pronator quadratus

Abductor pollicis brevis
Flexor pollicis brevis
Opponens pollicis
First and second lumbricals

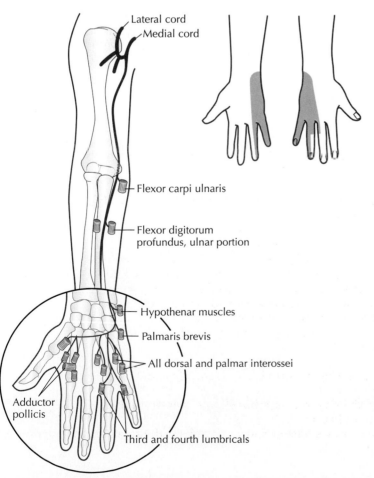

Lateral cord
Medial cord

6-17: Muscular and cutaneous distributions of the ulnar nerve.

Flexor carpi ulnaris

Flexor digitorum profundus, ulnar portion

Hypothenar muscles
Palmaris brevis
All dorsal and palmar interossei

Adductor pollicis

Third and fourth lumbricals

c. **Deep branch of ulnar nerve**
  (1) Passes through hypothenar muscles and runs with **deep palmar arterial arch** deep to long flexor tendons
  (2) Supplies **hypothenar muscles, adductor pollicis, palmar and dorsal interosseous muscles, and medial two lumbricals**
4. **Cutaneous innervation of dorsum of hand**
  a. Primarily by **superficial branch of radial nerve** to lateral 3½ digits and **dorsal branch of ulnar nerve** to medial 1½ digits
  b. By **median nerve** over distal phalanges of lateral 3½ digits
5. **Cutaneous innervation of palm**
  • By **palmar cutaneous** and **palmar digital branches of median and ulnar nerves**

C. **Arteries of Wrist and Hand (Figure 6-18)**
  1. **Radial artery**
    a. From dorsum of hand enters palm by passing between heads of **first dorsal interosseous muscle**
    b. Anastomoses with **deep branch of ulnar artery** to form **deep palmar arch**
    c. Dorsal carpal, **princeps pollicis**, and **radialis indicis branches**
  2. **Deep palmar arch**
    a. Direct continuation of **radial artery** that anastomoses with **deep branch of ulnar artery**
    b. Lies on **interosseous muscles** deep to long flexor tendons
    c. Gives rise to **palmar metacarpal arteries**
  3. **Ulnar artery**
    • Terminates by giving a **deep palmar branch** and then continuing as **superficial palmar arch**
  4. **Superficial palmar arch**
    a. Continuation of **ulnar artery**, which usually anastomoses with superficial **palmar branch of radial artery**
    b. Lies immediately deep to **palmar aponeurosis**
    c. Gives rise to **common** and **proper palmar digital arteries**

Control of palmar arch bleeding may require brachial artery compression.

Laceration of the superficial and/or deep **palmar arches** results in **profuse bleeding,** which may not be controllable by compression of either the ulnar or radial artery alone because of abundant anastomoses. The **brachial artery** may have to be compressed—for example, by a pneumatic tourniquet. This also may be done to obtain a bloodless operating field for hand surgery.

6-18: Arteries of the wrist and palm.

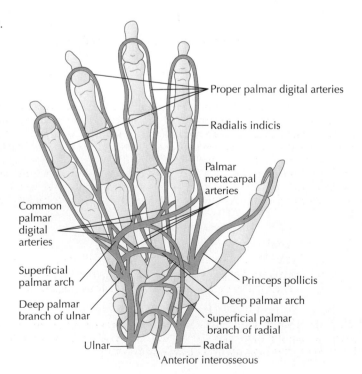

Proper palmar digital arteries

Radialis indicis

Palmar metacarpal arteries

Common palmar digital arteries

Superficial palmar arch

Deep palmar branch of ulnar

Princeps pollicis

Deep palmar arch

Superficial palmar branch of radial

Ulnar

Radial

Anterior interosseous

5. **Dorsal carpal arterial arch**
   a. Formed by anastomosis of **dorsal carpal branches of ulnar and radial arteries**
   b. Gives rise to **dorsal metacarpal** and **dorsal digital arteries**

Raynaud phenomenon is a peripheral vascular disorder characterized by bilateral, symmetrical **vasospasm** in the hands on exposure to cold or emotional stress. It is marked by pallor followed by cyanosis of the fingers and often numbness or pain. The condition occurs frequently in young females and in males who regularly use vibrating tools (e.g., chain saws). It is also common in connective tissue diseases such as **systemic sclerosis (scleroderma)** and **CREST syndrome,** a limited variant of systemic sclerosis.

Raynaud phenomenon is symmetrical vasospasm in both hands due to cold or stress.

Shoulder-hand syndrome is a form of **reflex sympathetic dystrophy (complex regional pain syndrome)** with severe burning pain, hyperesthesia, swelling, and trophic skin changes in the hand associated with ipsilateral restricted shoulder motion and pain. It may follow hand, neck, or shoulder injuries or myocardial infarction.

D. **Other Features of Wrist and Hand (Figure 6-19)**
   1. **Palmar aponeurosis**
      a. Thickened **deep fascia** of palm between thenar and hypothenar eminences
      b. Continuous proximally with tendon of **palmaris longus** (when present) and distally with **fibrous flexor sheaths** of fingers
      c. **Protects** superficial palmar arterial arch, digital nerves, and underlying long flexor tendons

Dupuytren contracture is localized **fibrosis and shortening** of the **palmar aponeurosis,** pulling the metacarpophalangeal (and proximal interphalangeal) joint of finger 4, and perhaps finger 5 and others, into flexion. Distal interphalangeal joints are *not* involved.

Dupuytren contracture is fibromatosis of palmar aponeurosis, drawing the fingers into permanent flexion.

   2. **Flexor retinaculum (transverse carpal ligament)**
      a. Tough, fibrous connective tissue bridging carpal arch to form **carpal tunnel**
      b. Attached to tubercles of **scaphoid and trapezium** laterally and to **hook of hamate and pisiform** medially
      c. Keeps long **flexor tendons** from "bowstringing" when wrist is flexed
   3. **Carpal tunnel (Figure 6-20)**
      a. Formed by **carpal arch** and **flexor retinaculum**
      b. Confined space with rigid walls that contains **median nerve** and **long flexor tendons**

Carpal tunnel syndrome—median nerve compression at the wrist—is the most common entrapment neuropathy.

Tinel sign is paresthesia from tapping over a damaged or regenerating nerve.

Carpal tunnel syndrome, which is compression of the **median nerve** within the carpal tunnel, is the most common **entrapment neuropathy.** It is commonly associated with **repetitive motion** affecting the long flexor tendon sheaths, **pregnancy** primary hypothyroidism, and chronic inflammatory diseases such as **rheumatoid arthritis.** Paresthesias and pain, often worse at night, occur in the cutaneous distribution of the median nerve to the palm and lateral 3½ digits. Tapping over the patient's carpal tunnel frequently reproduces the symptoms **(Tinel sign).** The motor innervation to thenar and first two lumbrical muscles may be affected in severe cases, resulting in weakness and atrophy (see Section VII.G). If conservative treatment fails, the flexor retinaculum may have to be surgically divided.

   4. **Flexor synovial sheaths (Figure 6-21)**
      a. **Facilitate movement** of long flexor tendons in hand
      b. Consist of **three separate synovial sheaths at wrist**—ulnar bursa, radial bursa, and bursa for flexor carpi radialis—and **four digital synovial sheaths**

Infection can travel to the **carpal tunnel** by the **ulnar and radial bursae** from finger 5 and the thumb, respectively. Infection may then spread into the fascial space between the flexor digitorum profundus and pronator quadratus and move into the forearm.

Infection from the little finger or thumb spreads to the carpal tunnel via the flexor synovial sheaths.

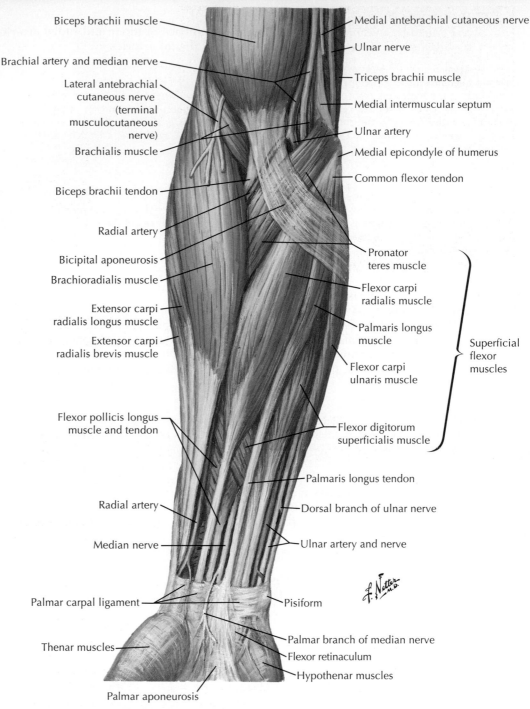

Biceps brachii muscle

Brachial artery and median nerve

Lateral antebrachial cutaneous nerve (terminal musculocutaneous nerve)

Brachialis muscle

Biceps brachii tendon

Radial artery

Bicipital aponeurosis

Brachioradialis muscle

Extensor carpi radialis longus muscle

Extensor carpi radialis brevis muscle

Flexor pollicis longus muscle and tendon

Radial artery

Median nerve

Palmar carpal ligament

Thenar muscles

Palmar aponeurosis

Medial antebrachial cutaneous nerve

Ulnar nerve

Triceps brachii muscle

Medial intermuscular septum

Ulnar artery

Medial epicondyle of humerus

Common flexor tendon

Pronator teres muscle

Flexor carpi radialis muscle

Palmaris longus muscle

Flexor carpi ulnaris muscle

Flexor digitorum superficialis muscle

Superficial flexor muscles

Palmaris longus tendon

Dorsal branch of ulnar nerve

Ulnar artery and nerve

Pisiform

Palmar branch of median nerve

Flexor retinaculum

Hypothenar muscles

6-19: Superficial structures of forearm flexor compartment and anterior wrist. Structures in the distal forearm are relatively superficial and are commonly lacerated. The radial artery pulse is typically taken just lateral to the flexor carpi radialis tendon. The palmar carpal ligament is a thickened band of antebrachial fascia superficial to the proximal part of the flexor retinaculum and does *not* participate in formation of the carpal tunnel. *(From Netter, F H: Atlas of Human Anatomy, 4th ed. Philadelphia, Saunders, 2006, Plate 446.)*

5. **Long flexor tendons**
   a. Overview
      (1) Surrounded by **synovial sheath** in each finger to facilitate movement within **fibrous digital sheath**
      (2) Connected to dorsal part of their synovial sheath by synovial folds called **vincula longus** and **brevis,** which carry blood supply

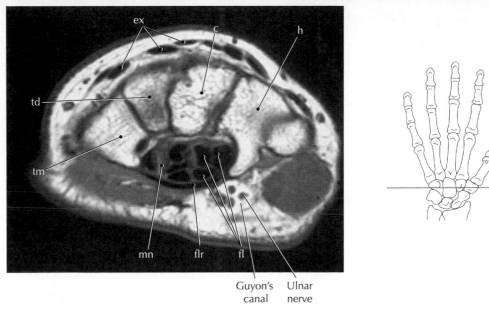

6-20: Axial, T1-weighted MRI of wrist showing contents of the carpal tunnel. Note that the ulnar nerve traverses Guyon canal superficial to the flexor retinaculum. Flr = flexor retinaculum; median nerve = mn; flexor digitorum superficialis and profundus tendons = fl; trapezium = tm; trapezoid = td; capitate = c; hamate = h; extensor tendons = ex. *(From Kelley, L, Petersen, C: Sectional Anatomy for Imaging Professionals, 2nd ed. Mosby, 2007, Figure 9.119.)*

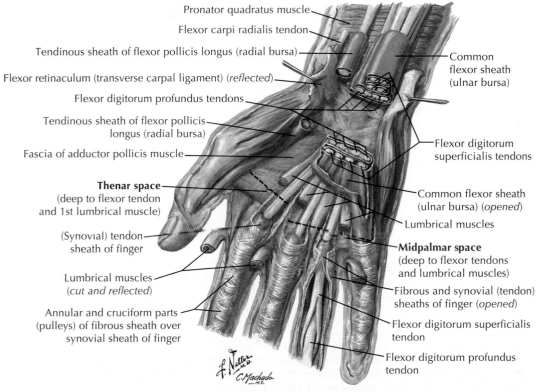

6-21: Synovial sheaths of the long flexor tendons of the wrist and hand. Infections can reach the carpal tunnel from the little finger and thumb via the ulnar bursa and radial bursa, respectively. The thenar and midpalmar spaces are potential spaces in the palm deep to the long flexor tendons. They may become infected and distended with fluid. *(From Netter, F H: Atlas of Human Anatomy, 4th ed. Philadelphia, Saunders, 2006, Plate 462.)*

Trigger finger (stenosing tenosynovitis) is a narrowing of the fibrous flexor tendon sheath at the metacarpophalangeal joint and/or a thickening of the long flexor tendon proximal to the fibrous tunnel. The patient may be unable to actively extend the finger, but it can be passively extended with a "snap." Flexion of the extended digit is possible with snapping similar to the action of a trigger.

Trigger finger is stenosing tenosynovitis of a finger or thumb fibrous flexor sheath.

b. **Flexor digitorum superficialis tendon**
   (1) Splits around tendon of flexor digitorum profundus
   (2) Inserts on lateral sides of base of **middle phalanx** of fingers 2-5
c. **Flexor digitorum profundus tendon**
   (1) Passes through split of **flexor digitorum superficialis tendon**
   (2) Inserts into base of **distal phalanx** of fingers 2-5
6. **Fascial spaces of palm**
   a. **Potential spaces** deep to long flexor tendons
   b. Separated into **thenar and midpalmar spaces** by midpalmar (oblique) fascial septum from palmar aponeurosis to third metacarpal

The flexor digitorum superficialis tendon splits to allow flexor digitorum profundus passage.

Swelling on the dorsum of the hand may be from a palmar infection.

Thenar and **midpalmar spaces** can become infected and distended with fluid from **acute tenosynovitis, a penetrating wound,** or hematogenous spread. Painful swelling is usually more evident on the dorsum of the hand, where the fascia is thinner.

7. **Pulp spaces of fingers**
   • Fat tightly packed between fibrous septa over terminal phalanx

Untreated finger pad infection may result in osteomyelitis or soft tissue necrosis.

The finger pad is vulnerable to minor trauma that may cause infection (felon). **Edema** in **pulp spaces** from the resulting inflammation produces severe pain. The infection may spread to the flexor synovial sheath or the terminal phalanx (osteomyelitis) or may impair venous drainage. Without treatment, tissues in the tip of the digit undergo necrosis.

8. **Extensor retinaculum**
   a. Thickening of dorsal **antebrachial fascia** that attaches laterally to distal radius and medially to styloid process of ulna and to triquetrum and pisiform
   b. Binds extensor tendons into place in one of six compartments over wrist

De Quervain disease is tenosynovitis of the abductor pollicis longus and extensor pollicis brevis tendons.

De Quervain disease is a stenosing tenosynovitis involving the **abductor pollicis longus and extensor pollicis brevis tendons** in the first dorsal wrist compartment. There is pain, tenderness, and swelling over the radial styloid process. The pain may radiate down to the thumb or up the forearm. De Quervain is frequently seen in middle-aged women and in new mothers who use repetitive hand movements.

9. **Extensor expansion (dorsal hood)**
   a. Triangular **expansion of extensor digitorum tendons** beginning over metacarpophalangeal joints
   b. Receives insertions of **lumbrical and interosseous muscles**
   c. Divides into **central band** to middle phalanx and **lateral bands** to distal phalanx

Mallet finger deformity: DIP joint flexion due to extensor tendon avulsion

Sudden forceful flexion of the DIP joint with the **extensor digitorum tendon** under tension may avulse the tendon's insertion into the distal phalanx or rupture the tendon. The DIP joint remains flexed and *cannot* be actively extended **(mallet finger).**

Boutonniére deformity: PIP joint flexion and DIP joint hyperextension

Swan neck deformity: PIP joint hyperextension and DIP joint flexion

With **rupture of the central band of the extensor expansion** attaching to the middle phalanx, the PIP joint becomes flexed as the DIP joint is hyperextended by the lateral bands. This **Boutonniére deformity** occurs commonly in **rheumatoid arthritis.** The PIP joint is hyperextended and the DIP joint is flexed in **swan neck deformity,** which is also seen in rheumatoid arthritis as well as following intrinsic muscle spasm or a palmar ligament (volar plate) injury.

10. **Skin of dorsum**
   • Loose, allowing fluid to easily collect beneath it

Infection in the palm often causes swelling of the dorsum of the hand, which masks the primary site of infection.

11. **Anatomical snuffbox**
   a. **Depression** on lateral surface of wrist when thumb is extended
   b. Defined anteriorly by **abductor pollicis longus** and **extensor pollicis brevis** and posteriorly by **extensor pollicis longus** tendons
   c. Floor formed by **styloid process of radius, scaphoid,** and **trapezium**
   d. Crossed superficially by cephalic vein and superficial branch of radial nerve
   e. Contains **radial artery** as it passes to dorsum of hand

The anatomical snuffbox is bounded by the abductor pollicis longus and extensor pollicis brevis anteriorly and by the extensor pollicis longus posteriorly.

VI. Innervation of Upper Extremity
A. Motor Innervation by Nerve
   1. **Musculocutaneous nerve (Figure 6-22)**
      • Flexor compartment of arm

Anterior view

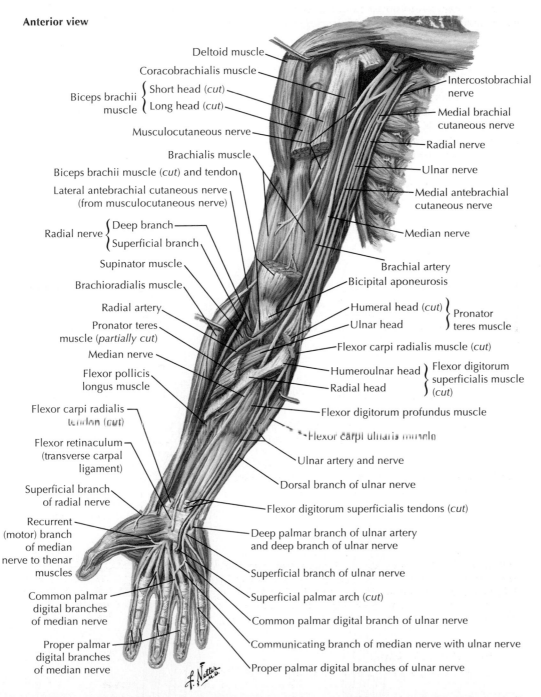

Deltoid muscle
Coracobrachialis muscle
Biceps brachii muscle { Short head (*cut*)
                        Long head (*cut*)
Musculocutaneous nerve
Brachialis muscle
Biceps brachii muscle (*cut*) and tendon
Lateral antebrachial cutaneous nerve (from musculocutaneous nerve)
Radial nerve { Deep branch
              Superficial branch
Supinator muscle
Brachioradialis muscle
Radial artery
Pronator teres muscle (*partially cut*)
Median nerve
Flexor pollicis longus muscle
Flexor carpi radialis tendon (*cut*)
Flexor retinaculum (transverse carpal ligament)
Superficial branch of radial nerve
Recurrent (motor) branch of median nerve to thenar muscles
Common palmar digital branches of median nerve
Proper palmar digital branches of median nerve

Intercostobrachial nerve
Medial brachial cutaneous nerve
Radial nerve
Ulnar nerve
Medial antebrachial cutaneous nerve
Median nerve
Brachial artery
Bicipital aponeurosis
Humeral head (*cut*) } Pronator teres muscle
Ulnar head
Flexor carpi radialis muscle (*cut*)
Humeroulnar head } Flexor digitorum superficialis muscle (*cut*)
Radial head
Flexor digitorum profundus muscle
Flexor carpi ulnaris muscle
Ulnar artery and nerve
Dorsal branch of ulnar nerve
Flexor digitorum superficialis tendons (*cut*)
Deep palmar branch of ulnar artery and deep branch of ulnar nerve
Superficial branch of ulnar nerve
Superficial palmar arch (*cut*)
Common palmar digital branch of ulnar nerve
Communicating branch of median nerve with ulnar nerve
Proper palmar digital branches of ulnar nerve

6-22: Nerves of the upper limb, anterior view. Note the musculocutaneous nerve piercing the coracobrachialis to supply muscles of the flexor compartment of the arm and then continuing as the lateral antebrachial cutaneous nerve to supply the skin of the anterolateral forearm. (*From Netter, F H: Atlas of Human Anatomy, 4th ed. Philadelphia, Saunders, 2006, Plate 473.*)

    2. **Median nerve (see Figure 6-16)**
      a. Flexor compartment of forearm (*except* flexor carpi ulnaris and medial/ulnar half of flexor digitorum profundus)
      b. Thenar muscles
      c. First and second lumbricals
    3. **Ulnar nerve (see Figure 6-17)**
      a. Flexor carpi ulnaris and ulnar half of flexor digitorum profundus in forearm
      b. Hypothenar muscles
      c. Adductor pollicis
      d. Dorsal and palmar interossei
      e. Third and fourth lumbricals
    4. **Radial nerve (Figure 6-23)**
      • Extensor compartment muscles of arm and forearm

B. **Muscle Function and Main Segmental Innervations**
    1. **Shoulder**
      a. **Flexion, lateral rotation, and abduction: C5**
      b. **Medial rotation and adduction: C6-8**
    2. **Elbow**
      a. **Flexion: C5, C6**
      b. **Extension: C7, C8**
    3. **Forearm**
      a. **Pronation: C7, C8**
      b. **Supination: C6**
    4. **Wrist**
      • **Flexion and extension: C6, C7**

> Ulnar nerve: intrinsic hand muscles except the thenar compartment and the first two lumbricals
>
> The radial nerve does *not* innervate any intrinsic hand muscles.

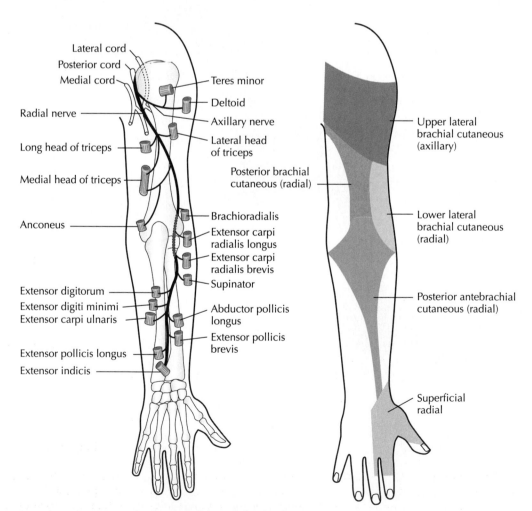

6-23: Muscular and cutaneous distributions of the radial and axillary nerves.

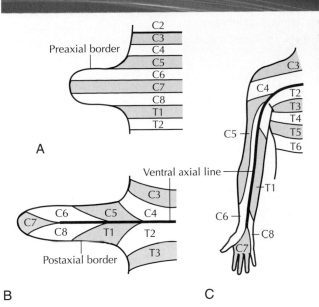

6-24: Dermatomes of the upper extremity. Simple dermatome pattern **(A)** changes with limb growth to definitive pattern **(B)**. **C**, C6 supplies the lateral forearm and thumb; C8 supplies the medial forearm, hand, and little finger; and T1 supplies the medial side of the limb above and below the elbow.

5. **Hand**
   - **Intrinsic muscles:** Mostly T1 with some C8
6. **Digits**
   - **Flexion and extension:** C7, C8
C. **Dermatomes of Upper Extremity (Figure 6-24)**

> **Supraclavicular nerves** (C3, C4) innervate the skin over the point of the shoulder and upper deltoid. **Inflammatory lesions** involving the **diaphragmatic pleura or peritoneum** may cause **referred pain** via the **phrenic nerve** (C3-5) to the shoulder.

VII. **Nerve Injuries of Upper Extremity**
   A. **Overview**
      1. Occur most commonly from **trauma** after a **penetrating injury** or **closed injury** (e.g., traction or compression) but may occur from **nontraumatic causes** (e.g., neoplasm, infection, radiation)

> Radiation-induced nerve damage may not appear until years later.

      2. Usually involve **more than one spinal nerve and peripheral nerve**
      3. Are **lower motor neuron lesions** that cause **flaccid paralysis** and **trophic atrophy** of affected muscles, often **cutaneous sensory loss**, and **loss of reflexes**
   B. **Injury of Upper Roots and Trunk (Erb-Duchenne Palsy)**
      1. Involves spinal nerves **C5 and C6**, usually when **shoulder is wrenched downward** and **head and neck are forced to opposite side** (e.g., violent fall in a motorcycle accident)
      2. May occur as **birth injury** from forceful pulling on infant's head during difficult delivery
      3. May occur from prolonged pressure on shoulder ("**backpacker's palsy**") or trauma by a football helmet ("**burner**" or "**stinger**"), but with recovery likely
      4. Causes **loss of abduction, flexion, and lateral rotation of shoulder and impaired supination of forearm**, resulting in "**waiter's tip position**" with arm hanging at side in medial rotation with forearm extended and pronated and wrist flexed **(Figure 6-25)**

> Upper brachial plexus injury: "waiter's tip position"

   C. **Injury of Lower Roots and Trunk (Klumpke Paralysis)**
      1. Involves damage to spinal nerves **C8 and T1**, which is less common than upper brachial plexus injury
      2. Often produced by **forcibly abducting arm above head** (e.g., grabbing for support during fall from height or as a birth injury)
      3. May occur in **thoracic outlet syndrome** with compression of lower trunk between clavicle and rib 1 or stretch over a cervical rib or fibrous band; compression by hypertrophied anterior scalene muscle is considered **scalenus anterior syndrome**

> Thoracic outlet syndrome is the compression of the lower brachial plexus or subclavian artery.

      4. May occur with **mass lesions** (e.g., **Pancoast tumor** or subclavian artery aneurysm)

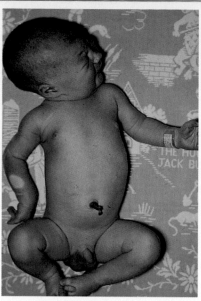

6-25: Right upper brachial plexus birth injury (Erb-Duchenne palsy) showing characteristic "waiter's tip" position. Arm is adducted and medially rotated with forearm pronated and wrist flexed. The elbow is usually extended. Difficult deliveries are a common cause of brachial plexus injuries. *(From Forbes, C D, Jackson, W F: Color Atlas and Text of Clinical Medicine, 3rd ed. Mosby Ltd., 2003, Figure 11.113.)*

Lower brachial plexus or ulnar nerve injury: clawhand deformity

5. Affects **intrinsic muscles of hand,** causing **clawhand deformity** from ulnar nerve loss; clawhand results from **hyperextension of metacarpophalangeal joints** because extensor digitorum is unopposed by lumbricals and interossei **(Figure 6-26)**
6. **Causes inability** to voluntarily flex DIP joints of **fingers 4-5** (ulnar half of flexor digitorum profundus)
7. Causes **impaired ulnar deviation** (adduction) and **flexion of wrist** (flexor carpi ulnaris)
8. May have associated **Horner syndrome** caused by interruption of preganglionic sympathetic nerve fibers by traction on **cervical sympathetic trunk**

Horner syndrome often is associated with a lower brachial plexus injury

Wristdrop: posterior cord or radial nerve injury

D. **Injury of Posterior Cord**
1. **Paralyzes extensor muscles of arm and forearm** with variable flexion at shoulder, elbow, wrist, and fingers
2. Causes **wristdrop (see Figure 6-26)** with consequent loss of effective finger function
3. May be caused by improperly fitted or incorrectly used axillary crutch (**"crutch palsy"**) or result from draping arm over back of chair or bench while inebriated (**"Saturday night palsy"**)

E. **Injuries of Individual Nerves**
 • May occur with penetrating or closed trauma or with disease of nerve's blood supply, the vasa nervorum (e.g., diabetic neuropathy)
1. **Injury to long thoracic nerve**
   a. **Paralyzes serratus anterior** muscle, which causes **inability to abduct or flex arm** above horizontal due to loss of scapular rotation
   b. Characterized by **"winged scapula"** when patient pushes forward against resistance (e.g., a wall)

Long thoracic nerve injury: "winged scapula"

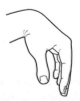

Radial nerve injury (wristdrop)

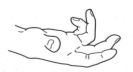

Dupuytren's contracture

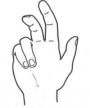

Median nerve injury (benediction hand)

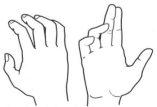

Ulnar nerve injury (clawhand)

6-26: Characteristic features of selected hand deformities.

2. **Injury to suprascapular nerve**
    a. May result from **entrapment in suprascapular foramen** or only in branch to infraspinatus at **spinoglenoid notch**
    b. Causes **difficulty initiating abduction of arm** (supraspinatus) and **weakness in lateral rotation** (infraspinatus)

3. **Injury to subscapular nerves**
    • Causes **weakness in medially rotating arm** (subscapularis and teres major)

4. **Injury to thoracodorsal nerve**
    a. Causes **decreased strength in adduction, extension, and medial rotation of arm** (latissimus dorsi)
    b. **Impedes walking with crutches and transferring from wheelchairs** from weakened shoulder depression (latissimus dorsi)

5. **Injury to musculocutaneous nerve (see Figure 6-22)**
    a. Greatly **weakens flexion of elbow** (biceps and brachialis) and **supination of forearm** (biceps)
    b. May be accompanied by **anesthesia over lateral aspect of forearm**

6. **Injury to axillary nerve (see Figure 6-23)**
    a. May result from **fracture of surgical neck of humerus or dislocation of shoulder joint**
    b. Causes **inability to abduct arm beyond first 15°** with flattening of shoulder contour (deltoid)
    c. Causes **loss of cutaneous sensation over deltoid**

F. **Injury to Radial Nerve**
1. Overview
    a. Causes **wristdrop** from **paralysis of wrist extensors (see Figure 6-26)**
    b. Produces **variable degree of paralysis of extensor muscles of arm and forearm** depending on level at which nerve is injured
    c. Because cutaneous nerves overlap, may cause only a **small area of sensory loss over first dorsal interosseous muscle**
    d. Does *not* prevent extension of interphalangeal joints when combined with metacarpophalangeal flexion from action of interossei and lumbricals
    e. Does *not* cause complete loss of supination because biceps brachii can partially compensate for paralysis of supinator

2. **Radial nerve injury in arm**
    a. Commonly caused by **fracture of humeral shaft**
    b. Usually **does *not* result in loss of extension at elbow** because branches to triceps arise proximal to **radial groove**

3. **Radial nerve injury at cubital fossa**
    a. May result from **hypertrophy or scarring of supinator muscle** (through which deep branch passes) or from **fracture of neck of radius**
    b. **Does *not* cause wristdrop** because branches to extensor carpi radialis longus and brevis arise proximal to this point; does cause **loss of MP joint extension**

G. **Injury to Median Nerve (see Figure 6-16)**
    • Commonly caused by a **supracondylar fracture of humerus, laceration at wrist, or compression in carpal tunnel**

1. **Median nerve injury at wrist**
    a. Paralyzes thenar muscles with **inability to oppose thumb** and **weakened flexion of thumb** at first metacarpophalangeal joint; laceration of superficially placed **recurrent branch** in palm has same effect.
    b. **Wasting of thenar eminence** from muscle atrophy
    c. Paralyzes first and second lumbricals with impaired movement of fingers 2-3
    d. Causes debilitating **sensory loss over lateral palm and lateral 3½ digits** (Note: Sensation over proximal palm is spared due to palmar cutaneous branch)
    e. Frequently is caused by **carpal tunnel syndrome**; paresthesias may be elicited by tapping over flexor retinaculum **(Tinel sign)**

2. **Median nerve injury at elbow**
    a. Causes **loss of forearm pronation** and **weakened wrist flexion and abduction**
    b. Causes **inability to flex thumb and fingers 2 and 3 at interphalangeal joints (benediction hand) (see Figure 6-26)**
    c. May occur in entrapment between heads of pronator teres **(pronator teres syndrome)** or supracondylar humeral fracture

---

Margin notes:

Crutch walking and wheelchair transfers are hindered by latissimus dorsi paralysis.

Radial nerve injury from a midhumeral fracture spares elbow extension but results in wristdrop.

Deep radial nerve injury at the supinator does *not* produce wristdrop.

Posterior and anterior interosseous nerve lesions cause no sensory loss.

Recurrent branch of median nerve lesion: loss of thumb opposition

Median nerve injury at elbow: benediction hand when trying to make a fist

d. May involve only **anterior interosseous branch** with **loss of interphalangeal flexion of thumb and DIP flexion of fingers 2-3 and weakened pronation (anterior interosseous syndrome)**

e. Includes **deficits present in injury at wrist**

H. Injury to Ulnar Nerve (see Figure 6-17)

- Frequently caused by **fracture of medial epicondyle or laceration at wrist** and less frequently by **compression in cubital tunnel or Guyon canal**

1. **Ulnar nerve injury at wrist**

The ulnar nerve innervates the adductor pollicis but not the other short thumb muscles.

   a. **Paralyzes intrinsic muscles of hand** except those of thenar eminence and first and second lumbricals
   b. Causes **inability to abduct or adduct fingers** (interosseous muscles) **or to adduct thumb (adductor pollicis)**
   c. Causes **inability to simultaneously flex metacarpophalangeal joints and extend interphalangeal joints of fingers 2-5** (lumbrical and interosseous muscles)
   d. Causes **clawhand** characterized by wasted hypothenar eminence, hyperextended MP joints, and flexed PIP and DIP joints
   e. Produces **variable paralysis in some individuals who have median-ulnar communications in forearm (Martin-Gruber anastomoses)**

2. **Ulnar nerve injury at elbow**

An ulnar nerve injury at the medial epicondyle affects most intrinsic hand muscles.

   a. May occur **posterior to medial epicondyle** or where **ulnar nerve passes between two heads of flexor carpi ulnaris muscle (cubital tunnel)**
   b. **Impairs ulnar deviation and flexion at wrist** because flexor carpi ulnaris function is lost
   c. Causes **inability to flex DIP joints of fingers 4-5** because ulnar portion of flexor digitorum profundus muscle is lost
   d. Includes **deficits present in injury at wrist**

VIII. Limb Development

A. Overview

1. Development of upper and lower extremities is similar, except that lower extremity lags behind that of upper.
2. Begins during week 4 with appearance of **limb buds,** opposite **cervical somites,** consisting of somatic mesoderm-derived mesenchyme covered by ectoderm

B. Apical Ectodermal Ridge

1. Ectodermal thickening that induces differentiation of limb buds
2. Promotes **proximodistal differentiation** of limb
3. Induces expression of limb growth factors, including fibroblast growth factors, bone morphogenetic proteins, and *HOX* genes

C. Zone of Polarizing Activity

1. Promotes **craniocaudal differentiation** of hand or foot through production of **sonic hedgehog (Shh)** peptide
2. Through Shh induces expression of **growth factors** including fibroblast growth factors, bone morphogenetic proteins, and *HOX* genes

D. *Wnt* Genes

- Associated with **dorsoventral patterning** of limbs

E. Digital Rays

- Condensations of mesenchyme with intervening regions that are broken down by **apoptosis** (programmed cell death) to form digits in **hand plates**

F. Developmental Defects of Limbs

Maternal thalidomide or vitamin A use during weeks 4 and 5 are associated with severe limb malformations.

- Include fusion of fingers (**syndactyly**), extra fingers (**polydactyly**), and total (**amelia**) or partial (**meromelia**) absence of limb

G. Endochondral Ossification

1. Forms long bones of limbs and limb girdles except clavicle
2. Involves development of **hyaline cartilage models** that are replaced by bone, except at **epiphyseal plates** (until growth ceases) and **articular cartilages**

H. Intramembranous Ossification

1. Forms clavicle
2. Characterized by direct ossification of mesenchyme
3. Lacks a cartilaginous precursor

CHAPTER 7
THE NECK

I. Triangles of Neck (Figure 7-1)
- Anterior and posterior triangles separated by **sternocleidomastoid muscle**
A. Anterior Cervical Triangle
1. **Submandibular triangle**
   a. **Floor** formed by **mylohyoid** and **hyoglossus** muscles
   b. Contains **submandibular salivary gland** (superficial part) and **lymph nodes, facial vein and artery, nerve to the mylohyoid, and submental artery**

> Enlarged lymph nodes in the **submandibular triangle** (e.g., from tongue cancer or infection) can be mistaken for an **enlarged submandibular gland.** Correct identification of the nodes can often be made by bimanual palpation with one finger on the floor of the oral cavity. During excision of the submandibular gland for a **tumor, the cervical and mandibular branches of the facial nerve** are at risk. Cutting the mandibular branch causes facial deformity because the lower lip and chin muscles are paralyzed.

2. **Submental triangle**
   a. **Floor** formed by **mylohyoid** muscles meeting in median fibrous raphe
   b. Unpaired median triangle above **hyoid bone** between **anterior bellies of digastric muscles**
   c. Contains **submental lymph nodes,** which receive lymph from apex of tongue and middle of lower lip
3. **Carotid triangle**
   - Contains **common, internal,** and **external carotid arteries, internal jugular vein,** and **vagus** and **hypoglossal nerves**
4. **Muscular triangle**
   a. **Floor** formed by **sternohyoid** and **sternothyroid** (infrahyoid) muscles
   b. **Anterior jugular vein** descends in fascia superficial to triangle
B. Posterior Cervical Triangle
1. Overview
   a. **Floor** formed by **prevertebral fascia** overlying splenius capitis, levator scapulae, posterior and middle scalene muscles
   b. Subdivided by **inferior belly of omohyoid muscle** into superior **occipital** and inferior **subclavian (omoclavicular) triangles**
2. Contents
   a. **Spinal accessory nerve**
   b. Roots and trunks of **brachial plexus**
   c. **Subclavian artery** crossing rib 1
   d. **Supraclavicular nerves** (C3,4) descending in fascial roof of triangle
   e. **Suprascapular, dorsal scapular, and long thoracic nerves**
   f. **Transverse cervical and suprascapular arteries** from thyrocervical trunk
II. Cervical Fasciae (Figure 7-2)
A. Superficial Cervical Fascia
- **Subcutaneous connective tissue** containing **platysma muscle,** superficial veins, cutaneous nerves, and variable amount of fat
B. Deep Cervical Fascia
- Forms series of cylindrical compartments descending through neck

---

Enlarged submandibular lymph nodes may be confused with an enlarged gland.

Damage to the mandibular branch of VII during submandibular gland surgery causes lower facial paralysis.

Cancer from the tip of the tongue and the lower lip metastasizes to submental lymph nodes.

The carotid triangle is used for a surgical approach to the carotid arteries, internal jugular vein, and hypoglossal and vagus nerves.

Subclavian artery compression against the first rib helps to control axillary and upper-extremity bleeding.

Pain carried by the phrenic nerve from the diaphragmatic pleura or peritoneum or from the pericardium may be referred to the shoulder via the supraclavicular nerves.

Laceration that penetrates platysma suggests a serious neck wound and requires further evaluation.

Cervical fasciae form cleavage planes that direct the spread of infection.

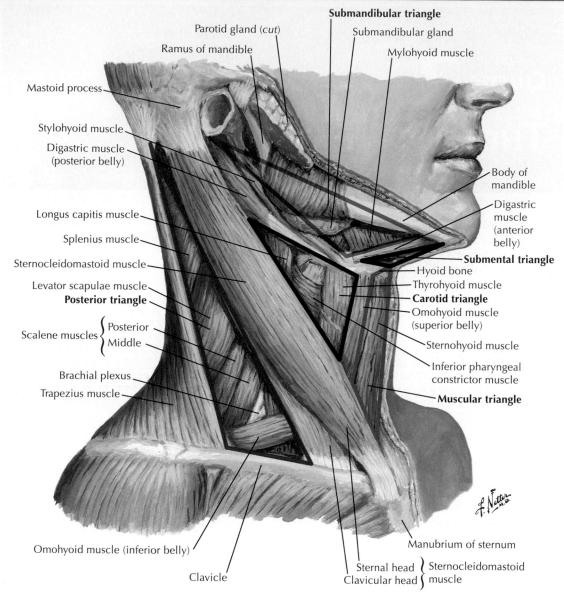

7-1: Triangles of neck viewed from right side. *(From Norton, N S: Netter's Head and Neck Anatomy for Dentistry. Philadelphia, Saunders 2007, p 113.)*

1. **Investing layer of deep cervical fascia**
   a. Cylindrical layer deep to superficial fascia forming roof of anterior and posterior triangles and splitting to invest **sternocleidomastoid** and **trapezius muscles**
   b. Attached superiorly to cranium and mandible and inferiorly to shoulder girdle and manubrium
2. **Pretracheal fascia**
   a. Lies deep to infrahyoid muscles anterior to **larynx, thyroid gland,** and **trachea**
   b. Splits to enclose **thyroid gland** and fuses on each side with **carotid sheath**
   c. Attaches superiorly to **thyroid cartilage** and inferiorly blends with connective tissue of **anterior mediastinum**

Swelling from pretracheal space infection may cause dyspnea, dysphagia, and hoarseness.

Infection can spread from the **neck into the mediastinum** through the potential **pretracheal space** between the **pretracheal fascia** and the trachea, causing fatal **mediastinitis**. Swelling from the infection may compress the trachea and esophagus, causing **hoarseness** and difficulty breathing **(dyspnea)** and swallowing **(dysphagia)**.

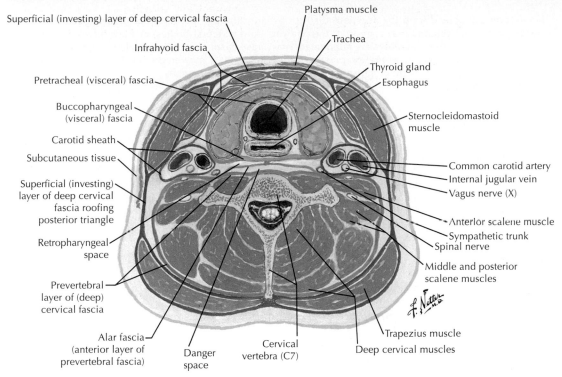

Superficial (investing) layer of deep cervical fascia

Platysma muscle

Infrahyoid fascia

Trachea

Pretracheal (visceral) fascia

Thyroid gland

Esophagus

Buccopharyngeal (visceral) fascia

Sternocleidomastoid muscle

Carotid sheath

Subcutaneous tissue

Common carotid artery

Internal jugular vein

Superficial (investing) layer of deep cervical fascia roofing posterior triangle

Vagus nerve (X)

Retropharyngeal space

Anterior scalene muscle

Sympathetic trunk

Spinal nerve

Prevertebral layer of (deep) cervical fascia

Middle and posterior scalene muscles

Alar fascia (anterior layer of prevertebral fascia)

Danger space

Cervical vertebra (C7)

Deep cervical muscles

Trapezius muscle

7-2: Horizontal section of neck at the level of the C7 vertebra showing cervical fasciae. Note the "danger space" between the anterior (alar) and posterior layers of prevertebral fascia and the retropharyngeal space between the alar fascia and buccopharyngeal fascia. These spaces are two pathways for the spread of infection into the mediastinum. *(From Netter, F H: Atlas of Human Anatomy, 4th ed. Philadelphia, Saunders, 2006, Plate 35.)*

3. **Carotid sheath**
   - Encloses **common** and **internal carotid arteries, internal jugular vein,** and **vagus nerve** from base of skull to root of neck
4. **Buccopharyngeal fascia**
   a. Covers pharyngeal constrictor and buccinator muscles
   b. Sometimes described as **posterior part of pretracheal fascia**
5. **Pharyngobasilar fascia**
   - Well-developed fascia in pharyngeal wall between mucosa and pharyngeal constrictor muscles

Pharyngeal mucosa is tightly bound to the underlying **pharyngobasilar fascia, and inflammation of the pharyngeal wall** with fluid accumulation is painful because swelling stretches the mucosa. Gargling with hypertonic saline solution removes excess fluid from the wall, relieving discomfort. **Group A streptococcal pharyngitis** has the potential to cause **acute rheumatic fever** with damage to heart valves, **glomerulonephritis,** and **toxic shock syndrome.**

Streptococcal pharyngitis may cause rheumatic fever with mitral valve damage.

6. **Prevertebral fascia**
   a. Cylindrical layer enclosing vertebral column and covering **prevertebral, scalene, and intrinsic back muscles**
   b. Over front of cervical vertebrae divides into **anterior and posterior layers**

The space between the anterior **(alar)** and posterior layers of prevertebral fascia has been called the **"danger space"** because it provides a **route for the spread of infection** from the base of the skull all the way to the respiratory diaphragm.

Retropharyngeal space is located between the buccopharyngeal and prevertebral fascia.

Retropharyngeal infection may spread into the mediastinum, causing fatal mediastinitis.

7. **Retropharyngeal space**
   - Between **prevertebral fascia** posteriorly and **buccopharyngeal fascia** anteriorly, extending from base of skull into mediastinum at **T3 or T4 vertebra**

A retropharyngeal abscess may cause dyspnea, dysphagia, aspiration pneumonia, carotid hemorrhage, or jugular thrombosis.

Infection can spread from the neck into the mediastinum through the **retropharyngeal space**. A **retropharyngeal abscess** may arise from the pharynx, from vertebral bodies, or from infected deep cervical lymph nodes. The abscess, if untreated, may cause **dyspnea** and **dysphagia** or rupture into the pharyngeal cavity, causing **aspiration pneumonia**. Alternatively, it may erode into the carotid artery to produce a fatal **hemorrhage** or cause **internal jugular venous thrombosis.**

The cervical pleura and apex of the lung may be injured in wounds to the base of the neck.

8. **Suprapleural membrane**
   • Thickening of **endothoracic fascia** that covers cupola and apex of lung and separates thoracic cavity from neck

The cervical pleura (cupola) and **apex of the lung** are vulnerable in a **penetrating injury to the posterior triangle** or when inserting a subclavian venous catheter. **Pneumothorax** or hemothorax is possible in these instances.

III. Muscles of Neck
A. Sternocleidomastoid
1. Laterally flexes head to same side and rotates face toward opposite side and acts as accessory muscle of respiration
2. Innervated by **spinal accessory nerve** (CN XI) with proprioceptive fibers from C3-4

Congenital or spasmodic torticollis mimics spasming sternocleidomastoid.

Torticollis (wryneck) is muscle shortening that reproduces the position of a strongly contracting **sternocleidomastoid.** It may be **congenital** (usually from a birth injury) or **spasmodic** (usually psychogenic).

B. Scalene Muscles
1. Anterior, middle, and posterior scalenes descend from transverse processes of cervical vertebrae to rib 1 or 2.
2. Stabilize neck and act as accessory muscles of respiration

A cervical rib or hypertrophied anterior scalene muscle causes thoracic outlet syndrome.

Collateral circulation between the subclavian and external carotid arteries occurs via their costocervical and occipital branches.

Roots of the brachial plexus and the subclavian artery pass into the posterior triangle between the anterior and middle scalenes. An elongated transverse process on vertebra C7 **(cervical rib, Figure 7-3)** or hypertrophy of the scalene muscles may stretch or compress the **subclavian artery** and/or lower trunk of the **brachial plexus** (C8, T1) to produce **thoracic outlet syndrome.** It is characterized by **pain, numbness,** and **muscular weakness** of the upper extremity, most commonly in the distribution of the **ulnar nerve.**

IV. Arteries of Neck
A. Subclavian Artery (Figure 7-4; Table 7-1)
1. On right side arises from **brachiocephalic trunk** and on left side arises from **arch of aorta**
2. Arches laterally over **cervical pleura** and **apex of lung** and grooves **rib 1** between **anterior** and **middle scalene muscles**
3. Becomes **axillary artery** at lateral border of rib 1
4. Divided into **three parts** in relation to **anterior scalene**

The distal subclavian artery often can be safely ligated due to collateral circulation around the scapula.

The carotid pulse can be felt in the angle between the sternocleidomastoid and thyroid cartilage.

The **axillary artery** is **vulnerable to traumatic injury** in the posterior triangle. Compressing the **third part of the subclavian artery** against rib 1 may control **hemorrhage** in the axilla or upper extremity. **Aneurysms** of the subclavian artery usually involve the third part and may compress the **lower trunk of the brachial plexus.** The distal subclavian artery often can be **ligated** without adversely affecting the upper extremity because of extensive **anastomoses around the scapula** between subclavian and axillary artery branches.

B. Common Carotid Artery (see Figures 7-4 and 7-5)
1. Overview
   a. Arises from **brachiocephalic trunk** on right and from **arch of aorta** on left

Cervical Ribs and Related Anomalies

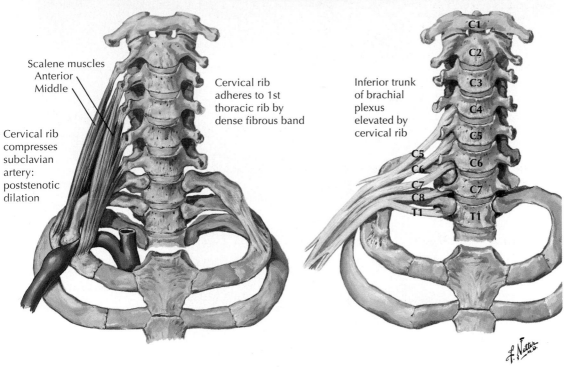

Scalene muscles
Anterior
Middle

Cervical rib
compresses
subclavian
artery:
poststenotic
dilation

Cervical rib
adheres to 1st
thoracic rib by
dense fibrous band

Inferior trunk
of brachial
plexus
elevated by
cervical rib

7-3: Cervical rib may stretch or compress lower trunk of brachial plexus or subclavian artery in thoracic outlet syndrome. *(From Netter, F H: Netter's Atlas of Human Anatomy, 3rd ed. Icon Learning Systems, 2003, Plate 181.)*

    b. Divides into **internal** and **external carotid** arteries at **superior border of thyroid cartilage (level of C4)**

> Ligation of the common carotid artery may be possible because of excellent **collateral circulation** between the external **carotid branches of the two sides** to the face and scalp; between the **superior and inferior thyroid arteries** and the **occipital and deep cervical arteries** connecting the external carotid and subclavian arteries; and from **vertebral artery contributions to the cerebral arterial circle**.
>
> **Extracranial carotid aneurysms** are uncommon and may present as asymptomatic, pulsatile swellings or cause symptoms such as **dyspnea, dysphagia, hoarseness,** tongue weakness, and **Horner syndrome**.

The common carotid artery divides at the superior border of the thyroid cartilage.

    2. **Internal carotid artery**
      • Normally has no branches in neck

> Partial **occlusion** of the **internal carotid artery** through **atherosclerosis** may reduce flow through the middle cerebral artery, with impaired sensory and motor function on the opposite side of the body. The **central artery of the retina** may also be affected, causing ipsilateral visual symptoms. A **carotid endarterectomy** may be performed to **remove plaque**, usually from the internal carotid artery at its origin.

The internal carotid artery has no branches in the neck.

A carotid endarterectomy removes internal carotid plaque to reduce stroke risk.

    3. **External carotid artery (Table 7-2)**
      a. Gives **eight branches,** four or five of which arise in carotid triangle
      b. Ends within **parotid gland** by dividing into **maxillary** and **superficial temporal** arteries

> To **control bleeding** from an inaccessible branch such as the middle meningeal, sphenopalatine, or lingual artery, the **external carotid artery can be ligated. Collateral circulation** occurs across the midline between external carotid branches and occurs also with branches of the internal carotid that originate intracranially.

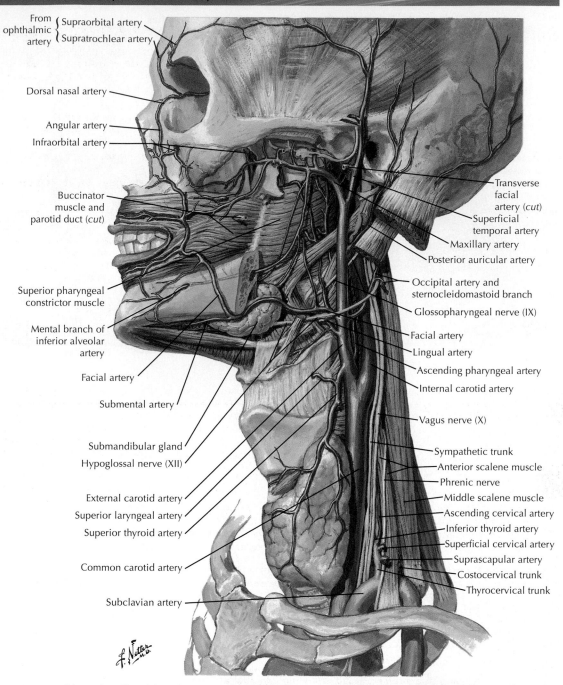

From ophthalmic artery { Supraorbital artery
Supratrochlear artery

Dorsal nasal artery

Angular artery

Infraorbital artery

Buccinator muscle and parotid duct (cut)

Superior pharyngeal constrictor muscle

Mental branch of inferior alveolar artery

Facial artery

Submental artery

Submandibular gland

Hypoglossal nerve (XII)

External carotid artery

Superior laryngeal artery

Superior thyroid artery

Common carotid artery

Subclavian artery

Transverse facial artery (cut)

Superficial temporal artery

Maxillary artery

Posterior auricular artery

Occipital artery and sternocleidomastoid branch

Glossopharyngeal nerve (IX)

Facial artery

Lingual artery

Ascending pharyngeal artery

Internal carotid artery

Vagus nerve (X)

Sympathetic trunk

Anterior scalene muscle

Phrenic nerve

Middle scalene muscle

Ascending cervical artery

Inferior thyroid artery

Superficial cervical artery

Suprascapular artery

Costocervical trunk

Thyrocervical trunk

7-4: Arteries of the neck and head, lateral view. Ramus of mandible has been removed to expose maxillary artery in infratemporal fossa of deep face. *(From Netter, F H: Atlas of Human Anatomy, 4th ed. Philadelphia, Saunders, 2006, Plate 69.)*

4. **Carotid sinus and carotid body**
   - Innervated mainly by carotid sinus branch of **glossopharyngeal nerve (IX)**
   a. **Carotid sinus**
      (1) Dilated terminal portion of common carotid artery and/or first part of **internal carotid**
      (2) Functions as **baroreceptor** for arterial **blood pressure**

External pressure on carotid sinus slows heartbeat and lowers blood pressure, causing some individuals to faint.

Some individuals develop hypersensitivity to **external pressure on the carotid sinus,** which may cause fainting **(carotid sinus syncope).** Care should be exercised, especially with cardiac patients, when taking the carotid pulse near the superior border of the thyroid cartilage.

TABLE 7-1. BRANCHES OF SUBCLAVIAN ARTERY

	SUPPLIES	COMMENTS
First Part		Medial to anterior scalene muscle
Vertebral artery	Spinal nerve roots, spinal cord, brainstem	Ascends transverse foramina of C1-C6, crosses posterior arch of atlas to enter foramen magnum; medullary branches reinforce blood flow to spinal arteries
Thyrocervical trunk		Three main branches
Inferior thyroid	Thyroid, parathyroid gland, larynx, esophagus	Main supply to parathyroid glands; forms collateral circulation with external carotid via anastomosis with superior thyroid artery
Transverse cervical	Trapezius, levator scapulae, and rhomboid muscles	Superficial branch on deep surface of trapezius; deep branch deep to rhomboids
Suprascapular	Supraspinatus and infraspinatus muscles	Crosses posterior triangle behind clavicle to pass above superior transverse scapular ligament
Internal thoracic	See Chapter 2	
Second Part		Posterior to anterior scalene muscle
Costocervical trunk		Runs posteriorly over cervical pleura dividing into deep cervical and superior intercostal branches
Deep cervical	Posterior neck muscles	Forms collateral circulation between subclavian and external carotid via anastomosis with occipital artery
Superior intercostal	First two intercostal spaces	Gives first two posterior intercostal arteries
Third Part		Between lateral borders of anterior scalene and rib 1
Dorsal scapular	Levator scapulae and rhomboid muscles	Variably present; replaces deep branch of transverse cervical when present

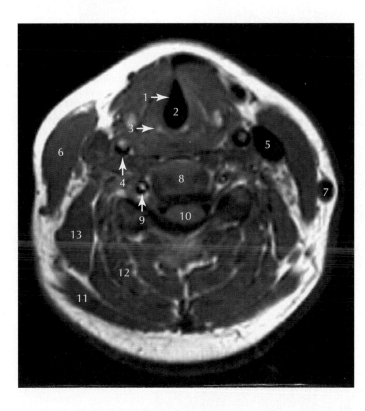

7-5: Axial MRI at level of larynx. Vocal fold = 1; rima glottidis = 2; arytenoid cartilage = 3; common carotid artery = 4; internal jugular vein = 5; sternocleidomastoid muscle = 6; external jugular vein = 7; vertebral body = 8; vertebral artery = 9; spinal cord = 10; trapezius muscle = 11; semispinalis muscle = 12; levator scapulae muscle = 13. *(From Weir, J, Abrahams, P: Imaging Atlas of Human Anatomy, 3rd ed. London, Mosby Ltd., 2003, p 23, f.)*

  b. **Carotid body**
    (1) Small structure deep to carotid bifurcation
    (2) Functions as **chemoreceptor** for blood gases reflexly changing heart rate, blood pressure, and respiration

V. **Veins of Neck and Superficial Head (Figure 7-6)**
  A. **Retromandibular Vein**
    1. Formed in parotid gland by union of **maxillary** and **superficial temporal veins**
    2. Splits into **anterior division** and **posterior division**
  B. **Facial Vein**

Carotid sinus: blood pressure receptor. Carotid body: blood gases receptor

TABLE 7-2. BRANCHES OF EXTERNAL CAROTID ARTERY

ARTERY	SUPPLIES	COMMENTS
Superior thyroid	Larynx, infrahyoid muscles, and thyroid gland	Travels with external laryngeal nerve
Lingual	Tongue, palatine tonsil, sublingual gland, and floor of mouth	Passes deep to hyoglossus muscle
Facial	Face, soft palate, palatine tonsil, and submandibular muscles	May arise in common with lingual artery
Ascending pharyngeal	Pharynx, palatine tonsil, and meninges	
Occipital	Posterior scalp, sternomastoid, and meninges	Parallels greater occipital nerve in scalp
Posterior auricular	Scalp, auricle, and facial nerve	
Maxillary	Muscles of mastication, temporomandibular joint, meninges, nasal cavity, palate, mandibular and maxillary teeth, and face	Terminal branch described with infratemporal and pterygopalatine fossae
Superficial temporal	Parotid gland, face, and scalp	Terminal branch described with face; ascends with auriculotemporal nerve

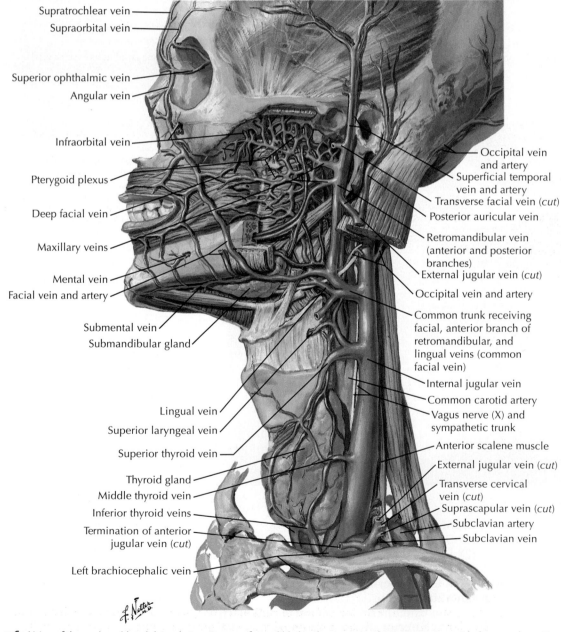

7-6: Veins of the neck and head, lateral view. Ramus of mandible has been removed to expose pterygoid plexus and maxillary veins in infratemporal fossa. Most of sternocleidomastoid muscle and overlying external jugular vein have been removed. *(From Netter, F H: Atlas of Human Anatomy, 4th ed. Philadelphia, Saunders, 2006, Plate 70.)*

1. Begins at medial angle of eye as **angular vein** and descends on face with **facial artery**
2. Below mandible joins **anterior division of retromandibular vein** to form **common facial vein,** which ends in internal jugular vein

C. **External Jugular Vein (see Figure 7-6)**
1. Formed by union of **posterior auricular vein** and **posterior division of retromandibular vein**
2. Descends obliquely across **sternocleidomastoid** to empty into **subclavian vein**

The **external jugular vein** can be easily cannulated. In the recumbent patient, the vein is normally distended and can usually be made more prominent by increasing intrathoracic pressure (e.g., holding one's breath). If the vein is **lacerated** where it penetrates the **investing layer of deep cervical fascia,** the fascial attachment prevents its collapse so that air sucked into the vein travels to the right side of the heart and may obstruct blood flow **(venous air embolism).**

> A venous air embolism from a cut external jugular vein may obstruct blood flow through the right heart.

D. **Anterior Jugular Vein**
1. Begins in **submental region,** descends near anterior midline, and drains into **external jugular vein**
2. Just above jugular notch may be connected to opposite vein by **jugular venous arch**

The **jugular venous arch** is in danger during a **tracheostomy.**

E. **Internal Jugular Vein (see Figure 7-6)**
1. Begins in **superior bulb** at **jugular foramen** as continuation of **intracranial sigmoid dural venous sinus**
2. Ends in **inferior bulb** that joins **subclavian vein** to form **brachiocephalic vein**

> The internal jugular vein is the continuation of the sigmoid sinus.

To **catheterize** the **internal jugular vein,** a needle can be inserted into the triangular interval formed by the clavicle and the clavicular and sternal heads of the **sternocleidomastoid** (central approach). **Venous air embolism** is a possible complication of **catheterization** or **laceration** of the internal jugular vein.

Deep cervical lymph nodes may **adhere to the internal jugular vein** because of **inflammation** or **malignancy,** with the vein tearing during surgical removal of the nodes. The vein is removed during block dissection of the neck for metastatic carcinoma.

> The internal jugular vein may be removed during radical neck dissection for cancer.

F. **Subclavian Vein**
1. Begins at **lateral border of rib 1** as continuation of **axillary vein**
2. Passes **anterior** to anterior **scalene muscle** and joins **internal jugular vein** to form **brachiocephalic vein**
3. Receives **external jugular vein** as its only constant tributary

> Basilic + brachial veins → axillary vein → subclavian vein

> The internal jugular and subclavian veins are used for central venous lines.

To enter the **subclavian vein** for **central venous line** placement, a needle can be directed medially and superiorly from below the junction of the middle and medial thirds of the clavicle (infraclavicular approach). Potential complications include **arterial puncture** and **pneumothorax.**

The subclavian vein may be **obstructed** as it crosses rib 1 by a **hypertrophied subclavius muscle** or **fibrous extension of the anterior scalene** insertion. **Obstruction** may cause **venous thrombosis** or intermittent **upper-extremity edema.** Venous thrombosis may also occur due to trauma in the costoclavicular space from repeated upper extremity movements **(effort thrombosis),** possibly resulting in **pulmonary embolism.**

> A misdirected needle during subclavian vein puncture may cause pneumothorax.

VI. **Lymphatics in Neck (Table 7-3)**
A. **General Arrangement**
- Lymph may drain first to one of several **regional groups** of nodes, some of which form a **circular collar** around the junction of the head and neck, but all drain eventually into **deep cervical lymph nodes.**

TABLE 7-3. LYMPH NODES OF NECK AND HEAD

Horizontal Group	Arranged in circular collar at junction of head and neck
Occipital	Back of scalp and neck
Mastoid	Posterior scalp, auricle, and external auditory meatus
Parotid	Anterior scalp, external and middle ear, and parotid gland
Submandibular	Scalp, face, upper lip, and side of tongue
Submental	Tip of tongue, floor of mouth, lower lip, and chin
Vertical Group	Most deep structures
Tracheal	Trachea, larynx, thyroid, and superficial neck below hyoid
Retropharyngeal	Nasopharynx, auditory tube, and middle ear
Superficial cervical (along external jugular vein)	Lower parotid, auricle, mastoid, and angle of mandible
Deep cervical (along internal jugular vein)	Entire head and neck, either directly or through regional lymph nodes
Superior group with jugulodigastric node	Palatine tonsil and posterior third of tongue, larynx, and pharynx
Inferior group with jugulo-omohyoid node	Anterior two-thirds of tongue, larynx, pharynx, and thyroid gland

B. Destination
- Lymph reaches **jugular lymph trunk,** which on **left** usually joins **thoracic duct** and on **right** either joins **right lymphatic duct** or empties directly into junction of internal jugular and subclavian veins (right venous angle)

Supraclavicular lymph node enlargement is often the first sign of thoracic or abdominal cancer.

Enlarged lymph nodes above the clavicle (**supraclavicular nodes**) are often the first indication of malignant disease in thoracic and abdominal organs and have been called **sentinel nodes.**

All head and neck lymphatics drain directly or indirectly into the deep cervical lymph nodes.

VII. Nerves of Neck
- **A. Cervical Plexus (Figure 7-7; Table 7-4)**
  - Formed by **anterior rami** of spinal nerves **C1-C4**
  1. **Phrenic nerve (C3,4,5 but mostly from C4)**
     - Descends on anterior scalene muscle passing behind subclavian vein

On x-rays, the paralyzed hemidiaphragm paradoxically elevates during inspiration.

Intractable **hiccups,** which are spasmodic contractions of the diaphragm, may be treated by **crushing or sectioning** the **phrenic nerve** as it lies on the anterior scalene. A damaged phrenic nerve will paralyze the hemidiaphragm, which may show symptoms only during exertion. On x-rays, the paralyzed hemidiaphragm is elevated during inspiration (**paradoxical movement**).

C3,4,5 keep the diaphragm alive.

Spinal cord transection or **compression at C4 or above** compromises the phrenic nerve and is **incompatible with unaided breathing.**

  2. **Supraclavicular nerves (C3,4)**
     - Supply skin over clavicle and shoulder and over upper thorax

When evaluating **cervical spinal cord injuries,** it is important to remember that cord damage at **C5** will not affect the upper cervical nerves but will **compromise the function** of all spinal nerves **below C5.** Some sensation over the upper thorax typically remains because innervation is by the **supraclavicular nerves** and not the thoracic spinal nerves. The effect on respiration will vary, depending on spinal cord levels contributing to the phrenic nerve.

Assessment of spinal cord injuries must consider cutaneous innervation of the upper thorax by the cervical plexus.

The four cutaneous branches of the cervical plexus emerge at the midpoint of the posterior border of the sternocleidomastoid. Local **anesthetic** infiltrated at this point will anesthetize most **skin of the neck.**

- **B. Brachial Plexus Branches in Neck (see Figure 6-10)**
  1. **Dorsal scapular nerve**
     - Arises from **C5** root to supply **levator scapulae, rhomboid major,** and **rhomboid minor**

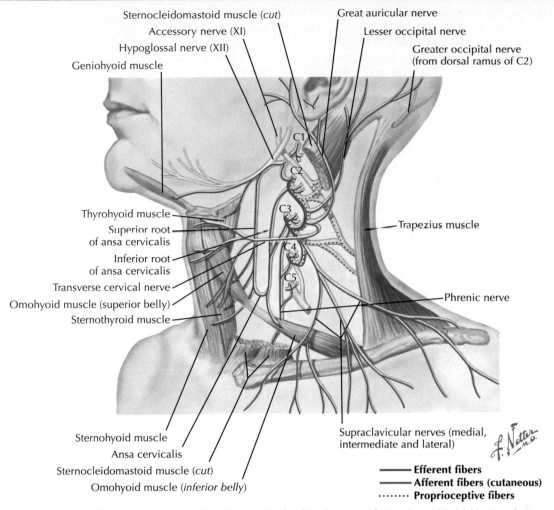

Sternocleidomastoid muscle (cut)
Accessory nerve (XI)
Hypoglossal nerve (XII)
Geniohyoid muscle
Great auricular nerve
Lesser occipital nerve
Greater occipital nerve
(from dorsal ramus of C2)
C1
C2
C3
C4
C5
Thyrohyoid muscle
Superior root
of ansa cervicalis
Inferior root
of ansa cervicalis
Transverse cervical nerve
Omohyoid muscle (superior belly)
Sternothyroid muscle
Trapezius muscle
Phrenic nerve
Sternohyoid muscle
Ansa cervicalis
Sternocleidomastoid muscle (cut)
Omohyoid muscle (inferior belly)
Supraclavicular nerves (medial,
intermediate and lateral)

Efferent fibers
Afferent fibers (cutaneous)
Proprioceptive fibers

7-7: Cervical plexus of nerves. *(From Norton, N S: Netter's Head and Neck Anatomy for Dentistry. Philadelphia, Saunders, 2007, p 151.)*

TABLE 7-4. CERVICAL PLEXUS OF NERVES

	SUPPLIES	COMMENTS
Cutaneous Nerves		Emerge near middle of posterior border of sternocleidomastoid
Lesser occipital (C2)	Scalp behind ear	
Great auricular (C2, C3)	Skin over auricle, parotid gland and angle of mandible, and mastoid process	
Transverse cervical (C2, C3)	Skin over anterior triangle	
Supraclavicular (C3, C4)	Skin over root of neck, shoulder, and upper thorax	May refer pain to shoulder from phrenic nerve distribution
Mixed Motor Nerves		
Phrenic (C3, **C4**, C5)	Motor to diaphragm, sensory to pericardium, mediastinal pleura, diaphragmatic pleura and peritoneum	Accessory phrenic nerve from C5 usually from nerve to subclavius
Ansa cervicalis (C1-3)	Motor to infrahyoid muscles (except thyrohyoid)	Nerve loop anterior to carotid artery
Superior root (C1) (descendens hypoglossi)		Appears to branch from hypoglossal nerve
Inferior root (C2, C3) (descendens cervicalis)		
Direct muscular branches with somatic nerve fibers	Geniohyoid, thyrohyoid, prevertebral, levator scapulae, and scalene muscles	Segmental supply by branches directly from the roots; contain all functional components of typical spinal nerve
Muscular branches without somatic motor fibers	Sternocleidomastoid (C2, C3) and trapezius (C3, C4)	Contain all components of spinal nerve except general somatic efferent fibers, which are from accessory nerve (CN XI)

2. **Long thoracic nerve**
   • Arises from **C5,6,7** roots to supply **serratus anterior**
3. **Suprascapular nerve**
   a. Arises from **upper trunk (C5,6)** of brachial plexus
   b. Supplies **supraspinatus and infraspinatus muscles** and glenohumeral joint
4. **Nerve to subclavius**
   a. Arises from **upper trunk (C5)** of brachial plexus to supply subclavius muscle
   b. Frequently gives rise to **accessory phrenic nerve (C5)**

Nerve to subclavius may give rise to accessory phrenic nerve.

Roots, trunks, and divisions of the **brachial plexus** lie superior to the clavicle in the posterior triangle and may be **damaged** there by **trauma** or a **tumor**.

C. **Cranial Nerves in Neck**
   1. **Hypoglossal nerve (CN XII)**
      a. Loops below posterior belly of digastric muscle ascending into **tongue** to supply its **muscles**
      b. **Superior root of ansa cervicalis** and **nerve to thyrohyoid** muscle (both from **C1**) travel with and **appear to branch** from hypoglossal nerve
   2. **Spinal accessory nerve (CN XI)**
      • Supplies **sternocleidomastoid** and then crosses **posterior cervical triangle** to supply **trapezius**

The inability to shrug the shoulder indicates spinal accessory nerve injury.

The relatively superficial **spinal accessory nerve** can be **damaged by surgery** or a **penetrating wound** in the posterior triangle. Injury produces **paralysis and wasting of the trapezius,** causing asymmetry in the slope of the neck, drooping of the shoulder, and weakness lifting the arm above the horizontal.

The vagus nerve supplies most of the muscles of the soft palate, pharynx, and larynx.

3. **Vagus nerve (CN X)**
   • Descends within **carotid sheath** posteriorly between **internal jugular vein** and **carotid artery**
   a. **Pharyngeal branch**
      • Special visceral efferent (SVE) fibers to most **muscles of pharynx and soft palate** via **pharyngeal plexus**
   b. **Superior laryngeal nerve**
      • Divides into **internal** and **external laryngeal nerves** for sensory supply (general visceral afferent [GVA]) of upper larynx and piriform recess and motor innervation (SVE) of **cricothyroid** muscle, respectively
   c. **Cardiac branches**
      • Convey **preganglionic parasympathetic (GVE)** and GVA fibers to cardiac plexuses of thorax
   d. **Recurrent laryngeal nerve**
      • Ends as **inferior laryngeal nerve** to supply SVE fibers to **intrinsic laryngeal muscles,** except cricothyroid, and GVA fibers to larynx below vocal fold

The recurrent laryngeal nerve supplies the muscles that control the size of the airway for respiration and phonation.

The glossopharyngeal nerve supplies taste and general sensation to the posterior one-third of the tongue.

4. **Glossopharyngeal nerve (CN IX)**
   a. From jugular foramen curves around **stylopharyngeus muscle,** accompanying it between superior and middle pharyngeal constrictors
   b. Courses through **bed of palatine tonsil** to posterior third of tongue
   c. Provides SVE fibers to **stylopharyngeus, general sensation (GVA)** to pharyngeal wall and posterior third of tongue, and **taste sensation** (special visceral afferent [SVA]) to posterior third of tongue

D. **Sympathetic Nerves in Neck**
   1. **Cervical sympathetic trunk**
      • Contains **ascending preganglionic sympathetic fibers (GVE)** from cell bodies in upper thoracic spinal cord segments and GVA fibers from cell bodies in dorsal root ganglia at same levels
   2. **Superior cervical ganglion**

All sympathetic fibers in the head are postganglionic and arise from cell bodies in the superior cervical ganglion.

   a. **All postganglionic sympathetic fibers to the head** via **internal** and **external carotid periarterial plexuses**
   b. **Gray rami communicantes** to spinal nerves C1-C4
   c. **Superior cervical sympathetic cardiac nerve** to thoracic cardiac plexus

3. **Middle cervical ganglion**
    a. **Gray rami communicantes** to spinal nerves C5-C6
    b. **Middle cervical sympathetic cardiac nerve**
    c. Branches to **periarterial plexus** around **inferior thyroid artery**
4. **Inferior cervical ganglion**
    a. Often fuses with ganglion of T1 to form **cervicothoracic** (stellate) **ganglion**
    b. **Gray rami communicantes** to spinal nerves **C7-C8**
    c. **Inferior cervical sympathetic cardiac nerve**
    d. Branches to **periarterial plexus** around **vertebral** and **subclavian** arteries
5. **Cervicothoracic (stellate) ganglion**
    • Fusion of inferior cervical and T1 sympathetic ganglia over neck of rib 1

> **Horner syndrome** is drooping of the upper eyelid **(ptosis)**, constriction of the pupil **(miosis)**, absence of sweating **(anhidrosis)**, and facial flushing and warmth due to **vasodilation**. Penetrating **injury** to the neck, **Pancoast** (apical lung) **tumor**, or **thyroid carcinoma** may cause Horner syndrome by interrupting the ascending preganglionic sympathetic fibers anywhere between their origin in the upper thoracic spinal cord and their synapse in the superior cervical ganglion. In **sympathectomies** for excess vasoconstriction in the upper extremity, Horner syndrome is avoided by sparing the stellate ganglion.

Horner syndrome is ptosis, miosis, anhidrosis, and vasodilation following injury to the cervical sympathetic trunk.

Unexplained Horner syndrome requires screening for a Pancoast tumor.

VIII. **Pharynx (Figures 7-8 and 7-9)**
    • Wall consists of **mucosa** and **pharyngeal musculature** that is lined internally by **pharyngobasilar fascia** and externally by **buccopharyngeal fascia**
A. **Nasopharynx**
    • Extends from base of skull to soft palate
    1. **Pharyngeal tonsil**
        • Embedded in upper **posterior wall** of nasopharynx but usually regresses after puberty

Nasopharynx: skullbase to soft palate. Oropharynx: soft palate to epiglottis. Laryngopharynx: epiglottis to bottom of cricoid cartilage

Adenoids are enlarged pharyngeal tonsils that may block nasal breathing, impair hearing, and spread infection to the tympanic cavity.

> **Adenoids** is hypertrophy of the **pharyngeal tonsil** and may obstruct airflow through the nasopharynx in children, causing chronic **mouth breathing**. A blocked auditory tube may impair hearing. **Adenoiditis** is common and readily spreads infection to the tympanic cavity through the auditory tube in children, causing **otitis media**, in part because of the tube's more horizontal orientation and shorter length.

2. **Auditory tube**
    a. Overview
        (1) Connects **nasopharynx** to **tympanic cavity,** allowing both equalization of pressure in middle ear and spread of infection
        (2) Covered by mucosa at its opening into pharynx to form **torus tubarius**
    b. **Cartilaginous part**
        (1) **Anterior two-thirds** that opens into nasopharynx
        (2) Normally closed but opens upon **swallowing** or **yawning** because of traction from **levator and tensor veli palatini muscles**
    c. **Bony part**
        (1) **Posterior third** that opens into tympanic cavity
        (2) Lies within **petrous temporal bone** and is always open
B. **Oropharynx**
    1. Extends from **soft palate** to superior border of **epiglottis**
    2. Related anteriorly to **oral cavity** and posterior third of tongue
    3. **Palatine tonsil (Figures 7-10 and 7-11)**
        a. Lymphoid tissue in **tonsillar fossa** between anterior **palatoglossal** and posterior **palatopharyngeal folds** but regresses after puberty
        b. Capsule of pharyngobasilar fascia separated by loose connective tissue (peritonsillar space) from superior pharyngeal constrictor
        c. Related at its lower pole to **glossopharyngeal nerve** as it descends to posterior third of tongue
        d. Receives main blood supply from tonsillar branch of facial artery
        e. Drained by **lymph vessels** mainly to **jugulodigastric lymph node,** which is body's most frequently enlarged lymph node

Otitis media is more common in infants due to the more horizonal auditory tube.

The palatine tonsil occupies the tonsillar fossa between the palatoglossal and palatopharyngeal folds.

The jugulodigastric node is called the tonsillar node due to its frequent enlargement during tonsillitis.

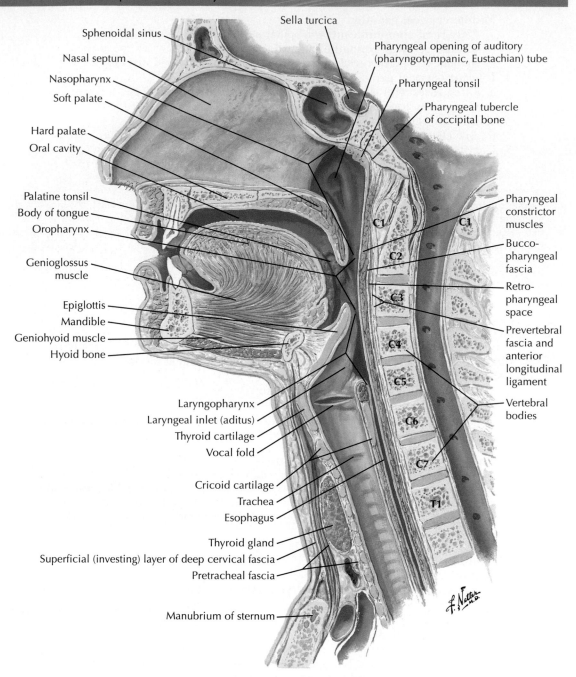

Sella turcica

Sphenoidal sinus

Nasal septum

Nasopharynx

Soft palate

Hard palate

Oral cavity

Palatine tonsil

Body of tongue

Oropharynx

Genioglossus muscle

Epiglottis

Mandible

Geniohyoid muscle

Hyoid bone

Laryngopharynx

Laryngeal inlet (aditus)

Thyroid cartilage

Vocal fold

Cricoid cartilage

Trachea

Esophagus

Thyroid gland

Superficial (investing) layer of deep cervical fascia

Pretracheal fascia

Manubrium of sternum

Pharyngeal opening of auditory (pharyngotympanic, Eustachian) tube

Pharyngeal tonsil

Pharyngeal tubercle of occipital bone

Pharyngeal constrictor muscles

Bucco-pharyngeal fascia

Retro-pharyngeal space

Prevertebral fascia and anterior longitudinal ligament

Vertebral bodies

C1, C2, C3, C4, C5, C6, C7, T1

7-8: Midsagittal section through the head and neck showing relationships of the alimentary and respiratory tracts. *(From Netter, F H: Atlas of Human Anatomy, 4th ed. Philadelphia, Saunders, 2006, Plate 63.)*

A peritonsillar abscess (quinsy) is a life-threatening complication of acute tonsillitis.

Peritonsillar abscess (quinsy), a life-threatening **complication of acute tonsillitis,** mainly affects adolescents and young adults. The soft palate and uvula are edematous and displaced toward the unaffected side. Sore throat, dysphagia, muffled voice, and trismus may be present.

Tonsillectomy may cause loss of taste and general sensation from the posterior third of the tongue.

During **palatine tonsillectomy,** the peritonsillar space facilitates tonsil removal, except after capsular adhesion to the superior constrictor in chronic tonsillitis. If the **glossopharyngeal nerve** is injured, taste and general sensation from the posterior third of the tongue are lost. **Hemorrhage** may occur, usually from the **tonsillar branch of the facial artery** or **paratonsillar (external palatine) vein;** if the superior constrictor is penetrated, a **tortuous internal carotid artery** may be injured with fatal consequences.

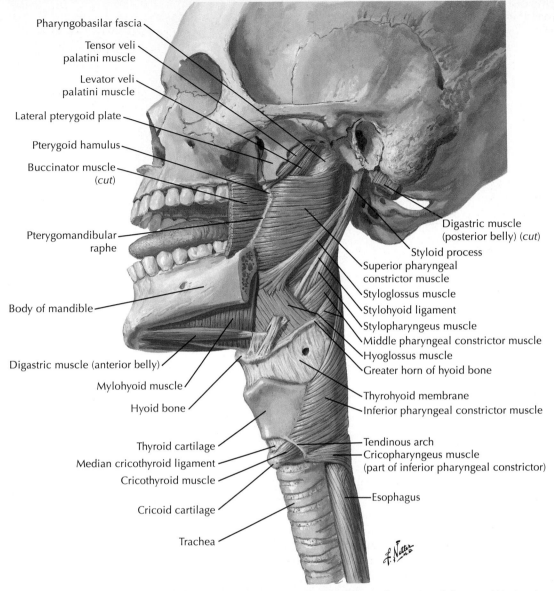

Pharyngobasilar fascia

Tensor veli palatini muscle

Levator veli palatini muscle

Lateral pterygoid plate

Pterygoid hamulus

Buccinator muscle (cut)

Pterygomandibular raphe

Body of mandible

Digastric muscle (anterior belly)

Mylohyoid muscle

Hyoid bone

Thyroid cartilage

Median cricothyroid ligament

Cricothyroid muscle

Cricoid cartilage

Trachea

Digastric muscle (posterior belly) (cut)

Styloid process

Superior pharyngeal constrictor muscle

Styloglossus muscle

Stylohyoid ligament

Stylopharyngeus muscle

Middle pharyngeal constrictor muscle

Hyoglossus muscle

Greater horn of hyoid bone

Thyrohyoid membrane

Inferior pharyngeal constrictor muscle

Tendinous arch

Cricopharyngeus muscle (part of inferior pharyngeal constrictor)

Esophagus

7-9: Pharyngeal constrictor muscles and their anterior attachments, lateral view. The ramus of the mandible has been removed. (From Netter, F H. Atlas of Human Anatomy, 4th ed. Philadelphia, Saunders, 2006, Plate 68.)

7-10: Oral cavity and palatal arches.

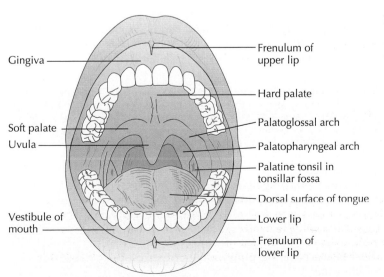

Gingiva

Soft palate

Uvula

Vestibule of mouth

Frenulum of upper lip

Hard palate

Palatoglossal arch

Palatopharyngeal arch

Palatine tonsil in tonsillar fossa

Dorsal surface of tongue

Lower lip

Frenulum of lower lip

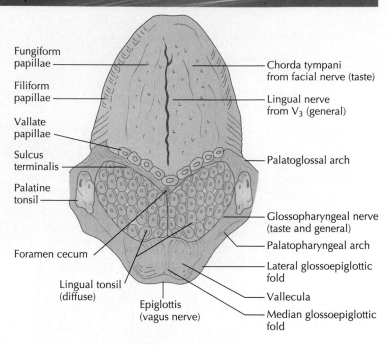

7-11: Oral (*gray*) and pharyngeal (*red*) parts of tongue and epiglottis, superior view.

Fungiform papillae

Filiform papillae

Vallate papillae

Sulcus terminalis

Palatine tonsil

Foramen cecum

Lingual tonsil (diffuse)

Chorda tympani from facial nerve (taste)

Lingual nerve from V₃ (general)

Palatoglossal arch

Glossopharyngeal nerve (taste and general)

Palatopharyngeal arch

Lateral glossoepiglottic fold

Vallecula

Median glossoepiglottic fold

Epiglottis (vagus nerve)

C. **Laryngopharynx**
1. Related to larynx and extends from superior border of **epiglottis** to inferior border of **cricoid cartilage**
2. Piriform recesses related to internal laryngeal nerves just deep to mucous membrane

> The internal laryngeal nerve can be topically anesthetized in piriform recess.

> **Sharp foreign objects** (e.g., bone fragments) may lodge in the **piriform recess**. The object or attempts to remove it may damage the **internal laryngeal nerve**.

D. **Muscles of Pharynx (Figure 7-12; see Figure 7-9)**
- Include three pairs of **circularly arranged** pharyngeal constrictor muscles outside three pairs of **longitudinal** muscles
1. **Pharyngeal constrictor muscles**
   a. Designated **superior, middle,** and **inferior**
   b. Bony and cartilaginous attachments anteriorly but are attached posteriorly only at median **pharyngeal raphe**
   c. Sequential contractions move food bolus inferiorly into esophagus
   d. **Gap between superior** and **middle constrictors** traversed by **stylopharyngeus muscle** and **glossopharyngeal nerve**

> The cricopharyngeus muscle is the upper esophageal sphincter, and its inability to relax during swallowing causes dysphagia.

> The cricopharyngeus is a common site of pharyngeal diverticula.

> The **cricopharyngeus region of the inferior pharyngeal constrictor** functions as the **upper esophageal sphincter** and remains tonically contracted except during swallowing. Its **spasm** may cause **dysphagia** and require **myotomy. Impaired contraction** may result in **aspiration** of regurgitated stomach contents in gastroesophageal reflux disease.
>
> **Pouches or diverticula** may develop at the sites of relative **weakness in the pharyngeal wall** where constrictors do not overlap. They most commonly arise in the **cricopharyngeus region.** Food may fill the pouch and cause **dysphagia** or be regurgitated and inhaled into the respiratory passages, inducing **aspiration pneumonia** and/or choking.

2. **Longitudinally arranged muscles**
   a. **Palatopharyngeus, salpingopharyngeus,** and **stylopharyngeus**
   b. Arise near base of skull and descend between pharyngeal constrictors and pharyngobasilar fascia to insert into wall of pharynx and thyroid cartilage
   c. Elevate pharynx to receive bolus of food
E. **Pharyngeal Plexus**
- Lies in **buccopharyngeal fascia** covering **pharyngeal constrictors** and receives contributions from the following:
1. **Vagus nerve**

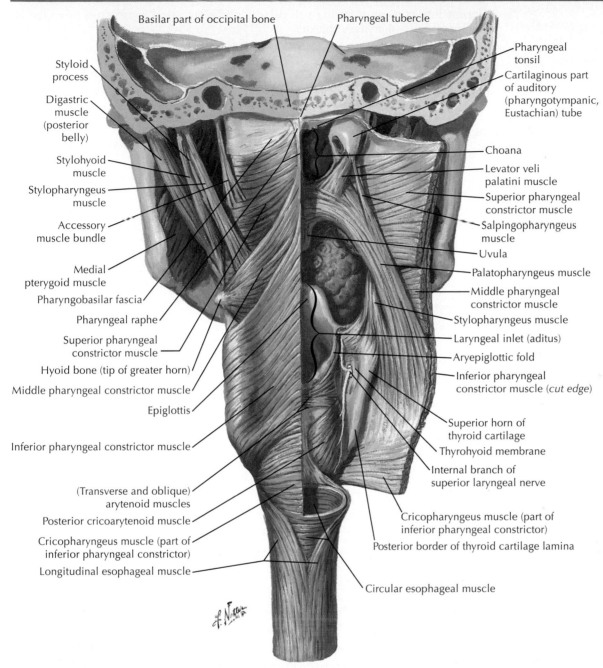

7-12: Pharyngeal muscles, posterior view. Right side of posterior pharyngeal wall has been reflected laterally to show longitudinally arranged pharyngeal muscles. *(From Netter, F H: Atlas of Human Anatomy, 4th ed. Philadelphia, Saunders, 2006, Plate 67.)*

- SVE fibers to **muscles** of pharynx and soft palate
2. **Glossopharyngeal nerve**
   - GVA fibers from **mucosa** of oropharynx
3. **Superior cervical sympathetic ganglion**
   - Postganglionic sympathetic fibers to **blood vessels** and **glands** of pharynx
F. **Blood Supply of Pharynx**
   1. Mainly from **ascending pharyngeal branch** of **external carotid artery**
   2. Also receives small branches of facial and maxillary arteries and superior and inferior thyroid arteries
G. **Deglutition (Swallowing)**
   1. Initiated voluntarily but completed by reflex; therefore, ***both*** **afferent and efferent innervation must be intact for normal swallowing**
   2. **Afferent innervation** of mucosa of posterior tongue and oropharynx provided by **glossopharyngeal nerve**

Stroking the mucosa of the pharynx elicits the gag reflex that tests the integrity of cranial nerves IX and X.

3. **Efferent innervation** of levator veli palatini and pharyngeal constrictors provided by **vagus nerve** via pharyngeal plexus

Pharyngeal neoplasm may cause otalgia.

Pharyngeal neoplasms may irritate cranial nerves IX and X. Pain that occurs when **swallowing** is then referred to the ear **(otalgia)** because both nerves also contribute sensory innervation to the external ear canal.

Vertebral levels: Hyoid bone: C3. Thyroid cartilage: C4-5. Cricoid cartilage: C6

IX. Larynx
A. Laryngeal Skeleton (Figure 7-13)
- Cartilaginous framework that moves superiorly and inferiorly with hyoid bone

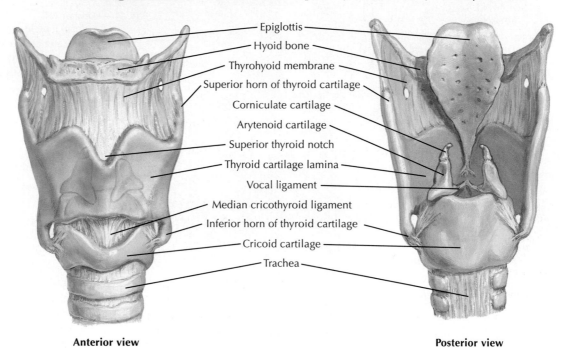

Epiglottis
Hyoid bone
Thyrohyoid membrane
Superior horn of thyroid cartilage
Corniculate cartilage
Arytenoid cartilage
Superior thyroid notch
Thyroid cartilage lamina
Vocal ligament
Median cricothyroid ligament
Inferior horn of thyroid cartilage
Cricoid cartilage
Trachea

Anterior view

Posterior view

Epiglottis
Hyoid bone
Thyrohyoid membrane
Thyroid cartilage lamina
Oblique line
Laryngeal prominence
Corniculate cartilage
Arytenoid cartilage
Muscular process
Vocal process
Vocal ligament
Median } Lateral }
Cricothyroid ligament
Cricoid cartilage
Cricothyroid joint
Trachea

Right lateral view

Medial view, median (sagittal) section

7-13: Laryngeal skeleton. In the median sagittal section (*lower right*) the vocal ligament, which is the superior free border of the cricothyroid ligament (conus elasticus), is seen extending between the vocal process of the arytenoid cartilage and the thyroid cartilage. (*From Netter, F H: Atlas of Human Anatomy, 4th ed. Philadelphia, Saunders, 2006, Plate 77.*)

1. **Thyroid cartilage**
   - Paired **laminae** fused anteriorly at **laryngeal prominence**
2. **Cricoid cartilage**
   a. Shaped like a signet ring with posterior shield (**lamina**) and narrow anterior **arch**
   b. Articulates with inferior horns of thyroid cartilage at **cricothyroid joints** and with arytenoid cartilages at **cricoarytenoid joints**
3. **Arytenoid cartilage**
   a. Paired cartilage articulating with superior edge of cricoid lamina
   b. **Vocal process** provides attachment for **vocal ligament**
   c. **Muscular process** provides attachment for **lateral cricoarytenoid** and **posterior cricoarytenoid muscles**
4. **Epiglottic cartilage**
   - Leaf-shaped cartilage posterior to root of tongue and anterior to laryngeal aditus
5. **Corniculate and cuneiform cartilages**
   - Small cartilages embedded within **aryepiglottic folds** that produce nodules seen through **laryngoscope**

B. **Laryngeal Cavity and Folds (Figures 7-14 and 7-15)**
   1. **Vestibular fold (false vocal cord)**
      a. Superior fold containing **vestibular ligament** and separated from opposite fold by **rima vestibuli**
      b. Apposes opposite fold to protect airway during swallowing and in **Valsalva maneuver**

> The **Valsalva maneuver** is attempted forced expiration against an airway closed by tightly adducted vocal and vestibular folds (e.g., during a cough). Strong anterolateral abdominal muscle contractions and a relaxed diaphragm result in **increased intrathoracic pressure, impeding venous return** to the right atrium. Therefore, **elderly and cardiac patients** are reminded to **not** hold their breath when straining, as during heavy lifting. The Valsalva maneuver is sometimes used to help **diagnose cardiac abnormalities** and may help arrest **supraventricular tachycardia.**

The Valsalva maneuver is attempted forced expiration against a closed airway.

The Valsalva maneuver is dangerous in cardiac patients.

   2. **Vocal fold (true vocal cord) (see Figures 7-5, 7-8, and 7-14)**
      a. Inferior fold containing **vocal ligament** and **vocalis muscle**
      b. Separated from opposite fold by rima glottidis, which is narrower than rima vestibuli; the glottis is the vocal folds plus the rima glottidis
   3. **Vestibule (supraglottic compartment)**
      - Laryngeal cavity superior to vestibular folds

Vocal folds are more medial than vestibular folds, so both are visible on laryngoscopy.

The cough reflex (X) attempts to expel foreign objects from the larynx or trachea.

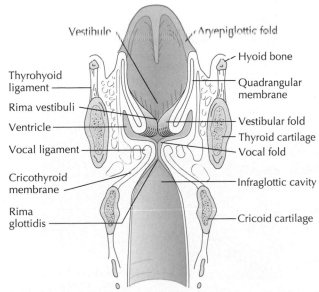

7-14: Coronal section of larynx showing internal features and their relationships to the laryngeal skeleton.

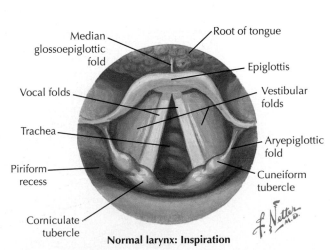

Normal larynx: Inspiration

7-15: Larynx during inspiration viewed through laryngoscope. (From Norton, N S: Netter's Head and Neck Anatomy for Dentistry. Philadelphia, Saunders 2007, p 458.)

The mucosa of the **vestibule** is sensitive to the entrance of **foreign objects,** resulting in vigorous coughing to expel the object **(cough reflex).** The **vagus nerve** mediates both afferent and efferent limbs of the reflex arc.

Epiglottitis is a life-threatening mucosal swelling of the airway in children.

Epiglottitis (supraglottitis) is a **life-threatening airway obstruction** caused by acute mucosal swelling over the epiglottis and other supraglottic structures, historically due to *Haemophilus influenzae* type B. The swollen epiglottis is visible as a **thumbprint-shaped** structure on lateral radiographs **(Figure 7-16).** Attempts to examine the larynx of young children with epiglottitis may precipitate sudden airway obstruction.

4. **Ventricle**
   a. Lateral recess between vestibular fold and vocal fold containing glands that lubricate vocal fold
   b. May expand superiorly and anteriorly as **saccule** of variable size
5. **Infraglottic cavity**
   • Laryngeal cavity inferior to vocal fold and continuous with trachea

In cricothyrotomy, the infraglottic cavity is entered below the obstruction at the vocal folds.

Aspirated foreign bodies ("cafe coronary") or **edema** in the **laryngeal mucosa** may obstruct the laryngeal airway. An emergency airway below the vocal folds may be made through the cricothyroid membrane **(cricothyrotomy)** or the trachea **(tracheostomy,** tracheotomy). In cricothyrotomy, the incision or needle passes successively through the skin, superficial fascia, investing layer of deep cervical fascia, pretracheal fascia, and median cricothyroid ligament. A **tracheostomy** may cause bleeding from the anterior jugular veins or jugular venous arch, inferior thyroid vein(s), isthmus of the thyroid gland, or if present, a thyroid ima artery. In a young child, the left brachiocephalic vein is also in danger due to the shorter neck. Incisions made too deeply, especially in a child, may damage the esophagus.

Tracheostomy incision may cause bleeding from midline vascular structures.

C. **Ligaments and Membranes of the Larynx (see Figures 7-13 and 7-14)**
   1. **Thyrohyoid membrane**
      a. Connects superior border of thyroid cartilage to inferior border of hyoid bone
      b. Pierced by **internal laryngeal nerve** and **superior laryngeal artery**

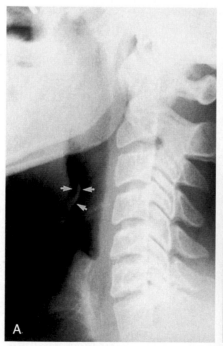
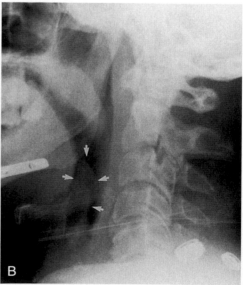

7-16: Lateral radiograph showing delicate curved structure of normal epiglottis (*arrows*) in **A** and thumbprint-shaped swollen epiglottis of epiglottitis in **B**. Notice the reduced size of the airway in the epiglottitis patient. (*From Mettler, F A: Essentials of Radiology, 2nd ed. Philadelphia, Saunders, 2004, Figure 2-34.*)

2. **Cricothyroid membrane (conus elasticus)**
   - Extends from cricoid cartilage upward deep to thyroid cartilage
3. **Vocal ligament**
   a. Thickened **superior free margin of conus elasticus** forming core of **vocal fold**
   b. Attached to **thyroid cartilage** and **vocal process of arytenoid cartilage**
4. **Quadrangular membrane**
   - Connects arytenoid and epiglottic cartilages in lateral wall of vestibule with superior and inferior free margins forming cores of **aryepiglottic** and **vestibular folds,** respectively

D. **Actions of Selected Intrinsic Laryngeal Muscles**
   1. **Posterior cricoarytenoid muscles**
      - **Abduct** vocal folds by rotating arytenoid cartilages laterally
   2. **Lateral cricoarytenoid muscles**
      - **Adduct** vocal folds by rotating arytenoid cartilages medially
   3. **Cricothyroid muscles**
      - **Lengthen and tense** vocal cords by tilting thyroid cartilage forward on cricoid cartilage
   4. **Vocalis muscles**
      - Lie in vocal folds to adjust **thickness** and **tension** of vocal ligaments

E. **Innervation of Larynx (Table 7-5)**
   1. **External laryngeal nerve**

In **thyroidectomy,** the **external laryngeal nerve** ("high note nerve") is vulnerable because of its intimate relationship to the superior thyroid artery. **Damage to the nerve** affects the cricothyroid muscle, with a resulting inability to lengthen the vocal cord. Loss of tension on one cord causes a **monotonous, easily fatigued voice.**

   2. **Recurrent laryngeal/inferior laryngeal nerve**

Goiters, tumors, or **thyroidectomy** may **damage** the **recurrent laryngeal/inferior laryngeal nerves.** In thyroidectomy, the nerve is vulnerable because of its intimate relationship to the inferior thyroid artery. **Nerve damage** causes **hoarseness. Unilateral nerve involvement** is more likely on the left because of the longer left recurrent laryngeal nerve, which can be affected by **thoracic lesions** (e.g., bronchial cancer or aortic aneurysm). If only one nerve is involved, speech may not be permanently affected because of compensation by the opposite functional vocal cord. With **bilateral nerve damage,** the vocal cords become fixed in position, causing **impaired speech** and **breathing.**

F. **Blood Supply of Larynx**
   1. **Superior laryngeal artery**
      a. Branch of **superior thyroid artery** from external carotid
      b. Pierces **thyrohyoid membrane** with internal laryngeal nerve to supply upper larynx
   2. **Inferior laryngeal artery**
      a. Branch of **inferior thyroid artery** from thyrocervical trunk of subclavian
      b. Accompanies inferior laryngeal nerve to supply larynx below vocal folds

Only posterior cricoarytenoid muscles can abduct the vocal folds to open the airway.

During thyroidectomy, the external laryngeal nerve may be injured near the superior thyroid artery or the recurrent laryngeal nerve near the inferior thyroid artery.

The left recurrent laryngeal nerve is more often damaged due to its intrathoracic course.

TABLE 7-5. INNERVATION OF LARYNX

NERVE	ORIGIN	COURSE	SUPPLIES
Internal laryngeal	Superior laryngeal nerve from vagus	Pierces thyrohyoid membrane to lie deep to mucosa in piriform recess	Sensory to piriform recess and laryngeal mucosa above vocal folds
External laryngeal	Superior laryngeal nerve from vagus	Descends adjacent to superior thyroid artery	Cricothyroid muscle
Inferior laryngeal	Recurrent branch of vagus	Ascends in tracheoesophageal groove to reach larynx	Intrinsic muscles of larynx, except cricothyroid; sensory to laryngeal mucosa below vocal folds

X. **Thyroid Gland**

A. **Overview**

1. **Endocrine gland** secreting **hormones** that **regulate metabolic rate**
2. Has fibrous capsule, outside of which is **sheath of pretracheal fascia**

B. **Lateral Lobes**

1. Lie on sides of **larynx** and **trachea**
2. Covered superficially by **sternothyroid** and **sternohyoid** muscles

C. **Isthmus**

• Horizontally crosses **second and third tracheal rings** to connect lateral lobes

D. **Pyramidal Lobe**

1. Present in <50% of glands, extending superiorly from **isthmus** as remnant of embryonic **thyroglossal duct**
2. Attached to **hyoid bone** by fibrous band, connective tissue, and/or muscle fibers

The isthmus of thyroid is vulnerable during a tracheostomy.

The pyramidal lobe is a remnant of the thyroglossal duct.

A goiter may cause hoarseness, dysphagia, and dyspnea.

An enlargement of the thyroid gland **(goiter)** may compress the trachea (causing **dyspnea**), recurrent laryngeal nerves (causing **hoarseness**), and rarely the esophagus (causing **dysphagia**), and can also cause venous compression. Superior enlargement of the goiter is limited by attachment of the **sternothyroid muscle** to the oblique line of the thyroid cartilage, so it may grow inferiorly behind the sternum **(retrosternal goiter)**.

Fascial attachments of the thyroid gland to laryngeal cartilages cause it to move with the larynx during swallowing, a characteristic that helps distinguish swellings that are part of the thyroid from other pathology in the neck.

A thyroid mass moves superiorly with the larynx during swallowing.

E. **Blood Vessels of Thyroid Gland**

1. **Superior thyroid artery**

• Usually **first branch** of **external carotid artery** descending in relation to **external laryngeal nerve**

2. **Inferior thyroid artery**

a. Branch of **thyrocervical trunk**
b. Crosses **recurrent laryngeal nerve** near lower pole of gland

3. **Thyroid ima artery**

• Inconstant branch (10%) of brachiocephalic trunk or arch of aorta that ascends anterior to trachea

The thyroid ima artery may cause dangerous bleeding during thyroid surgery or tracheostomy.

The **thyroid ima artery** is vulnerable during **thyroid surgery** or **tracheostomy**. Cutting the artery is dangerous because the vessel may retract into the thorax.

4. **Thyroid veins**

a. **Superior and middle thyroid veins** drain to the internal jugular vein.
b. **Inferior thyroid vein** drains to left brachiocephalic vein

Ligation of the blood supply to the thyroid during a **thyroidectomy** endangers nerves closely related to the vessels. The **superior thyroid artery** is accompanied by the **external laryngeal nerve,** and the **inferior thyroid artery** crosses the **recurrent laryngeal nerve.** Damage to these nerves affects the laryngeal muscles.

F. **Thyroid Development (Figures 7-17 and 7-18)**

1. **Foramen cecum**

a. Site on base of tongue marking embryonic origin of thyroid from proliferation of foregut endoderm
b. If embryonic tissue remains at the foramen cecum, it is called a **lingual thyroid** and may contain the only functioning thyroid tissue.

2. **Thyroglossal duct**

• Temporary connection to tongue as developing thyroid migrates inferiorly in front of hyoid bone and thyroid and cricoid cartilages

The developing thyroid is temporarily connected to the tongue by the thyroglossal duct.

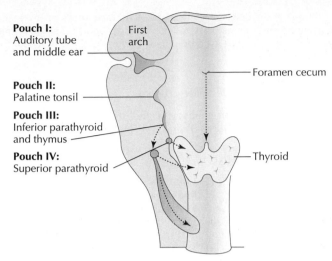

Pouch I:
Auditory tube and middle ear

First arch

Pouch II:
Palatine tonsil

Pouch III:
Inferior parathyroid and thymus

Pouch IV:
Superior parathyroid

Foramen cecum

Thyroid

7-17: Developmental origins of thyroid, parathyroid, and thymus glands. *Arrows,* pathways of migration.

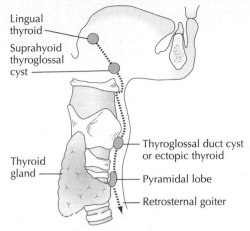

Lingual thyroid

Suprahyoid thyroglossal cyst

Thyroid gland

Thyroglossal duct cyst or ectopic thyroid

Pyramidal lobe

Retrosternal goiter

7-18: *Broken red line,* course of thyroglossal duct. *Red circles,* possible sites of ectopic thyroid tissue and thyroglossal duct remnants. *Arrow,* direction of thyroid migration.

Although the fully developed thyroid has no duct, remnants may be found along its migratory path as a **thyroglossal duct cyst.** Most cysts become apparent by age 5 as an anterior midline swelling that moves with the thyroid during swallowing or tongue protrusion. **Cystic infection** may cause pain and result in **sinus formation,** usually anterior to the laryngeal cartilages. **Ectopic thyroid tissue** may also be present along the migratory path. In rare cases, the ectopic tissue is the only thyroid gland present, and its surgical removal causes inadvertent thyroidectomy. **Lingual thyroid tissue** is common and usually asymptomatic; however, an enlarged lingual thyroid may cause **dysphagia, dyspnea,** and a "hot potato voice."

A thyroglossal duct cyst is a midline neck swelling that is usually apparent by age 5.

XI. Parathyroid Glands (see Figure 7-17)
A. Overview
1. Two to six small **endocrine glands** essential for life, usually two superior and two inferior, lying on or embedded in posterior aspect of thyroid gland
2. Supplied mainly by **inferior thyroid artery**
B. Superior Parathyroid Glands
- **Develop** from endoderm of **fourth pharyngeal pouches**
C. Inferior Parathyroid Glands
- **Develop** from endoderm of **third pharyngeal pouches** along with thymus

Inferior parathyroid glands vary in location from the level of thyroid cartilage to the superior mediastinum.

The relationship of the developing **inferior parathyroid glands** and **thymus** explains the variable location of the inferior parathyroids, which may be carried into the **lower neck** or **mediastinum** with the thymus. The inferior parathyroids may be difficult to find, but following the **inferior thyroid artery** may aid in locating them. **Total removal of the parathyroids,** which secrete **parathyroid hormone,** will **reduce plasma calcium,** producing a potentially fatal **tetany.**

Abnormal development of the third and fourth pharyngeal pouches occurs in **DiGeorge syndrome.** An **absent thymus** results in T cell deficiency and **absent parathyroid glands** result in hypoparathyroidism. Craniofacial anomalies are associated with **deficient neural crest cells.**

A total parathyroidectomy may result in fatal tetany.

XII. Trachea
A. Location
- Begins at **inferior border of cricoid cartilage** as inferior continuation of larynx and terminates by bifurcating into primary bronchi at level of **sternal angle**
B. Structure
- Kept patent by series of horseshoe-shaped hyaline **cartilage rings** completed posteriorly by smooth muscle **trachealis**

A thoracic mass may cause a deviation of the trachea in the neck.

Tumors and other space-occupying lesions easily displace the **trachea.** A thoracic mass or increased pressure in one hemithorax (e.g., tension pneumothorax) may cause the cervical portion of the trachea to shift position. A downward movement of the trachea synchronous with the heartbeat **(tracheal tug)** is often symptomatic of an **aortic arch aneurysm.**

XIII. Esophagus
    A. Muscular portion of digestive tract connecting pharynx and stomach
    B. In neck contains branchiomeric skeletal muscle innervated by SVE fibers from recurrent laryngeal nerves
    C. In neck supplied by branches of inferior thyroid arteries

An untreated esophageal perforation is rapidly fatal.

A cervical mass may compress the **esophagus,** resulting in **dysphagia.** Examples include an **enlarged thyroid gland** and anterior **osteophytes** of the cervical spine in **osteoarthritis** (spondylosis). **Perforation of the esophagus** iatrogenically (e.g., while passing a nasogastric tube), or rarely in blunt trauma, is a medical emergency and can be rapidly fatal.

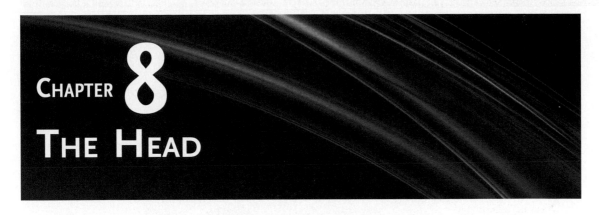

I. Skull (Figures 8-1 to 8-4)

- **Consists of neurocranium and viscerocranium**

A. Neurocranium

1. Overview
   a. Encloses **cranial cavity,** which houses brain and meninges
   b. Formed by **cranial base** and **cranial vault;** roof of cranial vault is **calvaria**
   c. Formed by **eight bones:** paired parietal and temporal bones and unpaired frontal, occipital, ethmoid, and sphenoid bones

2. **Temporal bones**
   a. **Squamous part**
      - Includes **mandibular fossa** and **articular tubercle** (articular eminence) for articulation at **temporomandibular joint**
   b. **Tympanic part**
      - Forms floor and anterior wall of **external acoustic meatus**
   c. **Mastoid part**
      (1) Contains **mastoid air cells**
      (2) Includes **mastoid process,** which develops after birth
   d. **Petrous part**
      - Contains **inner ear,** part of **middle ear,** and **carotid canal**

> **Fractures** of the **petrous portion of the temporal bone** often result in leakage of cerebrospinal fluid (CSF) from the ear **(CSF otorrhea)** and bruising over the mastoid process **(Battle sign).** The **facial and vestibulocochlear nerves** may be injured and hemorrhage may occur from a torn **internal carotid artery.**

The temporal bone is fractured in 75% of skull base fractures.

Petrous temporal bone fracture causes CSF otorrhea and the Battle sign.

3. **Frontal bone**
   a. Forms forehead and roof of orbit
   b. Contains paired **frontal sinuses**
   c. Develops as two bones separated by **metopic (interfrontal) suture,** which is usually fused by 8th year but remains in 8% of population

4. **Occipital bone**
   - Consists of basilar, squamous, and paired lateral parts enclosing **foramen magnum**
   a. **Basilar part** (basioccipital)
      - Articulates with body of sphenoid at former site of **sphenooccipital synchondrosis,** which is important in skull growth
   b. **Squamous part**
   c. **Lateral part**
      - Includes **occipital condyle, condylar fossa** and **canal,** and **hypoglossal canal**

5. **Ethmoid bone**
   a. **Cribriform plate**
      (1) Roof of **nasal cavity** and central floor of **anterior cranial fossa**
      (2) Perforated by **olfactory foramina** for **olfactory nerve fibers**
   b. **Perpendicular plate**
      - Projects inferiorly from cribriform plate to contribute to **nasal septum**

An unfused metopic suture between the frontal bones can be mistaken for a skull fracture.

The foramen magnum is the opening in the occipital bone where the spinal cord is continuous with the brainstem.

A fracture of the cribriform plate produces leakage of CSF from the nose (rhinorrhea).

The olfactory nerves traverse the cribriform plate to reach the nasal cavity.

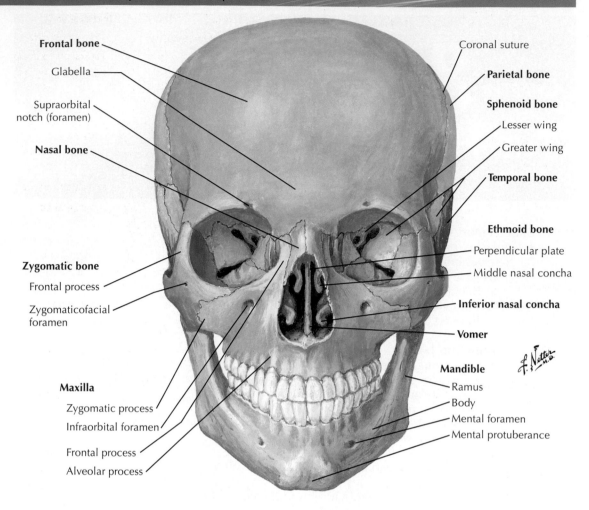

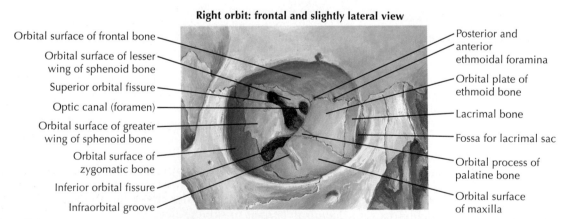

8-1: Skull, anterior view. *Lower figure* shows close-up view of right orbit with head rotated slightly toward left side. *(From Netter, F H: Atlas of Human Anatomy, 4th ed. Philadelphia, Saunders, 2006, Plate 2.)*

The sella turcica houses the pituitary gland.

   c. **Ethmoidal labyrinth**
- Encloses posterior, middle, and anterior **ethmoid air cells (see Figure 8-3)**
- Forms **superior and middle nasal conchae** on lateral wall of **nasal cavity** and **orbital lamina** on medial wall of **orbit**

6. **Sphenoid bone**
   a. **Body (see Figure 8-3)**
- Contains paired **sphenoidal sinuses** inferior to **sella turcica** of middle cranial fossa

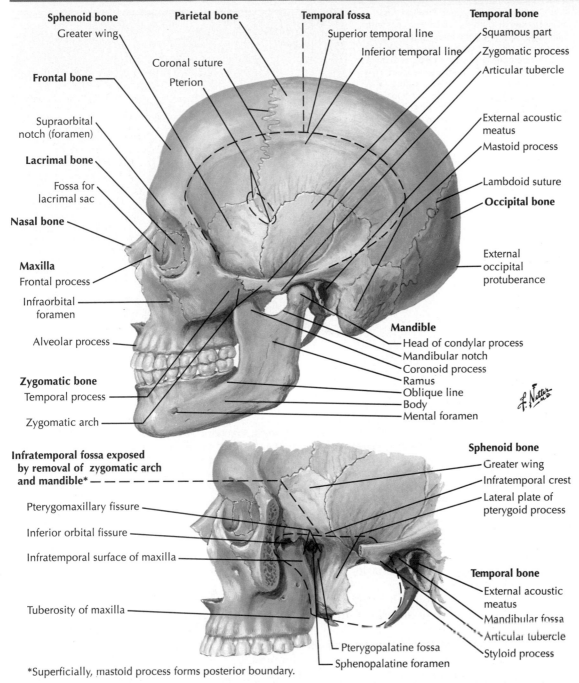

Sphenoid bone — Greater wing

Frontal bone

Parietal bone

Coronal suture

Pterion

Temporal fossa
Superior temporal line
Inferior temporal line

Temporal bone
Squamous part
Zygomatic process
Articular tubercle

External acoustic meatus

Mastoid process

Lambdoid suture

Occipital bone

Supraorbital notch (foramen)

Lacrimal bone
Fossa for lacrimal sac

Nasal bone

Maxilla
Frontal process

Infraorbital foramen

Alveolar process

Zygomatic bone
Temporal process

Zygomatic arch

External occipital protuberance

Mandible
Head of condylar process
Mandibular notch
Coronoid process
Ramus
Oblique line
Body
Mental foramen

Infratemporal fossa exposed by removal of zygomatic arch and mandible* ‑ ‑ ‑

Pterygomaxillary fissure

Inferior orbital fissure

Infratemporal surface of maxilla

Tuberosity of maxilla

Sphenoid bone
Greater wing
Infratemporal crest
Lateral plate of pterygoid process

Temporal bone
External acoustic meatus
Mandibular fossa
Articular tubercle
Styloid process

Pterygopalatine fossa
Sphenopalatine foramen

*Superficially, mastoid process forms posterior boundary.

8-2: Skull, lateral view. *Upper figure* shows temporal fossa outlined by *large oval dashed line*. Clinically important landmark pterion, which is outlined by *smaller oval dashed line*, is located within temporal fossa. *Lower figure* shows infratemporal fossa of deep face outlined by *dashed line* following removal of zygomatic arch and mandible. Infratemporal fossa communicates medially with pterygopalatine fossa through pterygomaxillary fissure (see Section VIII). *(From Netter, F H: Atlas of Human Anatomy, 4th ed. Philadelphia, Saunders, 2006, Plate 4.)*

b. **Lesser wing**
- Includes **optic canal, anterior clinoid process,** and **superior boundary of superior orbital fissure**

c. **Greater wing**
  (1) Contributes to roof of **infratemporal fossa** and floor of **middle cranial fossa**
  (2) Contains **foramina rotundum, ovale,** and **spinosum**

d. **Pterygoid process**
  (1) Consists of **medial** and **lateral pterygoid plates**
  (2) **Hamulus** from medial plate serves as pulley for **tensor veli palatini** muscle to tense soft palate and also gives attachment to **pterygomandibular raphe**

The skull may fracture opposite the site of impact.

8-3: Skull lateral radiograph. Pituitary fossa = 26 = 1; anterior clinoid process = 2; posterior clinoid process = 3; sphenoidal sinus = 4; ethmoidal air cells = 5; greater wing of sphenoid = 6; mastoid air cells = 7; frontal sinus = 8; grooves for middle meningeal vessels = 9; coronal suture = 10; lambdoid suture = 11; coronoid process of mandible = 12; palatine process of maxilla = 13; anterior arch of atlas = 14; dens of axis = 15. *(From Weir, J, Abrahams, P: Imaging Atlas of Human Anatomy, 3rd ed. London, Mosby Ltd., 2003, p 2, a.)*

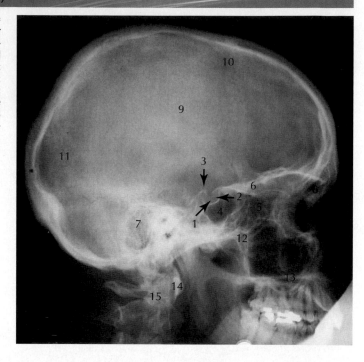

The skin is broken in a compound fracture with a danger of infection.

Skull fractures may occur opposite the point of impact. Skull fractures are frequent in the temporoparietal region because the bone there is thinnest. **Fractures at the pterion** may tear the **middle meningeal artery,** and a **depressed fracture** may compress the underlying brain. In most depressed fractures, the overlying scalp is lacerated **(compound fracture),** which predisposes to infection. A blow to the top of the head may **fracture the skull base,** with related cranial nerve injury, cerebrospinal fluid (CSF) leakage from a dura-arachnoid tear **(CSF fistula),** or **dural sinus thrombosis.** A **fracture of the petrous temporal bone** may cause blood or CSF to escape from the ear **(CSF otorrhea),** hearing loss, and facial nerve damage. **Fracture of the anterior cranial fossa** is suggested by anosmia, periorbital bruising **(raccoon eyes),** and CSF leakage from the nose **(CSF rhinorrhea).**

7. **Sutures and landmarks of neurocranium (see Figures 8-1 to 8-4)**
   a. **Bregma**
      (1) Point at which sagittal and coronal sutures meet in adult
      (2) Site of **anterior fontanelle,** the "soft spot" of an infant's head

The anterior fontanelle is used to assess ossification, hydration, and intracranial pressure.

   b. **Lambda**
      (1) Point at which sagittal and lambdoidal sutures meet
      (2) Site of neonate's **posterior fontanelle**
   c. **Pterion**
      • Site of anterolateral fontanelle where middle meningeal artery usually grooves internal surface of bone **(see Figures 8-3 and 8-5)**
8. **Development of skull**
   a. **Overview**
      (1) **Cranial base** (chondrocranium) develops mainly by **endochondral ossification.**
      (2) **Cranial vault** and **facial skeleton** develop by **intramembranous ossification**
      (3) **Sutures** are important sites of growth and allow bones to overlap (molding) during birth.

The skull deformity of craniosynostosis may cause increased intracranial pressure.

Premature sagittal suture fusion causes scaphocephaly, the most common form of craniosynostosis.

   b. **Craniosynostosis (Table 8-1)**
      (1) **Sutures fuse prematurely,** resulting in **skull deformity.**
      (2) Growth is restricted perpendicular to prematurely fused sutures, and **compensatory overgrowth** occurs at **open sutures.**
      (3) May produce **increased intracranial pressure** from skull deformity

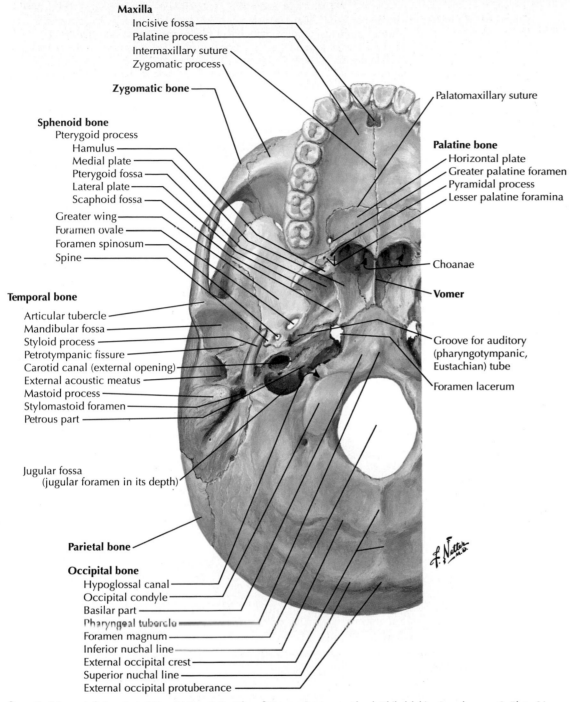

Maxilla
Incisive fossa
Palatine process
Intermaxillary suture
Zygomatic process

Zygomatic bone

Sphenoid bone
Pterygoid process
Hamulus
Medial plate
Pterygoid fossa
Lateral plate
Scaphoid fossa
Greater wing
Foramen ovale
Foramen spinosum
Spine

Temporal bone
Articular tubercle
Mandibular fossa
Styloid process
Petrotympanic fissure
Carotid canal (external opening)
External acoustic meatus
Mastoid process
Stylomastoid foramen
Petrous part

Jugular fossa
(jugular foramen in its depth)

Parietal bone

Occipital bone
Hypoglossal canal
Occipital condyle
Basilar part
Pharyngeal tubercle
Foramen magnum
Inferior nuchal line
External occipital crest
Superior nuchal line
External occipital protuberance

Palatomaxillary suture

Palatine bone
Horizontal plate
Greater palatine foramen
Pyramidal process
Lesser palatine foramina

Choanae

Vomer

Groove for auditory
(pharyngotympanic,
Eustachian) tube

Foramen lacerum

8-4: Skull base, inferior view. *(From Netter, F H: Atlas of Human Anatomy, 4th ed. Philadelphia, Saunders, 2006, Plate 8.)*

TABLE 8-1. SKULL DEFORMITIES IN CRANIOSYNOSTOSIS

DEFORMITY	SUTURE(S) INVOLVED	DESCRIPTION
Scaphocephaly	Sagittal suture	Long, narrow skull
Oxycephaly	Coronal suture, bilateral fusion	Short, tall, wide skull
Plagiocephaly	Coronal or lambdoid suture, unilateral fusion	Asymmetric skull with forehead protruding on one side and flattened on other
Trigonocephaly	Metopic suture	Wedge-shaped forehead

Synostotic plagiocephaly must be distinguished from reversible deformational plagiocephaly resulting from in utero factors or infant sleep position.

Craniosynostosis results in a permanent skull deformity that is correctible only by surgery. An asymmetric skull *not* resulting from premature suture fusion **(deformational or positional plagiocephaly)** and treatable by conservative means may result from in utero cramping, infant sleep position, or congenital torticollis. The recommendation to position sleeping infants on their backs to reduce the risk of **sudden infant death syndrome** (SIDS) has dramatically increased the incidence of deformational plagiocephaly.

    c. **Anterior fontanelle**
      (1) Present at birth; **closes at age 9-18 months**
      (2) **Diminished size or absence** at birth may indicate **craniosynostosis** or **microcephaly.**
    d. **Posterior fontanelle**
      (1) Present at birth; **usually closes by 2 months of age**
      (2) **Persistence** suggests underlying **hydrocephalus or congenital hypothyroidism.**
  9. **Major apertures of neurocranium (Figure 8-5; Table 8-2)**
B. Viscerocranium
  1. **Maxilla**
    a. Paired bone that joins at midline **intermaxillary suture** to form upper jaw
    b. Has **body** that contains **maxillary sinus** and contributes to walls of **nasal cavity, orbit,** and infratemporal fossa
  2. **Zygomatic bone**
    a. Paired bone that forms **prominence of cheek,** most of **lateral orbital margin,** and anterior boundary of **temporal fossa**
    b. Helps form zygomatic arch

A persistence of the anterior or posterior fontanelle may result from hydrocephalus, congenital hypothyroidism, or rickets.

Skull sectioned horizontally: superior view

Superior sagittal sinus (*cut*)
Falx cerebri (*cut*)
Superior ophthalmic vein
Anterior and posterior intercavernous sinuses
Cavernous sinus
Basilar venous plexus
Superior petrosal sinus
Inferior petrosal sinus
Tentorium cerebelli
Transverse sinus
Inferior sagittal sinus (*cut*)
Straight sinus
Falx cerebri (*cut*)
Confluence of sinuses
Superior sagittal sinus (*cut*)

Hypophysis (pituitary gland)
Optic nerve (II)
Internal carotid artery
Oculomotor nerve (III)
Sphenoparietal sinus
Trochlear nerve (IV)
Ophthalmic nerve (V₁)
Maxillary nerve (V₂)
Trigeminal ganglion
Mandibular nerve (V₃)
Middle meningeal artery
Abducent nerve (VI)
Facial nerve (VII), intermediate nerve, and vestibulocochlear nerve (VIII)
Glossopharyngeal (IX) and vagus (X) nerves
Jugular foramen
Sigmoid sinus (continuation of transverse sinus)
Accessory nerve (XI)
Hypoglossal nerve (XII)
Great cerebral vein (of Galen)

8-5: Cranial fossae and related major nerves and vessels, superior view. *Left,* Dural venous sinuses; *right,* nerves and arteries. *(From Netter, F H: Atlas of Human Anatomy, 4th ed. Philadelphia, Saunders, 2006, Plate 104.)*

TABLE 8-2. MAJOR APERTURES OF NEUROCRANIUM

APERTURE	COMMUNICATION BETWEEN	TRAVERSED BY
Cribriform plate	Nasal cavity and anterior cranial fossa	Olfactory nerves
Optic canal	Middle cranial fossa and orbit	Optic nerve, ophthalmic artery
Superior orbital fissure	Middle cranial fossa and orbit	Oculomotor, trochlear, ophthalmic, and abducens nerves; ophthalmic vein(s)
Foramen rotundum	Middle cranial fossa and pterygopalatine fossa	Maxillary nerve
Foramen ovale	Middle cranial fossa and infratemporal fossa	Mandibular nerve, accessory meningeal artery, lesser petrosal nerve
Foramen spinosum	Middle cranial fossa and infratemporal fossa	Middle meningeal artery, meningeal branch of mandibular nerve
Foramen lacerum	Middle cranial fossa and base of skull	Closed in life by cartilage transmitting only small vessels; sometimes defined as including opening of carotid canal
Carotid canal	Base of skull and middle cranial fossa	Internal carotid artery and plexus
Internal acoustic meatus	Posterior cranial fossa and facial canal	Facial nerve, nervus intermedius, vestibulocochlear nerve
Stylomastoid foramen	Facial canal and base of skull	Facial nerve
Jugular foramen	Posterior cranial fossa and base of skull	Glossopharyngeal, vagus, and accessory nerves; internal jugular vein, inferior petrosal sinus
Foramen magnum	Posterior cranial fossa and base of skull	Brainstem, vertebral arteries and veins, spinal arteries, spinal portion of accessory nerve
Hypoglossal canal	Posterior cranial fossa and base of skull	Hypoglossal nerve

3. **Lacrimal bone** (paired)
   - Contributes to **medial orbital wall** at **fossa for lacrimal sac**
4. **Palatine bone** (paired)
   a. **Horizontal plate** fuses anteriorly with palatine process of maxilla to form **bony palate**
   b. **Perpendicular plate** forms part of lateral wall of **nasal cavity,** medial wall of **pterygopalatine fossa,** and floor of **orbit**
5. **Inferior nasal concha** (paired)
   - Independent bone of lateral nasal wall overlying inferior meatus
6. **Vomer**
   - Forms posterior inferior part of **nasal septum** between **choanae**
7. **Mandible (Figure 8-6)**
   a. **Body**
      (1) Formed by two halves fused in midline at **mental symphysis**
      (2) **Alveolar process** to hold mandibular teeth
      (3) Mylohyoid line that separates sublingual and submandibular fossae
   b. **Ramus**
      (1) Superior coronoid and condylar processes separated by mandibular notch
      (2) Features **mandibular foramen** bordered by **lingula** on medial surface

II. **Scalp and Face**
   A. **Scalp (Figure 8-7)**
      1. **Skin**
      2. **Connective tissue**
         - Dense superficial fascia containing nerves and blood vessels
      3. **Aponeurosis**
         - Fibrous **epicranial aponeurosis** connecting **frontalis** and **occipitalis** parts of occipitofrontalis muscle
      4. **Loose connective tissue**
         - Allows three more superficial layers to move over skull surface
      5. **Pericranium**
         - Periosteum covering outer surface of bone

The SCALP acronym describes the five layers of the scalp.

The first three layers of the scalp detach together in scalping injuries.

In **scalping injuries,** the **loose connective tissue** layer is the **plane of separation** with the superficial three layers detaching together as a unit. The loose connective tissue allows **infection** to spread **across the calvaria** and potentially through **emissary veins** to the skull bones or intracranial dural venous sinuses, producing **meningitis** and/or **septicemia.** The **dense connective tissue** layer prevents retraction of lacerated blood vessels, resulting in **profuse bleeding** from the rich blood supply. Since the arteries supplying the scalp all ascend into it, bleeding can often be controlled by tying a string around the head above the ears. If the aponeurotic layer is cut in the coronal plane, **gaping** of the wound occurs due to the pull of the frontalis and occipitalis.

Scalp lacerations bleed profusely due to the lack of vessel retraction and abundant anastomoses.

Since arteries ascend into the scalp, bleeding may be controllable by tying a string around the head.

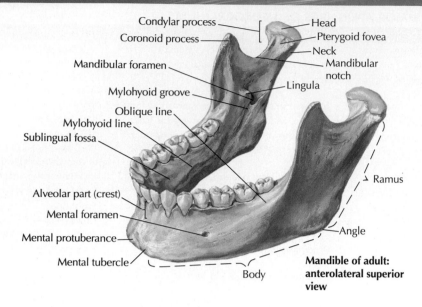

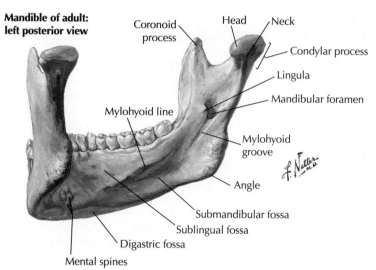

8-6: Mandible. Anterolateral superior view (*upper figure*). Left posteroinferior view (*lower figure*). (*From Norton, N S: Netter's Head and Neck Anatomy for Dentistry. Philadelphia, Saunders 2007, p 47.*)

B. Muscles of Face and Scalp

1. Subcutaneous voluntary muscles (**muscles of facial expression**) that move **skin of face** and **scalp**
2. Develop from mesoderm of **second pharyngeal arch** and are innervated by **facial nerve**

C. Nerves of Face and Scalp (Figure 8-8)

Cutaneous innervation of the face is from CN V. Motor innervation is from CN VII.

1. **Cutaneous innervation** of face and scalp is from **trigeminal nerve** (CN V) and **cervical spinal nerves** (C2, C3).
2. **Facial nerve** (CN VII)
   a. Exits **stylomastoid foramen** to enter parotid gland
   b. **Posterior auricular nerve** motor to posterior scalp muscles
   c. **Nerve to stylohyoid** and **posterior digastric** muscles
   d. **Branches within parotid gland**

To Zanzibar By Motor Car: temporal, zygomatic, buccal, mandibular, cervical branches of CN VII.

   (1) **Temporal** branches supply muscles of forehead and temple
   (2) **Zygomatic** branches supply orbicularis oculi and muscles of the upper lip and nose.
   (3) **Buccal** branches supply muscles of upper lip and angle of mouth
   (4) **Marginal mandibular** branch supplies muscles of lower lip and angle of mouth
   (5) **Cervical** branch supplies platysma muscle

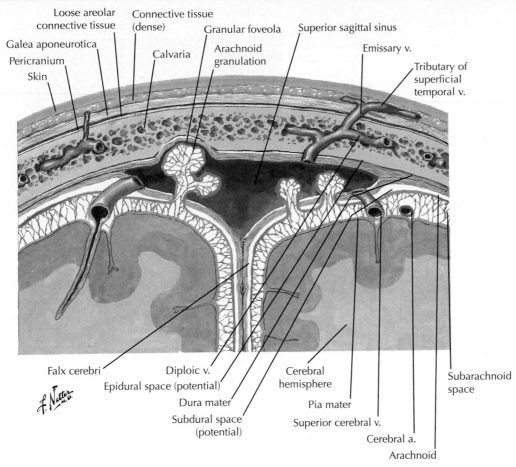

8-7: Layers of the scalp and the scalp's connection to intracranial structures (superior sagittal sinus) via emissary veins. *(From Norton, N S: Netter's Head and Neck Anatomy for Dentistry. Philadelphia, Saunders 2007, p 162.)*

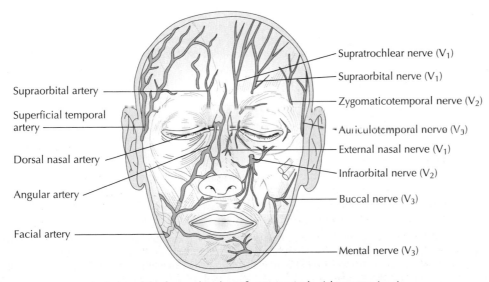

8-8: Cutaneous nerves and arteries of the face and scalp. *Left,* arteries *(red); right,* nerves *(gray).*

Terminal branches of **CN VII** may be injured by **parotid cancer** or by **surgery** to remove a parotid tumor **(Figure 8-9).** An infant's facial nerve may be injured during a **forceps delivery** because the mastoid process has not yet developed and the stylomastoid foramen is relatively superficial. **Bell palsy** is **idiopathic unilateral facial paralysis.**

The facial nerve is vulnerable to injury during forceps delivery of an infant or parotid surgery in an adult.

8-9: Axial CT showing tumor of left parotid gland. Parotid tumors or surgery to remove them may damage the facial nerve. *(From Drake, R, Vogl, W A, Mitchell, A: Gray's Anatomy for Students, 2nd ed. Philadelphia, Churchill Livingstone, 2010, Figure 8.57.)*

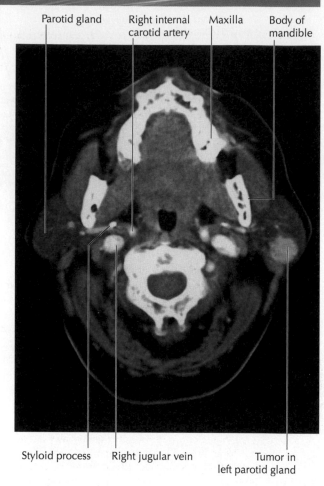

Parotid gland   Right internal carotid artery   Maxilla   Body of mandible

Styloid process   Right jugular vein   Tumor in left parotid gland

Bell palsy is unilateral paralysis of all the facial muscles from an idiopathic facial nerve lesion.

Symptoms associated with **lesions** of CN VII are determined by the location of the lesion. **Facial muscles** are always **paralyzed,** although the extent and severity vary. Of particular concern is the **inability to close the eyelids,** which may cause drying and ulceration of the cornea. A lesion within the facial canal will also affect **taste from the anterior two-thirds of the tongue** carried by the **chorda tympani.**

3. Cutaneous branches of trigeminal nerve

Intense, stabbing pain over the face, usually in the distribution of the **maxillary and/or mandibular divisions of the trigeminal nerve,** characterizes **trigeminal neuralgia** (tic douloureux). Attacks are precipitated by stimulation of **trigger zones.** Usual sensory and motor functions are unaffected in most patients. The cause may be compression of the sensory root by an aberrant blood vessel The pain may be alleviated by some anticonvulsant medications or by microvascular decompression, selective radiofrequency ablation of the trigeminal ganglion or sensory root, or glycerol injection.

Tic douloureux is intense paroxysms of pain along the maxillary and/or mandibular divisions of CN V.

Sweating and flushing of the skin along the distribution of the auriculotemporal nerve characterize **auriculotemporal nerve syndrome** (Frey syndrome). The syndrome is an abnormal response to eating that replaces salivation on the affected side due to anomalous regeneration of secretomotor fibers to sweat glands after parotid surgery.

The arteries of the face and scalp come mainly from the branches of the external carotid artery.

4. Cutaneous branches of cervical spinal nerves to head
  a. **Great auricular nerve** (anterior rami of C2, C3)
  b. **Lesser occipital nerve** (anterior ramus of C2)
  c. **Greater occipital nerve** (posterior ramus of C2)

D. Blood Vessels of Face and Scalp (see Figure 8-8)
1. **Superficial temporal artery**
   - Ascends anterior to auricle with **auriculotemporal nerve** (V_3)

Temporal arteritis is the most common vasculitis in adults, usually occurring after age 50. Blood flow is diminished. Inflammation of the superficial temporal artery causes pain overlying the vessel and pain when opening and closing the jaw as the inflamed vessel is stretched. The **ophthalmic artery** is also frequently involved, often resulting in **blindness.** Patients are placed on high doses of corticosteroids.

2. **Maxillary artery**
   - **Mental, buccal,** and **infraorbital** arteries are distributed with corresponding nerves.
3. **Facial artery**
   a. Passes deep to **submandibular gland** and over lower border of mandible to ascend toward **medial angle** of eye
   b. Branches in face include **superior and inferior labial, lateral nasal,** and **angular** arteries.
4. **Occipital artery**
   - Distributed to scalp with **greater occipital nerve**
5. **Posterior auricular artery**
   - Supplies back of auricle and scalp above and behind ear
6. **Ophthalmic artery**
   - Gives branches that become **cutaneous** around eye, including supraorbital, supratrochlear, lacrimal, and dorsal nasal arteries

Extensive **collateral circulation** exists between the branches of the **external carotid arteries** in the face and neck. Collateral circulation between the **internal** and **external carotid arteries** is provided by anastomosis of the **dorsal nasal artery** (from the ophthalmic artery) with the **angular artery** (from the facial artery).

7. **Facial vein** (see Figure 7-6)
   a. Begins as **angular vein** near medial angle of eye and parallels facial artery
   b. Connects with **cavernous sinus** via **ophthalmic veins** and **deep facial vein-pterygoid plexus**

The **middle third of the face** is a "danger area" because **infections** there may produce **thrombophlebitis of the facial vein** that can **spread to the cavernous venous sinus** via the pterygoid venous plexus or ophthalmic veins. Septicemia leads to **meningitis** and **cavernous sinus thrombosis,** both of which can cause neurological damage and are life-threatening.

III. Parotid, Temporal, and Infratemporal Regions
A. Parotid Gland
1. Overview
   a. Extends superficially over **ramus of mandible** and **masseter** (superficial lobe) and deep to ramus (deep lobe)
   b. Enclosed by tough **parotid fascia** from investing layer of deep cervical fascia
2. **Structures partially embedded within parotid gland**
   a. **Facial nerve** and its terminal branches
   b. **Retromandibular vein** and its originating tributaries
   c. **External carotid artery** and its terminal branches
   d. **Parotid lymph nodes**
3. **Parotid duct** (Stensen's duct)
   - Crosses **masseter** superficially and pierces **buccinator** and cheek **mucosa** to open opposite **upper second molar**

(margin notes)

Temporal arteritis is the most common vasculitis in adults.

The inferior border of the mandible anterior to the masseter is the pressure point to control facial artery bleeding.

The involvement of the ophthalmic artery in temporal arteritis may result in blindness.

The middle third of the face is a "danger area" because infection can spread to the cavernous sinus.

Salivary gland stones can cause painful glandular swelling while eating.

A **salivary gland stone** (sialolith) may **block** the **parotid duct,** causing painful swelling of the gland that is worse at mealtimes or after eating a sour pickle. Surgical removal of the calculus may be required. Parotid stones are less common than submandibular duct stones.

4. **Innervation of parotid gland**
    a. **Parasympathetic innervation** (secretomotor)
        (1) **Preganglionic parasympathetic fibers** traverse tympanic branch of **glossopharyngeal nerve** (CN IX), tympanic plexus, and lesser petrosal nerve to **otic ganglion**
        (2) **Postganglionic parasympathetic fibers** from otic ganglion are distributed to parotid gland via **auriculotemporal nerve** (V_3).
    b. **Sympathetic innervation** (vasomotor)
        • **Postganglionic sympathetic fibers** from **superior cervical ganglion** are distributed via periarterial **external carotid plexus**

Preganglionic parasympathetic fibers of IX to parotid gland synapse in the otic ganglion

Mumps may be complicated by orchitis, producing sterility.

Mumps is a highly contagious viral infection of the **parotid gland.** Swelling of the gland within its tough capsule causes intense pain, which is exacerbated by compression between the mandibular ramus and mastoid process during chewing. Infection may involve the testes **(orchitis),** resulting in sterility, or less commonly cause meningitis or pancreatitis. Since salivary glands contain **amylase,** serum amylase often is markedly increased in mumps.

B. **Temporal Fossa**
    1. Bounded by **temporal lines, frontal process of zygomatic bone** and **zygomatic process of frontal bone,** and **zygomatic arch**
    2. **Floor** formed by parts of greater wing of sphenoid, squamous temporal, frontal, and parietal bones meeting at **pterion**
    3. Contains **temporalis muscle, deep temporal nerves and vessels** (deep to temporalis **muscle), zygomaticotemporal** and **auriculotemporal nerves, temporal branch of facial nerve,** and **superficial temporal vessels**
C. **Infratemporal Fossa**
    1. Overview
        a. Bounded by **posterior surface of maxilla, greater wing of sphenoid, lateral pterygoid plate,** and **ramus of mandible**
        b. Communicates with orbit, pterygopalatine fossa, and middle cranial fossa
        c. Contains mandibular nerve (V_3), maxillary artery, pterygoid venous plexus, pterygoid muscles, temporalis tendon, chorda tympani, and otic ganglion
    2. **Muscles of mastication (Figure 8-10; Table 8-3)**
        • Develop from **first pharyngeal arch** and are innervated by **mandibular nerve** (V_3)
    3. **Temporomandibular joint (TMJ)**
        a. Paired **synovial joint** between **mandibular condyle (head)** and **articular tubercle** (articular eminence) of temporal bone

TMJ disorders are often due to grinding the teeth.

Temporomandibular joint disorders occur in 15% of the population. They often result from clenching the jaws and grinding the teeth **(bruxism)** due to stress, but the TMJ is also subject to the same diseases as other synovial joints, including rheumatoid arthritis, infection, and neoplasia.

    b. Joint cavity subdivided by **articular disc** into **upper compartment for gliding movements** and **lower compartment for hinge movements**
    c. Differs from other synovial joints in having articular surfaces covered by fibrous tissue rather than hyaline cartilage
    d. **Fibrous capsule** reinforced by **lateral temporomandibular ligament**
    e. Innervated by **auriculotemporal** and **masseteric nerves** (V_3)
    f. **Sphenomandibular ligament**
        (1) Thin band from **spine of sphenoid bone** to **lingula** of mandible
        (2) Remnant of **first pharyngeal arch cartilage** (Meckel cartilage)

The lateral pterygoid pulls the head of the mandible and articular disc forward onto the articular tubercle when opening the jaw.

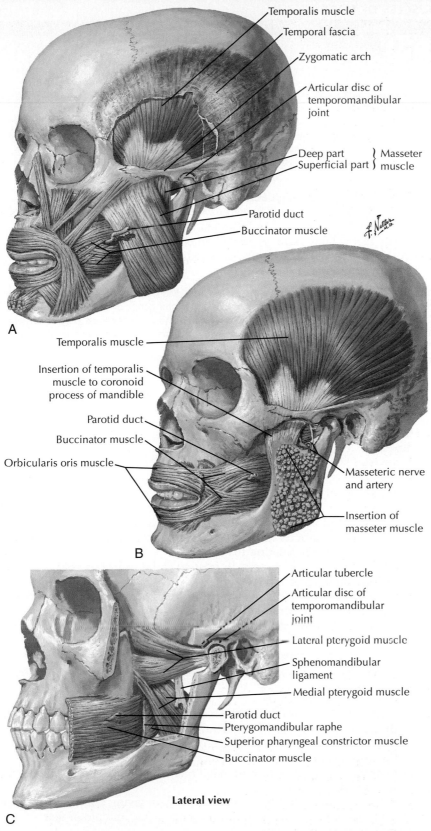

Temporalis muscle
Temporal fascia
Zygomatic arch
Articular disc of temporomandibular joint
Deep part ⎫ Masseter
Superficial part ⎰ muscle
Parotid duct
Buccinator muscle

A

Temporalis muscle
Insertion of temporalis muscle to coronoid process of mandible
Parotid duct
Buccinator muscle
Orbicularis oris muscle
Masseteric nerve and artery
Insertion of masseter muscle

B

Articular tubercle
Articular disc of temporomandibular joint
Lateral pterygoid muscle
Sphenomandibular ligament
Medial pterygoid muscle
Parotid duct
Pterygomandibular raphe
Superior pharyngeal constrictor muscle
Buccinator muscle

Lateral view

C

8-10: Muscles of mastication. **A,** Masseter and temporalis shown in lateral view. **B,** Masseter removed to show temporalis insertion. **C,** Masseter, temporalis, part of ramus of mandible, and zygomatic arch removed to show lateral and medial pterygoid muscles. *(From Netter, F H: Atlas of Human Anatomy, 4th ed. Philadelphia, Saunders, 2006, Plates 54 and 55.)*

TABLE 8-3. MUSCLES OF MASTICATION

MUSCLE	ORIGIN	INSERTION	ACTION
Temporalis	Temporal fossa and temporal fascia	Coronoid process and ramus of mandible	Elevates and retracts mandible
Masseter	Zygomatic arch	Lateral surface of ramus and angle of mandible	Elevates mandible
Lateral pterygoid	Greater wing of sphenoid and lateral pterygoid plate	Neck of mandible, capsule and disc of temporomandibular joint	Protracts and depresses mandible; deviation to opposite side
Medial pterygoid	Lateral pterygoid plate and maxilla	Medial surface of ramus and angle of mandible	Elevates mandible; deviation to opposite side

All muscles of mastication develop from the first pharyngeal arch and are innervated by its nerve, the mandibular division of the trigeminal nerve (CN V3).

g. **Stylomandibular ligament**
   (1) Thickened parotid fascia between **styloid process** and mandible near **angle,** separating parotid and submandibular salivary glands
   (2) Helps limit extreme protrusion of mandible and spread of infection between parotid and submandibular glands

> TMJ may dislocate if the condyle slides too far anteriorly over the articular tubercle.

Dislocation of the **temporomandibular joint** occurs when the condyle of the mandible slides too far anteriorly over the **articular tubercle** and cannot return to the condylar fossa. The jaw is then held in the dislocated position by action of the **muscles of mastication.** Dislocation may occur when the mouth is opened too far (as during yawning) or when the chin is struck while the mouth is open. A **blow to the chin** with the **mouth closed** can drive the head of the mandible posteriorly and superiorly, **fracturing** the bony **auditory canal** and/or the floor of the **middle cranial fossa.**

> The TMJ and the ear may refer pain to each other.

Ankylosis of the TMJ is unilateral or bilateral loss of movement. It may result from rheumatoid arthritis, infectious agents, neoplasia, or trauma. **Pain may be referred to the TMJ** by stimulation of abnormal muscle foci **(trigger points)** in the head and neck.

4. **Maxillary artery (Figure 8-11)**
   a. Overview
      (1) **Terminal branch of external carotid artery** within parotid gland
      (2) Traverses infratemporal fossa superficial or deep to lateral pterygoid muscle to enter **pterygopalatine fossa**
      (3) Divided into three parts in relation to **lateral pterygoid**
   b. **Middle meningeal artery**
      (1) Ascends between roots of **auriculotemporal nerve** to enter middle cranial fossa through **foramen spinosum**
      (2) Courses between bone and dura mater, supplying both
      (3) Anterior branch often grooves bone in region of **pterion**
   c. **Accessory meningeal artery**
      (1) Arises from maxillary *or* middle meningeal artery
      (2) Traverses **foramen ovale** to supply trigeminal ganglion and dura mater

> A skull fracture at pterion tears the middle meningeal artery to produce an epidural hematoma.

   d. **Inferior alveolar artery**
      • Distributed with inferior alveolar nerve to lower teeth, chin, and lower lip
   e. **Branches to muscles of mastication**
      • Arise from **second part** of maxillary artery
   f. **Posterior superior alveolar artery**
      • Enters posterior surface of maxilla to supply posterior maxillary teeth
   g. **Infraorbital artery**
      • Distributed with **infraorbital nerve** (V2), giving **anterior superior alveolar artery** to supply anterior maxillary teeth and middle of face
   h. **Sphenopalatine artery**
      (1) Passes medially into **nasal cavity** through **sphenopalatine foramen**
      (2) Major blood supply to **nasal cavity** and **paranasal sinuses**
   i. **Descending palatine artery**
      • Descends through **palatine canal,** dividing into **greater** and **lesser palatine arteries** to supply **hard** and **soft palates,** respectively

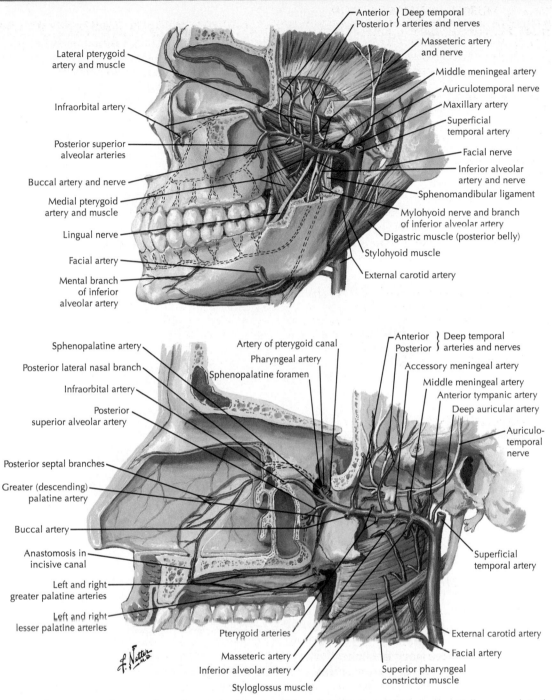

Anterior ⎫ Deep temporal
Posterior ⎬ arteries and nerves

Masseteric artery
and nerve

Middle meningeal artery

Auriculotemporal nerve

Maxillary artery

Superficial
temporal artery

Facial nerve

Inferior alveolar
artery and nerve

Sphenomandibular ligament

Mylohyoid nerve and branch
of inferior alveolar artery

Digastric muscle (posterior belly)

Stylohyoid muscle

External carotid artery

Lateral pterygoid
artery and muscle

Infraorbital artery

Posterior superior
alveolar arteries

Buccal artery and nerve

Medial pterygoid
artery and muscle

Lingual nerve

Facial artery

Mental branch
of inferior
alveolar artery

Sphenopalatine artery

Posterior lateral nasal branch

Infraorbital artery

Posterior
superior alveolar artery

Posterior septal branches

Greater (descending)
palatine artery

Buccal artery

Anastomosis in
incisive canal

Left and right
greater palatine arteries

Left and right
lesser palatine arteries

Artery of pterygoid canal

Pharyngeal artery

Sphenopalatine foramen

Anterior ⎫ Deep temporal
Posterior ⎬ arteries and nerves

Accessory meningeal artery

Middle meningeal artery

Anterior tympanic artery

Deep auricular artery

Auriculo-
temporal
nerve

Superficial
temporal artery

External carotid artery

Facial artery

Pterygoid arteries

Masseteric artery

Inferior alveolar artery

Styloglossus muscle

Superior pharyngeal
constrictor muscle

8-11: Maxillary artery. In the *upper figure* the ramus of the mandible and zygomatic arch have been partially removed. In the *lower figure* a paramedian sagittal section of the face and removal of the mandible show the course of maxillary artery branches to the nasal and oral cavities. The middle meningeal artery typically ascends between the roots of the auriculotemporal nerve as shown. *(From Netter, F H: Atlas of Human Anatomy, 4th ed. Philadelphia, Saunders, 2006, Plate 40.)*

5. **Pterygoid venous plexus**
   a. Formed around **maxillary artery** and **lateral pterygoid muscle**
   b. Receives tributaries corresponding to branches of maxillary artery
   c. Coalesces to form **maxillary vein,** which joins **superficial temporal vein** to form **retromandibular vein**
   d. Communicates with **facial vein,** with **inferior ophthalmic vein,** and with **cavernous sinus**

The pterygoid venous plexus may spread infection to the cavernous sinus from an abscessed tooth or the danger area of the face.

6. **Mandibular nerve (V₃) (Figure 8-12)**
   a. Overview
      (1) Passes from **trigeminal (semilunar) ganglion** through **foramen ovale**
      (2) Only division of trigeminal nerve to give motor innervation to skeletal muscles; small **motor root** joins **mandibular nerve** high in infratemporal fossa
      (3) Supplies **sensory** (general somatic afferent [GSA]) **innervation** to mandible, temporomandibular joint, face, cheek and tongue, and dura

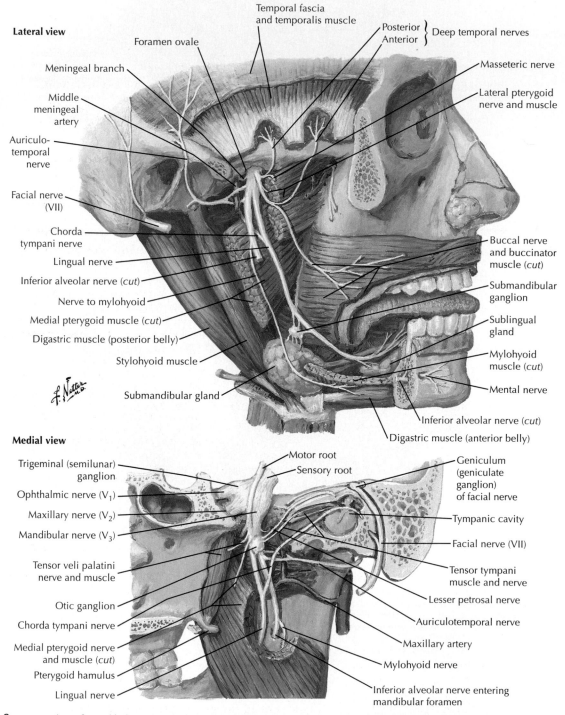

Lateral view

Temporal fascia and temporalis muscle
Foramen ovale
Posterior } Deep temporal nerves
Anterior }
Meningeal branch
Masseteric nerve
Middle meningeal artery
Lateral pterygoid nerve and muscle
Auriculo-temporal nerve
Facial nerve (VII)
Chorda tympani nerve
Buccal nerve and buccinator muscle (cut)
Lingual nerve
Inferior alveolar nerve (cut)
Submandibular ganglion
Nerve to mylohyoid
Sublingual gland
Medial pterygoid muscle (cut)
Digastric muscle (posterior belly)
Mylohyoid muscle (cut)
Stylohyoid muscle
Mental nerve
Submandibular gland
Inferior alveolar nerve (cut)
Digastric muscle (anterior belly)

Medial view

Motor root
Sensory root
Geniculum (geniculate ganglion) of facial nerve
Trigeminal (semilunar) ganglion
Ophthalmic nerve (V₁)
Maxillary nerve (V₂)
Tympanic cavity
Mandibular nerve (V₃)
Facial nerve (VII)
Tensor veli palatini nerve and muscle
Tensor tympani muscle and nerve
Otic ganglion
Lesser petrosal nerve
Chorda tympani nerve
Auriculotemporal nerve
Medial pterygoid nerve and muscle (cut)
Maxillary artery
Pterygoid hamulus
Mylohyoid nerve
Lingual nerve
Inferior alveolar nerve entering mandibular foramen

8-12: Branches of mandibular nerve. In the *upper figure* the ramus and part of the body of the mandible have been removed to give a lateral view of the mandibular nerve. Part of the inferior alveolar nerve was removed with the mandible. In the *lower figure* a medial view of the mandibular nerve is shown as it exits the cranial cavity via the foramen ovale to enter the infratemporal fossa. The otic ganglion is closely related to the mandibular nerve. (*From Netter, F H: Atlas of Human Anatomy, 4th ed. Philadelphia, Saunders, 2006, Plate 46.*)

b. **Motor branches**
   (1) Supply **motor** (special visceral efferent, branchial efferent) **innervation** to muscles that develop from **first pharyngeal arch**
   (2) Innervate four paired **muscles of mastication: temporalis, masseter, medial and lateral pterygoids**
c. **Meningeal branch**
   • Accompanies middle meningeal artery through **foramen spinosum** to supply **dura mater** of middle cranial fossa
d. **Buccal nerve**
   • Pierces **buccinator muscle,** supplying sensation to skin and mucous membrane of cheek and gums

The buccal branch of V is sensory, and the buccal branch of VII is motor.

e. **Auriculotemporal nerve**
   (1) Arises by **two roots** that encircle **middle meningeal artery**
   (2) Ascends in front of ear, supplying external ear and tympanic membrane, temporomandibular joint, and scalp of temporal region
   (3) Carries **postganglionic parasympathetic fibers** from **otic ganglion** to **parotid gland**
f. **Lingual nerve**
   (1) Carries **general sensation (GSA)** from **anterior two-thirds of tongue**
   (2) Joined by **chorda tympani** carrying **preganglionic parasympathetic** (general visceral efferent, GVE) fibers to **submandibular ganglion** and **taste** (special visceral afferent [SVA]) fibers from **anterior two-thirds of tongue**
   (3) Distal to **submandibular ganglion** carries postganglionic **parasympathetic fibers** to **sublingual salivary gland; submandibular gland** is supplied by direct **branches of ganglion**
g. **Inferior alveolar nerve**
   (1) Enters **mandibular foramen** after giving off **mylohyoid nerve** to supply **mylohyoid muscle** and **anterior belly of digastric muscle**
   (2) Gives **inferior dental** and **gingival branches** in **mandibular canal**
   (3) Divides into **incisive nerve** to canine and incisor teeth and **mental nerve** to chin and skin and mucosa of lower lip

Temporary facial paralysis may result from an errant inferior alveolar nerve block.

The **mandibular nerve** can be blocked in the infratemporal fossa just after it emerges from the **foramen ovale.** For dental procedures on the mandibular teeth, the **inferior alveolar nerve** is blocked as it enters the **mandibular foramen.** The **facial nerve** or **lingual nerve** may be blocked or injured by incorrect needle placement during an inferior alveolar injection. Temporary facial paralysis and tongue anesthesia, respectively, may result.

Four paired parasympathetic ganglia in head: otic, submandibular, pterygopalatine, and ciliary

7. **Otic ganglion (Table 8-4)**
   a. Closely related to **mandibular nerve** just below foramen ovale
   b. Receives **preganglionic parasympathetic** fibers from **glossopharyngeal nerve** via tympanic branch and **lesser petrosal nerve**
   c. Sends **postganglionic parasympathetic** fibers to **parotid gland** via **auriculotemporal nerve**
IV. **Cranial Cavity, Meninges, and Dural Venous Sinuses**
   A. **Meninges**
      1. **Pia mater**
         a. Fine vascular **inner layer** inseparable from surface of **brain**
         b. Forms **sheath** around **blood vessels** as they penetrate brain
         c. Normally a transparent membrane unless inflamed as in **meningitis**

Pia mater covers the surface of the brain.

      2. **Arachnoid mater**
         a. Transparent **intermediate layer** applied to inner surface of **dura mater**
         b. Separated from pia mater by **subarachnoid space** containing cerebrospinal fluid (CSF), but connected to it by delicate **arachnoid trabeculae**
         c. **Arachnoid granulations** pass CSF into venous blood of **superior sagittal sinus** and **lateral lacunae**

Hydrocephalus is excess CSF inside the cranial cavity due to obstructed flow or resorption.

TABLE 8-4. AUTONOMIC INNERVATION OF THE HEAD

PREGANGLIONIC CELL BODIES	PREGANGLIONIC NERVE FIBERS	POSTGANGLIONIC CELL BODIES	POSTGANGLIONIC NERVE FIBERS	STRUCTURES INNERVATED
Parasympathetic				
Edinger-Westphal nucleus	Oculomotor nerve, inferior division, motor root to ciliary ganglion	Ciliary ganglion	Short ciliary nerves	Ciliary muscle, sphincter pupillae muscle
Superior salivatory nucleus	Facial nerve, greater petrosal nerve, nerve of pterygoid canal	Pterygopalatine ganglion	Maxillary nerve branches and lacrimal branch of ophthalmic nerve	Lacrimal gland, nasal and palatine glands
Superior salivatory nucleus	Facial nerve, chorda tympani, lingual nerve	Submandibular ganglion	Direct branches of ganglion; lingual nerve	Submandibular gland, sublingual gland, and microscopic salivary glands
Inferior salivatory nucleus	Glossopharyngeal nerve, tympanic plexus, lesser petrosal nerve	Otic ganglion	Auriculotemporal nerve	Parotid gland
Sympathetic				
Intermediolateral cell column of upper thoracic spinal cord	White rami communicantes, thoracic and cervical sympathetic trunk	Superior cervical sympathetic ganglion	External and internal carotid arterial plexuses	Vascular smooth muscle, sweat glands, dilator pupillae, superior tarsal muscle

---

Communicating hydrocephalus: impaired CSF resorption. Noncommunicating hydrocephalus: obstructed CSF flow

Hydrocephalus ("water on the brain") is the accumulation of excess CSF inside the cranial cavity with possible **brain damage** due to compression from **increased intracranial pressure.** When arachnoid granulations are scarred (e.g., **bacterial meningitis**), CSF fluid collects in the subarachnoid space. This is called **communicating hydrocephalus** because CSF can flow through the brain ventricles and the subarachnoid space. **Noncommunicating hydrocephalus** occurs when CSF flow is obstructed and ventricles become dilated.

3. **Dura mater**
   a. Tough fibrous **outer layer** consisting of inner **meningeal** and outer **periosteal dura;** only meningeal layer is continuous with spinal dura

The meningeal layer of cranial dura mater, but not the periosteal layer, is continuous with the spinal dura.

   b. Encloses **dural venous sinuses** between the two layers or within infoldings of meningeal layer
B. **Spaces Related to Meninges**
   1. **Epidural space**
      • **Potential space** because dura forms **periosteum** lining cranial cavity

An epidural hematoma forms a biconvex mass, and a subdural hematoma forms a crescent-shaped mass on CT images.

An **epidural (extradural) hematoma** usually forms when the **middle meningeal artery** is **torn** after trauma near **pterion,** but it may also be caused by a **torn dural venous sinus. Unconsciousness and death are often rapid** because the bleeding dissects a wide space as it strips the dura from the inner surface of the skull, which puts pressure on the brain. An epidural hematoma forms a characteristic **biconvex hyperdense mass on CT images (Figure 8-13).**

   2. **Subdural space**
      • Not present normally because arachnoid is loosely attached to dura by dural border cell layer, and CSF pressure resists separation.

Torn cerebral veins can cause a subdural hematoma days to months after an injury.

A **subdural hematoma** creates an artifactual space by tearing the dura mater from the underlying arachnoid. The hematoma usually results when **cerebral veins** bridging the dura-arachnoid to a dural venous sinus are **torn** by **excessive anteroposterior movement** of the brain within the skull and may develop days to months after injury. Subdural hematomas are usually **crescent-shaped on CT images.** They can be spontaneous or follow a lumbar puncture and are more frequent in elderly people with **brain atrophy.**

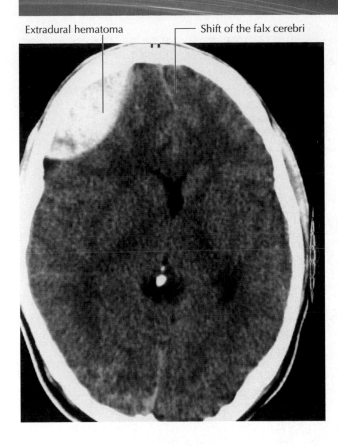

Extradural hematoma — | — Shift of the falx cerebri

8-13: Axial CT showing characteristic biconvex shape of epidural hematoma. *(From Drake, R, Vogl, W A, Mitchell, A: Gray's Anatomy for Students, 2nd ed. Philadelphia, Churchill Livingstone, 2010, Figure 8.45.)*

3. **Subarachnoid space**
   a. Space between **arachnoid** and **pia mater** in which **CSF** circulates
   b. Enlarged in regions known as **cisterns**

CSF circulates in the subarachnoid space around the brain and spinal cord.

The most common form of hydrocephalus is **obstructive (noncommunicating) hydrocephalus** with CSF accumulation within the ventricles of the brain. It may be **congenital** or acquired. **Stenosis of the cerebral aqueduct** is a common cause of congenital hydrocephalus. **Subarachnoid hemorrhage, trauma,** and **infection** cause **acquired hydrocephalus** due to blocked flow toward the superior sagittal sinus.

Sudden onset of a severe headache, nuchal rigidity, vomiting, and coma characterizes a **subarachnoid hemorrhage,** which is bleeding from a vessel that crosses the subarachnoid space. The bleeding may result from **trauma** or a **ruptured berry aneurysm** of the cerebral vessels related to the arterial circle or a bleeding **arteriovenous malformation.**

A hemorrhagic stroke of the cerebral arterial circle causes a subarachnoid hemorrhage; an ischemic stroke from artery occlusion does not.

C. **Folds of Cranial Dura Mater (Figure 8-14)**
   - Tough double-layered infoldings of **meningeal layer** that partition cranial cavity into **compartments**
   1. **Falx cerebri**
      a. Sickle-shaped, midline fold in **longitudinal cerebral fissure**
      b. Attached posteriorly to **tentorium cerebelli**
      c. Encloses **superior sagittal sinus** in its attached superior border and **inferior sagittal sinus** in its free inferior border
   2. **Tentorium cerebelli**
      a. Tentlike partition over posterior cranial fossa attached above to falx cerebri
      b. Encloses **straight sinus** in its junction with falx cerebri
      c. Free concave anterior border forms **tentorial notch** around midbrain

Increased intracranial pressure may cause fatal brain herniation.

Sagittal section

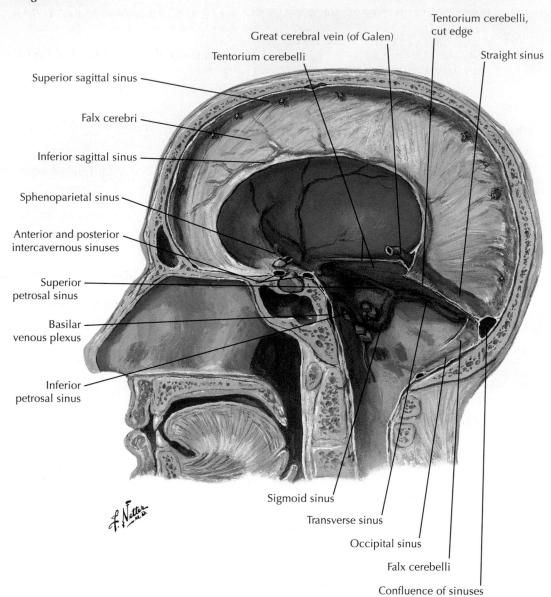

Superior sagittal sinus

Great cerebral vein (of Galen)

Tentorium cerebelli

Tentorium cerebelli, cut edge

Straight sinus

Falx cerebri

Inferior sagittal sinus

Sphenoparietal sinus

Anterior and posterior intercavernous sinuses

Superior petrosal sinus

Basilar venous plexus

Inferior petrosal sinus

Sigmoid sinus

Transverse sinus

Occipital sinus

Falx cerebelli

Confluence of sinuses

8-14: Dural venous sinuses in paramedian sagittal section of head. See Figure 8-5 for a superior view. *(From Netter, F H: Atlas of Human Anatomy, 4th ed. Philadelphia, Saunders, 2006, Plate 103.)*

Transtentorial herniation: ipsilateral dilated pupil and contralateral hemiparesis

Increased **intracranial pressure** may damage the brain through impaired cerebral perfusion or shifting of intracranial contents. Herniation of a cerebral hemisphere under the **falx cerebri** causes compression of the **anterior cerebral artery.** The tentorium cerebelli separates **supratentorial** and **infratentorial compartments,** which communicate through the **tentorial notch.** A **space-occupying lesion** in half of the supratentorial compartment may cause medial displacement and **herniation** of the **temporal lobe** into the infratentorial compartment (transtentorial herniation), usually compressing the ipsilateral **oculomotor nerve** (dilated pupil), **cerebral peduncle** (contralateral hemiparesis), and **posterior cerebral artery** (hemorrhagic infarction of the occipital lobe). A **mass** in the **posterior fossa** may cause **herniation** of one or both **cerebellar tonsils** through the foramen magnum, compressing the medulla and causing sudden respiratory arrest.

3. **Falx cerebelli**
   - Small sickle-shaped median fold **between cerebellar hemispheres** that encloses **occipital sinus** in its posterior attached border

4. **Diaphragma sellae**
   - Roof of **hypophyseal fossa** with opening in middle for passage of hypophyseal stalk (infundibulum)

D. Innervation of Cranial Dura Mater
- Supplied by meningeal branches of trigeminal nerve and fibers of cervical spinal nerves distributed with vagus and hypoglossal nerves

1. **Anterior cranial fossa dura**
   - Supplied by **anterior ethmoidal nerves** (V_1)
2. **Middle cranial fossa dura**
   - Supplied by branches of **maxillary** and **mandibular nerves,** which follow **middle meningeal artery** to also supply dura of calvaria
3. **Posterior cranial fossa dura**
   - Supplied by **spinal nerves C2** and **C3** directly or through meningeal branches of vagus and hypoglossal nerves
4. **Tentorium cerebelli and falx cerebri**
   - Supplied by **meningeal branch** of **ophthalmic nerve,** which arises in wall of cavernous sinus and passes posteriorly onto tentorium

E. Blood Supply of Cranial Dura Mater
1. **Middle meningeal artery**
   - Largest artery supplying meninges; arises from **maxillary artery** to supply dura on floor of **middle cranial fossa** and **calvaria**
2. Ethmoidal, accessory meningeal, ascending pharyngeal, and occipital arteries contribute to blood supply

F. Dural Venous Sinuses and Emissary Veins (see Figure 8-14)
1. Overview
   a. **Dural venous sinuses** empty directly or indirectly into **internal jugular vein**
   b. **Emissary veins** provide communication between venous sinuses and tributaries of jugular and facial veins.
2. **Cavernous sinus (Figures 8-14, *A* and 8-15)**
   a. Overview
      (1) Lateral to sella turcica, forming lateral wall of **hypophyseal fossa**
      (2) Receives sphenoparietal sinus, superior ophthalmic vein, central retinal vein, and superficial middle cerebral vein; drains via superior and inferior petrosal sinuses
   b. **Structures in lateral wall of sinus (see Figure 8-15)**
   c. **Structures that pass through sinus**

> Meningeal nerves mediate referred headache pain from eyestrain, neck strain, temporomandibular joint disease, or sinus infection.

> Cancer cells and infection may spread to the cranial dural venous sinuses from the pelvis, abdomen, and thorax through the vertebral venous plexus.

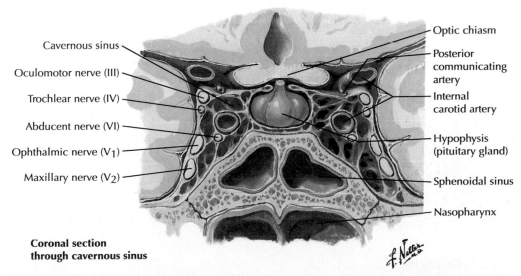

Cavernous sinus

Oculomotor nerve (III)

Trochlear nerve (IV)

Abducent nerve (VI)

Ophthalmic nerve (V_1)

Maxillary nerve (V_2)

Optic chiasm

Posterior communicating artery

Internal carotid artery

Hypophysis (pituitary gland)

Sphenoidal sinus

Nasopharynx

Coronal section through cavernous sinus

8-15: Cavernous sinuses, coronal section. *(From Netter, F H: Atlas of Human Anatomy, 4th ed. Philadelphia, Saunders, 2006, Plate 104.)*

• Separated from venous blood only by vascular endothelium
(1) **Internal carotid artery** and **internal carotid plexus**
(2) **Abducens nerve (CN VI)**

A carotid-cavernous fistula produces pulsating exophthalmos.

Traumatic **laceration of the internal carotid artery** in a basilar skull fracture or its **aneurysmal rupture** in the cavernous sinus causes an **arteriovenous (carotid-cavernous) fistula.** Arterial blood fills the cavernous sinus and its tributaries, resulting in **pulsating exophthalmos.** Pressure on related cranial nerves, usually CN VI first, may paralyze the extraocular muscles. A **pituitary tumor** or an **aneurysm** of the internal carotid artery within the sinus may also impinge on cranial nerves.

An internal carotid aneurysm in cavernous sinus may cause palsy involving CN III, CN IV, and CN VI.

3. **Emissary veins**
    a. Connect dural venous sinuses and veins outside cranial cavity
    b. Valveless veins allowing blood flow in either direction, potentially spreading infection into cranial cavity
4. **Venous communications of cavernous sinus**
    a. **Facial vein** via **superior ophthalmic vein**
    b. **Pterygoid venous plexus** via **sphenoidal emissary vein** and via communicating vein to inferior ophthalmic vein
    c. **Cavernous sinus** of other side via **intercavernous sinuses**
    d. **Sigmoid sinus** and **internal jugular vein** via **superior** and **inferior petrosal sinuses,** respectively

The emissary veins may carry infections from the face or scalp into the cranial cavity.

Infectious material may spread to the **cavernous sinus** from the **face, orbit, sphenoidal sinus, pterygoid venous plexus,** or **middle ear,** causing life-threatening **meningitis** and thrombosis. The **contralateral sinus** is usually involved from the spread of infection through the **intercavernous sinuses.**

Cavernous sinus thrombosis differs from orbital cellulitis by causing bilateral eye involvement, cranial nerve dysfunction, and mental status changes.

V. **Blood Supply of Brain (Figure 8-16)**
   • Derived from **internal carotid and vertebral arteries**
   A. **Vertebral Artery**
      1. Ascends from subclavian artery through **transverse foramina** of vertebrae **C1-C6** and passes medially on posterior arch of atlas to enter **foramen magnum**
      2. At lower border of pons unites with opposite artery to form **basilar artery**
      3. Gives rise to **spinal arteries** and **posterior inferior cerebellar artery**
   B. **Internal Carotid Artery**
      1. Enters **carotid canal** to traverse **petrous temporal** bone and reach middle cranial fossa above **foramen lacerum**

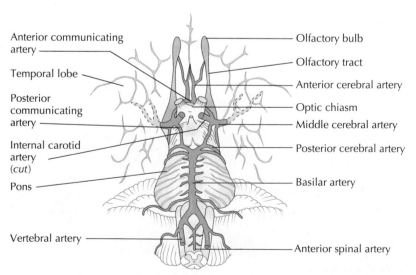

8-16: Cerebral arterial circle in inferior view of brain.

2. Runs **through cavernous sinus** and pierces its roof by curving superiorly and posteriorly (**carotid siphon** on arteriograms) medial to anterior clinoid process

3. Branches into **middle and anterior cerebral arteries**

4. Within **cavernous sinus,** related medially to hypophyseal fossa and sphenoidal sinus and related laterally to oculomotor, trochlear, abducens, V$_1$, and V$_2$ nerves

C. Cerebral Arteries

  1. **Posterior cerebral artery**
    • Supplies **medial surface** of **temporal** and **occipital lobes**

  2. **Anterior cerebral artery**
    • Supplies orbital surface of frontal lobe and medial surface of **frontal** and **parietal lobes**

  3. **Middle cerebral artery**
    • Runs upward and laterally through **lateral cerebral fissure** to supply **lateral surface of cerebral hemisphere**

D. **Cerebral Arterial Circle** (Circle of Willis) (see Figure 8-16)

  1. Potentially important **anastomotic connection** between terminal branches of **internal carotid** and **vertebral arteries** of two sides at base of brain

  2. Common site of **berry aneurysms,** particularly on **anterior communicating artery**

A sudden onset of neurological deficits resulting from impaired blood flow due to occlusion or hemorrhage from a cerebral artery is a **stroke** or **cerebrovascular accident. Ischemic strokes** are much more common than **hemorrhagic strokes.** Temporary neurological deficits may result from transient ischemia, called **transient ischemic attacks or TIAs,** which often precede strokes. Hemorrhage into the subarachnoid space most often results from rupture of a congenital berry (saccular) aneurysm in the cerebral arterial circle in the region of the **anterior communicating artery** and is associated with hypertension.

VI. **Orbit**

A. **Bony Orbit (see Figure 8-1)**

  1. **Roof**
    a. Formed by **orbital plate of frontal bone** and **lesser wing of sphenoid**
    b. Related to **frontal lobe** of brain in **anterior cranial fossa**

  2. **Floor**
    a. Formed by **orbital plate of maxilla, zygomatic bone,** and **orbital process of palatine bone** separating it from **maxillary sinus**
    b. Includes **infraorbital groove** and **canal**

A **blow-out fracture** is a fracture of the **orbital floor** or **medial wall** with no involvement of the orbital rim and is caused by blunt trauma to the orbital contents (e.g., by a handball). The infraorbital nerve in the orbital floor may prevent the orbital contents from being displaced into the maxillary sinus, but an injured infraorbital artery can cause **hemorrhaging. The inferior oblique** or **inferior rectus muscle** may be **entrapped,** limiting upward gaze. Blow-out fractures are rare in young children because the maxillary sinus is small and the orbital floor is not a weak point.

  3. **Medial wall**
    a. Formed by **orbital plate of ethmoid bone, lacrimal bone, frontal bone,** and to small degree by **body of sphenoid**
    b. Related to **ethmoidal air cells, sphenoidal sinus,** and **nasal cavity**
    c. Includes **fossa for lacrimal sac** and opening of **nasolacrimal canal**

  4. **Lateral wall**
    a. Formed by **zygomatic bone, greater wing of sphenoid,** and **frontal bone**
    b. Related through greater wing of sphenoid to **temporal lobe** of brain
    c. Doesn't extend as far anteriorly as medial wall, providing good **surgical access** to eye

  5. **Apex**
    • At **optic canal** just medial to superior orbital fissure

B. **Eyeball (Figure 8-17)**

  1. **Cornea**

The anterior and posterior cerebral arteries supply the medial surface of the cerebral hemisphere. The middle cerebral artery supplies the lateral surface of the cerebral hemisphere.

Collateral circulation through the cerebral arterial circle may prevent brain ischemia in gradual, but not sudden, occlusion.

A stroke in one cerebral hemisphere causes contralateral hemiplegia and sensory loss.

Ischemic strokes occur four times as often as hemorrhagic strokes.

TIAs are stroke like symptoms that last less than 24 hours.

Sharp objects can easily penetrate the roof of the orbit to enter the frontal lobe of the brain.

A blow to the eye may cause a blow-out fracture of the orbital floor or medial wall.

Fractures of the orbital floor may damage the infraorbital nerve and artery.

The thin medial wall of the orbit separates it from the ethmoidal air cells.

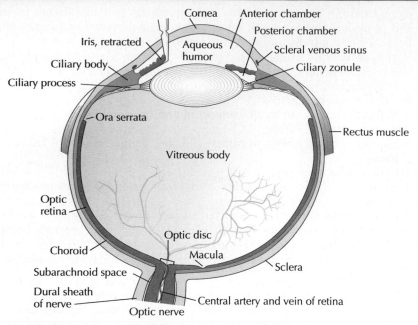

8-17: Right eyeball, horizontal section, superior view.

- Transparent, avascular **anterior component of outer layer** that functions as lens of fixed focal length to refract light entering the eye

2. **Pupil**
   a. Central **aperture of iris** with diameter adjustable by intrinsic smooth muscles
   b. Route for **aqueous humor** flow from **posterior chamber** to **anterior chamber**

> **Glaucoma with initial loss of peripheral vision** from **increased intraocular pressure** usually results from decreased drainage of aqueous humor from the anterior chamber of the eye through the scleral venous sinus (open angle glaucoma).

Glaucoma is increased intraocular pressure with a loss of peripheral vision.

   c. **Sphincter pupillae** of iris decreases aperture size under **parasympathetic control** (CN III)
   d. **Dilator pupillae** increases aperture size under **sympathetic control**

The pupil constricts under parasympathetic control and dilates under sympathetic control.

> A slightly unequal pupil size (physiological **anisocoria**) is considered normal, but such asymmetry should be consistent from bright to dim ambient light. Pupillary constriction (**miosis**) is characteristic of **Horner syndrome.** The pupil usually is *not* dilated in vascular third nerve palsy but *is* dilated (**mydriasis**) in compressive third nerve palsy because visceromotor fibers are superficially placed in the oculomotor nerve.

The pupil is usually dilated in compressive, but not vascular, oculomotor palsy.

3. **Lens**
   a. Transparent **biconvex disc** slightly flattened from tonic tension exerted by **ciliary body** and **suspensory ligament**
   b. Rounds slightly when tension is released by contraction of **ciliary muscle**

> Constriction of the pupil (sphincter pupillae muscle) and rounding of the lens (ciliary muscle) characterize **accommodation,** which is the reflex response that brings objects into focus for **near vision** (e.g., reading). Accommodation is mediated by **parasympathetic** components of the **oculomotor nerve** and the **ciliary ganglion.**

Accommodation is mediated by oculomotor parasympathetic fibers via the ciliary ganglion.

> **Elasticity** and **transparency** of the lens diminish with **age,** predisposing to difficulty with near vision (**presbyopia**) and the need for increased illumination. Additional risk factors for opaque lens (**cataract**) development include diabetes, exposure to some forms of radiation (e.g., ultraviolet light), and the use of corticosteroids. Cataracts may be surgically replaced with artificial lenses.

Cataracts often develop with age and have to be surgically replaced with artificial lenses.

4. **Retina**
   a. Overview
      (1) Inner layer of eyeball adjacent to **vitreous body**
      (2) Consists of posterior optic part of retina and anterior nonvisual part meeting at **ora serrata**
   b. **Optic retina** is formed by inner, light-receptive **nervous layer** and outer **pigmented layer**
      (1) **Macula lutea** is small yellowish area of nervous retina lateral to optic disc
      (2) **Fovea centralis** is central depression of macula lutea containing only **cones** to make it **area of greatest visual acuity**
   c. **Nonvisual retina** is continuation of pigmented layer over ciliary body and posterior surface of iris

> The retina develops from the embryonic **optic cup**, an outgrowth of the forebrain. The optic cup consists of an inner **nervous layer** and outer **pigmented layer** separated by an **intraretinal space** that later disappears. After birth the two layers may separate along the original intraretinal space to produce a **detached retina** and **blindness**. Risk factors for a detached retina include a **tear** through the nervous layer due to **posterior vitreous detachment** with age (allowing fluid to seep between the layers), **trauma** to the eye, **nearsightedness**, and **cataract surgery**. Patients often complain of painless **flashes of light** and a sudden increase in the number of **floaters** in the eye.

5. **Optic disc**
   a. Point on posterior retina where **ganglion cell axons** converge to form **optic nerve; blind spot** caused by absence of photoreceptor cells
   b. Site at which **central artery** enters eyeball to ramify over **retina**

C. **Extraocular Muscles (Figure 8-18; Table 8-5)**
   1. Develop from **preotic somites** and are **innervated by general somatic efferent fibers** in oculomotor, trochlear, and abducens nerves
   2. **Tested in cardinal directions of gaze,** not from anatomical position
      a. Move eyeball in fascial sheath (bulbar sheath) that forms socket; movement of artificial eye may be possible if fascial sheath is preserved
      b. Convergence of pupils by medial recti is involved in binocular vision for close viewing

D. **Nerves of Orbit**
   1. **Ophthalmic nerve (V₁) (Figure 8-19)**
      • Contains only **GSA** fibers
      a. **Frontal nerve**
         • Divides into cutaneous **supraorbital** and **supratrochlear nerves**
      b. **Lacrimal nerve**
         (1) Supplies lacrimal gland, conjunctiva, and upper eyelid
         (2) Receives branch from zygomaticotemporal nerve (V₂) carrying **postganglionic parasympathetic** secretomotor fibers from **pterygopalatine ganglion** for **lacrimal gland**
      c. **Nasociliary nerve**
         • Supplies eyeball, skin of face, mucosa of nasal cavity, and ethmoidal and sphenoidal sinuses; mediates **afferent limb of corneal reflex**
         (1) **Branch (sensory root) to ciliary ganglion**
         (2) **Long ciliary nerves** to the eyeball carry **sensory** fibers and may carry **postganglionic sympathetic** fibers.
         (3) **Posterior ethmoidal nerve** supplies sphenoidal and posterior ethmoidal sinuses.
         (4) **Anterior ethmoidal nerve** supplies anterior and middle ethmoidal air cells, dura mater of anterior cranial fossa, nasal cavity, and dorsum of nose (as external nasal nerve).
         (5) **Infratrochlear nerve**

> **Herpes zoster** (shingles) frequently affects the ophthalmic division of **CN V** (herpes zoster ophthalmicus) with periorbital and possibly ocular lesions. Corneal ulceration and scarring may occur. Reactivation of the varicella-zoster virus follows a period of dormancy within the trigeminal ganglion years to decades after chicken pox.

Photoreceptor cells: rods function in dim light and cones function for color vision and acuity.

The fovea centralis is the area of the greatest visual acuity.

A detached retina is a separation of the nervous layer from the pigmented layer, causing blindness.

The optic disc is the blind spot of the eye because it lacks rods and cones.

The extraocular muscles are tested clinically in the cardinal directions of gaze, not from the anatomical position.

The nasociliary nerve from V₁ is the sensory nerve of the eyeball tested in the corneal reflex; the pupillary light reflex tests CN II and CN III.

Herpes zoster ophthalmicus produces corneal ulceration and scarring.

Right lateral view

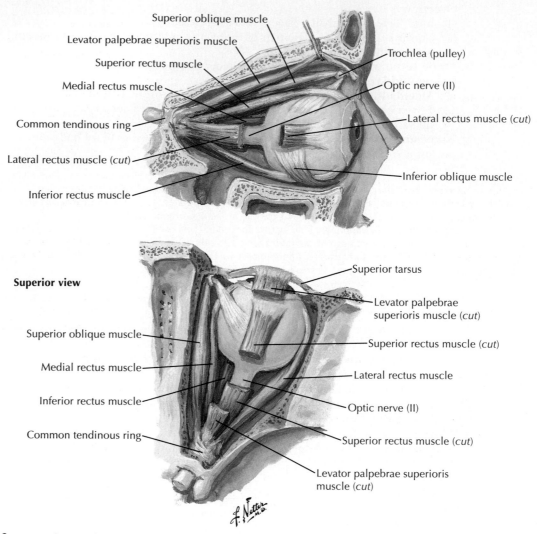

Superior view

8-18: Extraocular muscles. Lateral (*upper figure*) and superior (*lower figure*) views of right orbit. (*From Netter, F H: Atlas of Human Anatomy, 4th ed. Philadelphia, Saunders, 2006, Plate 84.*)

TABLE 8-5. EXTRAOCULAR MUSCLES

MUSCLE	ACTION*	INNERVATION	CLINICAL TEST
Superior rectus	Elevates and adducts pupil	CN III	Patient directed to look far laterally and then upward
Inferior rectus	Depresses and adducts pupil	CN III	Patient directed to look far laterally and then downward
Medial rectus	Adducts pupil	CN III	Patient directed to look far medially
Lateral rectus	Abducts pupil	CN VI	Patient directed to look far laterally
Superior oblique	Depresses and abducts pupil	CN IV	Patient directed to look far medially and then downward
Inferior oblique	Elevates and abducts pupil	CN III	Patient directed to look far medially and then upward
Levator palpebrae superioris	Elevates upper eyelid	CN III	Check for ptosis

*Action relates to eye moving from primary position (gaze is straight ahead).

Superior view

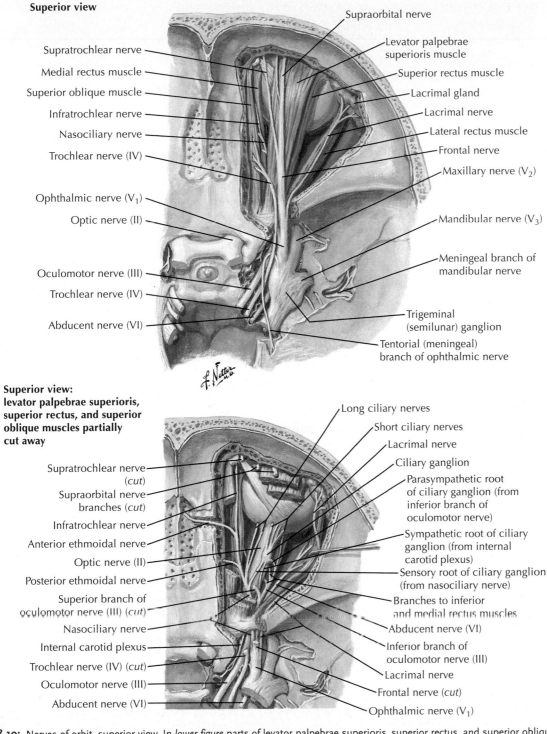

Supraorbital nerve

Supratrochlear nerve

Levator palpebrae superioris muscle

Medial rectus muscle

Superior rectus muscle

Superior oblique muscle

Lacrimal gland

Infratrochlear nerve

Lacrimal nerve

Nasociliary nerve

Lateral rectus muscle

Trochlear nerve (IV)

Frontal nerve

Maxillary nerve (V₂)

Ophthalmic nerve (V₁)

Optic nerve (II)

Mandibular nerve (V₃)

Oculomotor nerve (III)

Meningeal branch of mandibular nerve

Trochlear nerve (IV)

Abducent nerve (VI)

Trigeminal (semilunar) ganglion

Tentorial (meningeal) branch of ophthalmic nerve

Superior view: levator palpebrae superioris, superior rectus, and superior oblique muscles partially cut away

Long ciliary nerves

Short ciliary nerves

Lacrimal nerve

Ciliary ganglion

Supratrochlear nerve (cut)

Parasympathetic root of ciliary ganglion (from inferior branch of oculomotor nerve)

Supraorbital nerve branches (cut)

Infratrochlear nerve

Sympathetic root of ciliary ganglion (from internal carotid plexus)

Anterior ethmoidal nerve

Optic nerve (II)

Sensory root of ciliary ganglion (from nasociliary nerve)

Posterior ethmoidal nerve

Superior branch of oculomotor nerve (III) (cut)

Branches to inferior and medial rectus muscles

Nasociliary nerve

Abducent nerve (VI)

Internal carotid plexus

Inferior branch of oculomotor nerve (III)

Trochlear nerve (IV) (cut)

Lacrimal nerve

Oculomotor nerve (III)

Frontal nerve (cut)

Abducent nerve (VI)

Ophthalmic nerve (V₁)

8-19: Nerves of orbit, superior view. In *lower figure* parts of levator palpebrae superioris, superior rectus, and superior oblique muscles and frontal nerve have been removed. See also Figure 8-25. *(From Netter, F H: Atlas of Human Anatomy, 4th ed. Philadelphia, Saunders, 2006, Plate 86.)*

2. **Trochlear nerve (CN IV)**
   - Innervates **superior oblique** muscle
3. **Abducens nerve (CN VI)**
   - Innervates **lateral rectus** muscle
4. **Oculomotor nerve (CN III)**
   a. Innervates all extraocular muscles except superior oblique and lateral rectus and carries **preganglionic parasympathetic fibers**
   b. Sends **motor (parasympathetic) root** to **ciliary ganglion**

Diplopia (double vision) results from paralysis of one or more extraocular muscles.

Innervation of extraocular muscles: LR₆SO₄AO₃

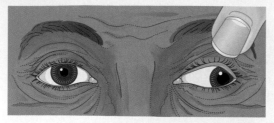
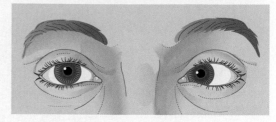

A   B

8-20: Ocular palsies. **A,** External strabismus in oculomotor nerve lesion. **B,** Internal strabismus in abducens nerve lesion. *(From Fitzgerald, M J T, Gruener, G, Mtui E: Clinical Neuroanatomy and Neuroscience, 5th ed. Saunders, 2007, Figure CP 23.1.1.)*

An oculomotor nerve lesion causes external strabismus; an abducens lesion causes internal strabismus.

Weakness or paralysis of extraocular muscles causes misalignment of the two eyes **(strabismus)**, which may be congenital or acquired **(Figure 8-20). Congenital strabismus** often is of unknown etiology. **Acquired strabismus** usually involves a nerve lesion. An **oculomotor nerve lesion** causes the pupil of the affected eye to remain abducted **(external strabismus, exotropia)** due to unopposed contraction of the lateral rectus muscle. The pupil may also be depressed by the superior oblique. A **lesion of the abducens nerve** leaves the eye turned inward **(internal strabismus, esotropia)** or unable to move laterally beyond the neutral position.

5. **Ciliary ganglion (see Table 8-4)**
   • Located posteriorly between **optic nerve** and **lateral rectus** muscle
   a. **Sensory root**
      • Carries **GSA** fibers from **nasociliary nerve** that pass through ganglion without synapsing
   b. **Motor root**
      • Carries **preganglionic parasympathetic** fibers from III that synapse in ganglion
   c. **Sympathetic root**
      • Carries **postganglionic sympathetic** fibers from internal carotid plexus and may join nasociliary nerve to reach ciliary ganglion; fibers traverse ganglion without synapsing
   d. **Short ciliary nerves**
      (1) **Postganglionic parasympathetic** fibers from cell bodies in ganglion
      (2) **GSA** fibers from cornea (V₁) that pass through ganglion without synapsing
      (3) **Postganglionic sympathetic** fibers that traverse ganglion without synapsing

Parasympathetic fibers synapse in the ciliary ganglion, but sympathetic and sensory fibers don't synapse.

An oculomotor nerve lesion produces complete ptosis; a sympathetic nerve lesion causes partial ptosis.

Ptosis may result from oculomotor *or* sympathetic damage. **Oculomotor nerve palsy** causes the inability to **voluntarily** raise the upper eyelid (complete ptosis) and may be associated with pupillary dilation from loss of parasympathetic innervation to the sphincter pupillae muscle. In **Horner syndrome,** partial ptosis from the loss of sympathetic innervation to the superior tarsal muscle is accompanied by pupillary constriction.

6. **Optic nerve (CN II)**
   a. Not a true peripheral nerve, but rather a **brain tract** formed by axons of retinal ganglion cells
   b. Carries **special somatic afferent (SSA)** fibers for **vision** and forms **afferent limb of pupillary light reflex**
   c. Enclosed by meninges and **subarachnoid space** to back of eyeball
   d. Pierced near eyeball by **central artery and vein of retina**
   e. Traverses **optic canal** to join opposite nerve at **optic chiasm,** which may be compressed by **pituitary tumor** or by cerebral arterial circle **aneurysm**

The optic nerve is enclosed by the meninges and subarachnoid space.

Papilledema is a sign of increased intracranial pressure.

Papilledema is optic disc swelling caused by **increased intracranial pressure.** Papilledema is a contraindication to **lumbar puncture** until an intracranial mass has been ruled out due to danger of fatal **brainstem herniation.** Orbital masses that compress CN II and intraocular pathology (e.g., central retinal vein occlusion) may also produce optic disc swelling.

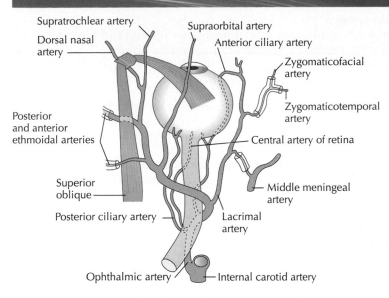

Supratrochlear artery
Dorsal nasal artery
Supraorbital artery
Anterior ciliary artery
Zygomaticofacial artery
Zygomaticotemporal artery
Posterior and anterior ethmoidal arteries
Central artery of retina
Superior oblique
Middle meningeal artery
Posterior ciliary artery
Lacrimal artery
Ophthalmic artery
Internal carotid artery

E. Blood Vessels of Orbit
1. **Ophthalmic artery (Figure 8-21)**
   - Arises from **internal carotid artery** medial to anterior clinoid process and enters orbit through **optic canal**

An **aneurysm** of the **ophthalmic artery** may compress **CN II** and cause **loss of vision**.

   a. **Central artery of retina**
      (1) Pierces **optic nerve** near eyeball to reach and supply **retina** except layer of rods and cones
      (2) A functional **end artery** lacking anastomoses with other arteries

Occlusion of the central artery of the retina produces sudden blindness in that eye.

Amaurosis fugax is the temporary loss of vision that may precede a stroke or myocardial infarction.

Blindness may result from **ischemia** caused by a retinal embolus from a diseased ipsilateral carotid artery, carotid artery insufficiency, or retinal vascular spasm. **Amaurosis fugax** is the transient loss of vision, usually resulting from brief obstruction of the retinal circulation but sometimes from neurologic or ocular problems. Amaurosis fugax of circulatory origin may precede a stroke or myocardial infarction.

   b. **Lacrimal artery**
      - Supplies lacrimal gland, eyelids, and conjunctiva
   c. **Short and long posterior ciliary arteries**
      - Enter back of eyeball to supply choroid, ciliary body, and iris
   d. **Anterior ethmoidal artery**
   e. **Dorsal nasal artery**
      - Supplies lacrimal sac, and dorsum of nose and anastomoses with **angular artery** from external carotid
2. **Central vein of retina**
   - May drain directly into cavernous sinus or superior ophthalmic vein

A **thrombus** in the **central vein of the retina** impairs venous return and causes slow, painless loss of vision.

3. **Ophthalmic veins**
   - Valveless veins permitting blood flow in **either direction**
   a. **Superior ophthalmic vein**
      (1) Passes through **superior orbital fissure** to **cavernous sinus**
      (2) Receives tributaries corresponding to branches of ophthalmic artery and inferior ophthalmic vein

b. **Inferior ophthalmic vein**
  (1) Communicates through inferior orbital fissure with **pterygoid plexus**
  (2) Drains into superior ophthalmic vein or directly into cavernous sinus
F. **Eyelids and Lacrimal Apparatus**
  1. **Eyelids**
    a. **Overview**
      (1) **Closed** by **orbicularis oculi** muscle innervated by **facial nerve**
      (2) **Opened** voluntarily by **levator palpebrae superioris** (CN III) and held open subconsciously by **superior tarsal muscle** (sympathetic)
    b. **Orbital septum**
      (1) Continues from **periorbita** at margins of orbit to attach to tarsal plates
      (2) Together with tarsal plates forms layer separating **orbital space** from subcutaneous layer of face **(periorbital space)**
    c. **Tarsal plates**
      • Thin plates of **fibrous tissue** that **support eyelids**

The orbital septum inhibits the spread of infection from the periorbital space into the orbit.

Orbital cellulitis is a life-threatening infection resulting most often from ethmoidal sinusitis.

Infection of the skin of the eyelid or surrounding area **(periorbital or preseptal cellulitis)** anterior to the curtain formed by the **orbital septum** and **tarsal plates** usually will not spread posteriorly into the orbit. Infection posterior to this curtain **(orbital cellulitis)** may spread intracranially to the cavernous sinus, meninges, and brain. Orbital cellulitis most commonly results from **ethmoidal sinusitis** but may also follow osteomyelitis, facial vein thrombophlebitis, and dental infections.

  2. **Lacrimal apparatus**
    a. **Lacrimal gland**
      (1) Secretes **lacrimal fluid** into superior fornix of **conjunctival sac**
      (2) Receives **preganglionic parasympathetic innervation** from facial nerve with **postganglionic fibers** carried from **pterygopalatine ganglion** by maxillary nerve (V_2)
    b. **Nasolacrimal duct**
      • Drains fluid from lacrimal sac into inferior nasal meatus

The "runny nose" when crying is caused by tears draining through the **nasolacrimal duct. Obstruction** of the drainage system predisposes to **infection** of the **nasolacrimal duct** and **conjunctiva.** In contrast, the "runny nose" associated with the flu or allergies is from sinus drainage directly into the nasal cavity.

VII. **Nasal Cavity and Paranasal Sinuses**
  A. **External Nose**
    • Consists of **bony part** formed by nasal bones and frontal processes of maxillae and **cartilaginous part** formed by alar and lateral nasal cartilages
  B. **Nasal Cavity (Figure 8-22)**
    • Paired chamber separated by **nasal septum** and extending from **naris** anteriorly to communication with nasopharynx at **choana** posteriorly
    1. **Subdivisions of nasal cavity**
      a. **Vestibule**
      b. **Olfactory region**
        • **Upper third** of nasal cavity lined with **olfactory mucosa** for sense of smell
      c. **Respiratory region**
        • **Lower two-thirds** of nasal cavity lined with highly vascular, glandular **respiratory mucosa** to **warm and humidify air**
    2. **Relationships of nasal cavity**
      a. **Roof**
        • Related anteriorly **to anterior cranial fossa** and posteriorly to **body of sphenoid** with **sphenoidal sinuses**
      b. **Floor**
        • **Hard palate** separating nasal cavity from oral cavity
      c. **Medial wall (Figure 8-23)**
        • Formed by **nasal septum** of **septal cartilage, perpendicular plate of ethmoid,** and **vomer**

CSF rhinorrhea from a cribriform plate fracture predisposes to meningitis.

Coronal section

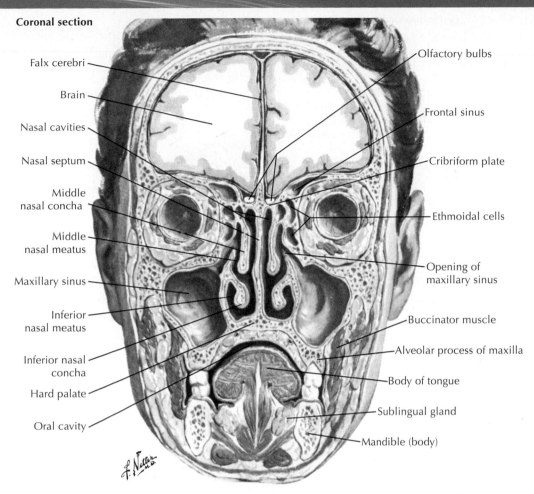

Falx cerebri

Brain

Nasal cavities

Nasal septum

Middle nasal concha

Middle nasal meatus

Maxillary sinus

Inferior nasal meatus

Inferior nasal concha

Hard palate

Oral cavity

Olfactory bulbs

Frontal sinus

Cribriform plate

Ethmoidal cells

Opening of maxillary sinus

Buccinator muscle

Alveolar process of maxilla

Body of tongue

Sublingual gland

Mandible (body)

8-22: Coronal section of head showing nasal cavity and paranasal sinuses. Note that high ostium of maxillary sinus in middle meatus provides inefficient drainage. *(From Netter, F H: Atlas of Human Anatomy, 4th ed. Philadelphia, Saunders, 2006, Plate 48.)*

8-23: Nasal septum, lateral view.

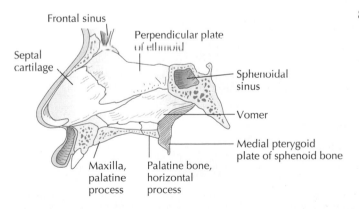

Frontal sinus

Perpendicular plate of ethmoid

Septal cartilage

Sphenoidal sinus

Vomer

Medial pterygoid plate of sphenoid bone

Maxilla, palatine process

Palatine bone, horizontal process

Deviation of the **nasal septum** may **obstruct** the **nasal airway** and **block** the openings of the **paranasal sinuses.** Nasal trauma and developmental defects are the most common causes. Direct **nasal trauma** may cause a "saddle nose deformity" from a loss of cartilage support, or a posttraumatic **septal hematoma** may become infected with the same result. Septal perforation from intranasal cocaine use or Hansen disease also can produce saddling.

Nasal deformities from direct trauma, an infection of posttraumatic hematoma, or medical conditions.

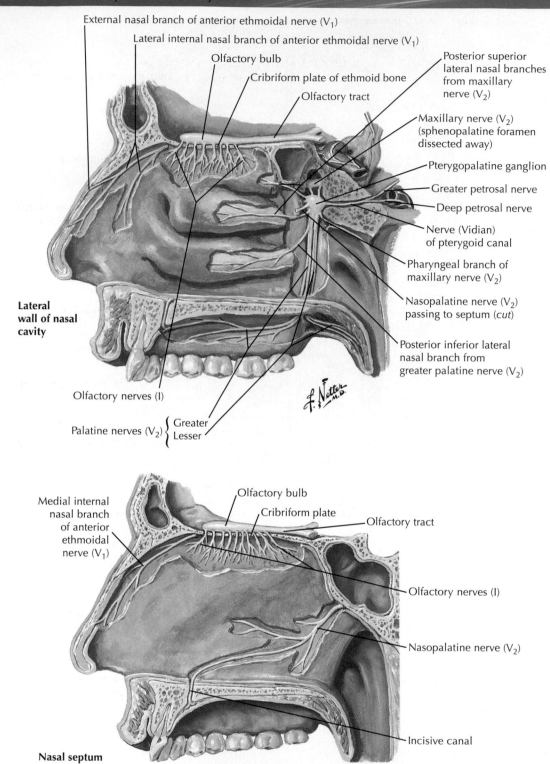

External nasal branch of anterior ethmoidal nerve (V₁)

Lateral internal nasal branch of anterior ethmoidal nerve (V₁)

Olfactory bulb

Cribriform plate of ethmoid bone

Olfactory tract

Posterior superior lateral nasal branches from maxillary nerve (V₂)

Maxillary nerve (V₂) (sphenopalatine foramen dissected away)

Pterygopalatine ganglion

Greater petrosal nerve

Deep petrosal nerve

Nerve (Vidian) of pterygoid canal

Pharyngeal branch of maxillary nerve (V₂)

Nasopalatine nerve (V₂) passing to septum (cut)

Posterior inferior lateral nasal branch from greater palatine nerve (V₂)

Lateral wall of nasal cavity

Olfactory nerves (I)

Palatine nerves (V₂) { Greater / Lesser

Medial internal nasal branch of anterior ethmoidal nerve (V₁)

Olfactory bulb

Cribriform plate

Olfactory tract

Olfactory nerves (I)

Nasopalatine nerve (V₂)

Incisive canal

Nasal septum

8-24: Innervation of nasal cavity. Lateral wall of nasal cavity is shown in *upper figure* with bone removed to expose pterygopalatine ganglion in pterygopalatine fossa. Nasal septum is shown in *lower figure*. (From Netter, F H: Atlas of Human Anatomy, 4th ed. Philadelphia, Saunders, 2006, Plate 43.)

    d. **Lateral wall (Figure 8-24)**
- Complicated structure formed by parts of lacrimal, ethmoid, maxillary, palatine, sphenoid, and inferior nasal concha bones
(1) **Superior** and **middle nasal conchae** of ethmoid bone
(2) **Inferior nasal concha,** a separate bone

(3) **Superior meatus**
  • Receives opening of posterior ethmoidal air cells
(4) **Middle meatus**
  (a) Contains **ethmoidal bulla** and **semilunar hiatus**
  (b) Receives openings of frontal and maxillary sinuses and anterior and middle ethmoidal air cells
(5) **Inferior meatus**
  • Receives opening of **nasolacrimal duct**

3. **Innervation of nasal cavity (see Figure 8-24)**
  a. Overview
    (1) **GSA** innervation to mucosa of nasal cavity supplied by branches of **ophthalmic** (V_1) and **maxillary** (V_2) **nerves**
    (2) **SVA** olfaction carried by **olfactory nerves**
    (3) **Preganglionic parasympathetic** innervation to glands derived from facial nerve with **postganglionic fibers** from cell bodies in **pterygopalatine ganglion** distributed through branches of maxillary nerve (V_2)
    (4) **Postganglionic sympathetic** innervation to **blood vessels** from cell bodies in **superior cervical ganglion** distributed through branches of maxillary nerve and also through perivascular plexuses
  b. **Nasopalatine nerve** (V_2)
    • Branch that descends on nasal septum and through **incisive canal**, supplying **septum** and anterior **hard palate**
  c. **Anterior ethmoidal nerve** (V_1)
    • GSA innervation to mucosa of **upper anterior** nasal cavity
  d. **Olfactory nerves**
    • Arise from neuron cell bodies in **olfactory mucosa** and pierce **cribriform plate** of ethmoid to reach olfactory bulb

> The nasal cavity receives GSA innervation from V_1 and V_2 and SVA innervation from CN I.

4. **Blood supply of nasal cavity**
  • Derived mostly from **sphenopalatine** and **anterior ethmoidal** arteries with contributions from greater palatine, superior labial, and posterior ethmoidal arteries
  a. **Sphenopalatine artery**
    (1) Arises in pterygopalatine fossa from **maxillary artery** and enters nasal cavity through **sphenopalatine foramen**
    (2) Supplies **posterior part** of nasal septum and lateral nasal wall
  b. **Anterior ethmoidal artery**
    (1) Arises from **ophthalmic artery** and traverses **ethmoidal labyrinth** and **anterior cranial fossa** before entering **nasal cavity**
    (2) Supplies **upper anterior part** of septum and lateral nasal wall

> The sphenopalatine artery is the major supply to the nasal cavity.

Epistaxis (nosebleed) most often occurs from the anterior nasal septum **(Kiesselbach area)**, where branches of the sphenopalatine, anterior ethmoidal, greater palatine, and superior labial (from facial) arteries converge. In severe cases, **ligation of the external carotid artery** may be necessary to **control hemorrhage.** Unfortunately, ligation might not be completely successful because of abundant collateral circulation and because the **ethmoidal arteries** arise from the **internal carotid** via the ophthalmic artery. For posterior hemorrhage, the pterygopalatine part of the **maxillary artery** may be approached through the maxillary sinus and **ligated.**

> A nosebleed usually occurs from Kiesselbach area on the anterior nasal septum.

C. **Paranasal Sinuses (Table 8-6)**
  1. **Overview**
    a. Develop as outgrowths of nasal mucosa into bones surrounding nasal cavity
    b. Innervated by **maxillary** and **ophthalmic** divisions of **trigeminal nerve**
    c. Reduce weight of skull, serve as resonating chambers for sound production, and increase surface area for warming and humidifying inspired air
  2. **Maxillary sinus (see Figure 8-22)**
    • Largest of paranasal sinuses and already present at birth

> Maxillary sinusitis frequently causes toothaches.

TABLE 8-6. PARANASAL SINUSES

PARANASAL SINUS	LOCATION	RELATIONSHIPS	DRAINAGE SITE IN NASAL CAVITY
Maxillary Sinus	Body of maxilla	Nasal cavity medially, orbit above	Semilunar hiatus
Sphenoidal Sinus	Body of sphenoid	Pituitary gland and optic chiasm above, nasopharynx below, cavernous sinuses laterally, brainstem posteriorly	Sphenoethmoidal recess
Ethmoidal Sinus (ethmoidal air cells)	Ethmoidal labyrinth	Nasal cavity medially, orbit laterally	
Anterior air cells			Semilunar hiatus
Middle air cells			Ethmoidal bulla
Posterior air cells			Superior meatus
Frontal Sinus	Squamous and orbital parts of frontal bone	Anterior cranial fossa posteriorly, orbit below	Middle meatus

In **maxillary sinusitis,** the sinus accumulates mucus. Because the **ostium** of the maxillary sinus is well above the level of its floor, its drainage is inefficient, particularly when inflamed. To facilitate drainage, an accessory opening may be created surgically, often into the inferior meatus. Only a thin layer of bone and mucoperiosteum or just mucous membrane may separate the **roots** of the **maxillary teeth** and the **superior alveolar nerves** from the sinus cavity, and sinusitis frequently produces a **toothache.** If only a thin layer of bone covers the roots of the molars, **extraction** may create a **fistula** between the sinus and oral cavity, resulting in infection.

3. Sphenoidal sinus (see Figure 8-3)

Relationships of the **sphenoidal sinus** are clinically important because of potential **injury during pituitary surgery** and the possible **spread of infection.** Pituitary adenomas frequently are removed via a nasal cavity approach **(endonasal transsphenoidal surgery).** Infection can reach the sinuses through their ostia from the nasal cavity or through their floor from the nasopharynx. Infection may erode the walls to reach the cavernous sinuses, pituitary gland, optic nerves, or brainstem.

4. Ethmoidal sinus (see Figures 8-3 and 8-22)

Infection in the **ethmoidal air cells** can erode the medial wall of the orbit, resulting in **orbital cellulitis** that can spread to the cranial cavity. Ethmoidal sinusitis is most commonly seen in children.

5. Frontal sinus (see Figures 8-3 and 8-23)

A frontal sinus infection may spread intracranially to cause meningitis.

Frontal sinusitis is usually accompanied by **maxillary sinusitis** because of the close relationship of the ostia in the middle meatus. **Frontal sinusitis** may erode the thin bone of the anterior cranial fossa, producing **meningitis** and/or brain abscess. Despite antibiotic therapy, sinusitis with intracranial spread is a significant source of morbidity and mortality.

VIII. Pterygopalatine Fossa
    A. Branches of Pterygopalatine Portion of Maxillary Artery (see Figure 8-11)
        1. Posterior superior alveolar artery
          • Enters posterior surface of maxilla to supply **upper molars and premolars**
        2. Infraorbital artery
          a. Accompanies infraorbital nerve to supply **middle face**
          b. Gives rise to **anterior superior alveolar artery**
        3. Sphenopalatine artery
        4. Descending palatine artery
          • Divides into **greater** and **lesser palatine arteries,** which exit greater and lesser palatine foramina to supply **hard** and **soft palates,** respectively

B. Maxillary Nerve (V₂) (Figure 8-25)

1. Overview
   a. Arises from **trigeminal ganglion** in middle cranial fossa and enters **pterygopalatine fossa** through **foramen rotundum**
   b. Supplies **nasal cavity** and **paranasal sinuses, palate and upper teeth, middle face** and **cheek**, and **dura mater**
2. **Functional components carried in branches of maxillary nerve**
   a. **GSA fibers** from cell bodies in **trigeminal ganglion**
   b. **Postganglionic parasympathetic (GVE) fibers (from CN VII)** from **pterygopalatine ganglion** to lacrimal gland and glands of nasal cavity and palate
   c. **Postganglionic sympathetic fibers** from **superior cervical ganglion** to blood vessels of nasal cavity and palate
   d. SVA taste and GVA fibers (from CN VII) to soft palate via greater petrosal nerve and nerve of pterygoid canal
3. **Branches of maxillary nerve trunk**
   a. **Meningeal branch** supplies dura of middle cranial fossa.
   b. **Posterior superior alveolar nerves** supply posterior maxillary teeth and the maxillary sinus.

The maxillary nerve supplies general sensation to the nasal cavity, palate, and maxillary teeth.

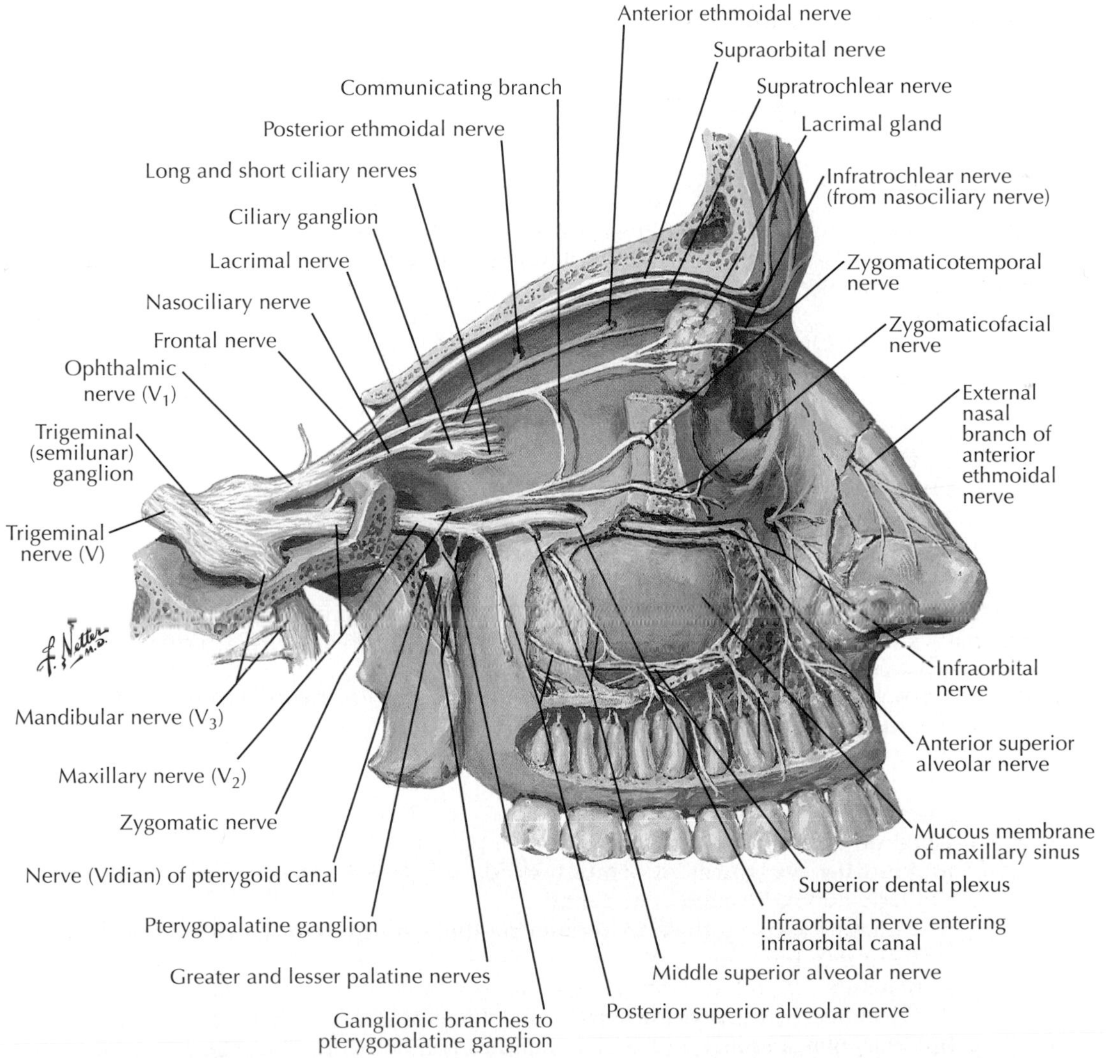

8-25: Ophthalmic (V1) and maxillary (V2) divisions of trigeminal nerve in lateral view with lateral walls of orbit and maxillary sinus removed. Note branches of maxillary nerve and pterygopalatine ganglion. For a medial view of pterygopalatine ganglion branches see Figure 8-24. (*From Netter, F H: Atlas of Human Anatomy, 4th ed. Philadelphia, Saunders, 2006, Plate 45.*)

Labels in figure:
Anterior ethmoidal nerve
Supraorbital nerve
Communicating branch
Supratrochlear nerve
Posterior ethmoidal nerve
Lacrimal gland
Long and short ciliary nerves
Infratrochlear nerve (from nasociliary nerve)
Ciliary ganglion
Zygomaticotemporal nerve
Lacrimal nerve
Zygomaticofacial nerve
Nasociliary nerve
Frontal nerve
External nasal branch of anterior ethmoidal nerve
Ophthalmic nerve (V₁)
Trigeminal (semilunar) ganglion
Trigeminal nerve (V)
Infraorbital nerve
Mandibular nerve (V₃)
Anterior superior alveolar nerve
Maxillary nerve (V₂)
Mucous membrane of maxillary sinus
Zygomatic nerve
Superior dental plexus
Nerve (Vidian) of pterygoid canal
Infraorbital nerve entering infraorbital canal
Pterygopalatine ganglion
Middle superior alveolar nerve
Greater and lesser palatine nerves
Posterior superior alveolar nerve
Ganglionic branches to pterygopalatine ganglion

    c. **Zygomatic nerve** gives **zygomaticotemporal** and **zygomaticofacial nerves** and communicating branch carrying postganglionic parasympathetic fibers for **lacrimal gland**

    d. **Infraorbital nerve** passes through **inferior orbital fissure, infraorbital groove** and **canal,** giving off **anterior superior alveolar nerves** before reaching **infraorbital foramen**

4. **Pterygopalatine ganglion (see Figures 8-24 and 8-25)**

    a. Overview

      (1) Suspended from maxillary nerve by **pterygopalatine nerves**

      (2) Contains cell bodies of **postganglionic parasympathetic neurons** for supply of **lacrimal gland** and **glands of nasal cavity** and **palate**

    b. **Pterygopalatine nerves**

      • **Sensory root** of ganglion carrying **GSA fibers** from V_2 that pass through ganglion **without synapse**

    c. **Nerve of pterygoid canal**

      (1) Formed by union of **greater petrosal** and **deep petrosal nerves**

      (2) **Motor root** of ganglion carrying **preganglionic parasympathetic fibers** in **greater petrosal branch** of facial nerve for synapse in ganglion

      (3) Carries **postganglionic sympathetic fibers** in **deep petrosal** branch of internal carotid plexus to be distributed with branches of ganglion

5. **Branches of pterygopalatine ganglion**

    • Contain mainly nerve fibers of maxillary nerve

    a. **Greater palatine nerve** descends through **greater palatine canal** and **foramen** to supply mucosa of hard palate, giving off posterior inferior lateral nasal branches

    b. **Lesser palatine nerve** descends through **lesser palatine canal** and **foramen** to supply mucosa of soft palate

    c. **Posterior superior lateral and medial nasal nerves** pass through **sphenopalatine foramen** to posterior lateral nasal wall and septum

    d. **Nasopalatine nerve** descends anteriorly on nasal septum and through **incisive canal,** supplying septum and hard palate anterior to incisive fossa

    e. **Pharyngeal nerve** passes through **palatovaginal canal** to supply mucosa of nasopharynx and sphenoidal sinus

IX. Oral Cavity

  A. Divisions of Oral Cavity (see Figure 7-10)

    1. **Vestibule**

      a. Bounded by lips and cheeks externally and by teeth and gums internally

      b. Receives opening of parotid duct at **parotid papilla** opposite **second maxillary molar**

    2. **Oral cavity proper**

      a. Bounded anteriorly and laterally by teeth and gums

      b. Roof formed by **hard** and **soft palates**

      c. Floor formed by **anterior two-thirds of tongue** and **sublingual sulcus** supported mainly by fused **mylohyoid muscles**

      d. Communicates posteriorly with **oropharynx** at **palatoglossal folds**

  B. Teeth

    1. Anchored individually in sockets **(alveoli)** in **alveolar processes** of maxillae and mandible by **periodontal ligament**

    2. Necessary for alveolar processes, which are resorbed in edentulous individual

  C. Palate

    • Separates nasal and oral cavities

    1. **Hard palate**

      a. **Anterior two-thirds of palate** formed by palatine processes of maxillae and horizontal parts of palatine bones

      b. Contains **incisive fossa** in anterior midline and **greater** and **lesser palatine foramina** posterolaterally on each side

    2. **Soft palate**

      a. Fibromuscular **posterior third** attached to posterior border of hard palate

      b. Projects posteriorly and is elevated into contact with pharyngeal wall and tensed during swallowing to close entrance into nasopharynx

      c. Formed by **palatine aponeurosis** and **muscles**

      d. Continuous inferiorly with **palatoglossal** and **palatopharyngeal folds**

3. **Muscles of soft palate**
  - Innervated by **vagus nerve** via **pharyngeal plexus,** except for **tensor veli palatini** supplied by mandibular nerve (V_3)
4. **Blood supply of palate**
  - Derived from **descending** and **ascending palatine arteries**
5. **Sensory nerves of palate** (see Figure 8-24)
  a. **Greater palatine nerve**
  b. **Lesser palatine nerve**
  c. **Nasopalatine nerve**

D. **Tongue**
  - Attached to hyoid bone, mandible, styloid process, soft palate, and pharynx
  1. **Dorsal surface of tongue** (see Figure 7-11)
    - Divided into oral and pharyngeal parts by V-shaped **sulcus terminalis**
    a. **Oral part (anterior ⅔) of dorsal surface**
      (1) Mucous membrane covered by numerous conical **filiform papillae** and scattered **fungiform papillae** bearing taste buds
      (2) V-shaped row of large, round **vallate papillae** with numerous taste buds lying anterior and parallel to sulcus terminalis
    b. **Oropharyngeal part (posterior ⅓) of dorsal surface**
      (1) Covered by lymphoid nodules of **lingual tonsil**
      (2) Connected to epiglottis by median and paired lateral **glossoepiglottic folds** with depressions **(valleculae)** between folds where foreign bodies sometimes lodge
    c. **Foramen cecum of tongue**
      - Apex of sulcus terminalis where **thyroid gland** began embryonic development

> A **lingual thyroid gland** may be present at the foramen cecum. It may be asymptomatic or enlarge in the child or young adult to cause difficulty swallowing **(dysphagia),** difficulty breathing **(dyspnea),** and a **"hot potato voice."** Rarely it may be a source of **hemorrhage.** Surgical excision and possible autotransplantation follow studies to determine if it is the only thyroid tissue present.

2. **Frenulum**
  a. Midline **mucosal fold** connecting tongue to floor of mouth
  b. Restricts movement of tongue in **ankyloglossia** (tongue-tie)
3. **Muscles of tongue** (Figure 8-26)
  a. Consist of **intrinsic muscles** that change shape of tongue and **extrinsic muscles** responsible for larger movements
  b. Develop from myoblasts that migrate from **occipital somites** and carry innervation from **hypoglossal nerve (CN XII)** with them

> A **lesion of CN XII** allows the contralateral, unparalyzed genioglossus muscle to push the protruded tongue toward the paralyzed side. In a supine **unconscious** individual or one under **general anesthesia,** relaxed genioglossus muscles allow the tongue to fall posteriorly and obstruct the airway, potentially causing **suffocation.**

4. **Summary of innervation of tongue**
  a. **General somatic efferent** motor innervation to muscles of tongue from **hypoglossal nerve**
  b. General (GSA) sensation from **anterior two-thirds** of tongue from **lingual nerve** (V_3)
  c. Taste (SVA) sensation from **anterior two-thirds** of tongue from **chorda tympani** (VII)
  d. General (GVA) and taste (SVA) sensation from **posterior third** of tongue from **glossopharyngeal nerve**
5. **Lingual artery** (Figure 8-27)
  - Arises near greater horn of hyoid bone and passes **deep to hyoglossus** muscle, which is used to divide it into **three parts**
  a. **Dorsal lingual arteries**
    - Two to three branches from **second part** that supply **dorsum of tongue**

The levator veli palatini elevates and the tensor veli palatini tenses the soft palate during swallowing to prevent food or drink from entering the nasopharynx.

The vallate and fungiform papillae of the tongue have taste buds.

Foreign objects may lodge in the valleculae.

A large lingual thyroid gland causes dysphagia, dyspnea, and hot potato voice.

The foramen cecum of tongue marks the embryonic origin of the thyroid gland.

A short lingual frenulum causes tongue-tie and may require frenectomy.

In a hypoglossal nerve lesion, the protruded tongue deviates toward the paralyzed side.

Taste in the anterior two-thirds of the tongue is from the chorda tympani (VII), and general sensation is from the lingual nerve (V_3).

Taste and general sensation in the posterior third of tongue are from CN IX.

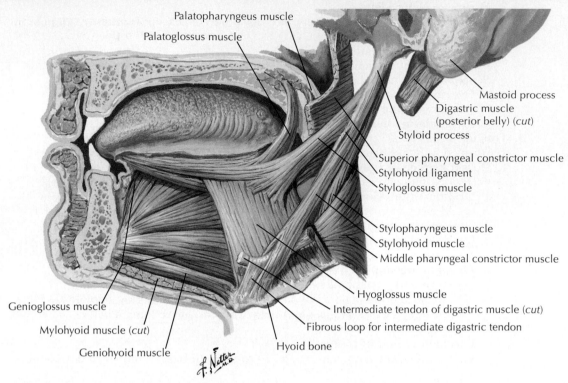

8-26: Extrinsic muscles of tongue, lateral view with left half of mandible removed. Closely related muscles of the pharynx are also shown. *(From Netter, F H: Atlas of Human Anatomy, 4th ed. Philadelphia, Saunders, 2006, Plate 59.)*

8-27: Branches of the lingual artery, lateral view.

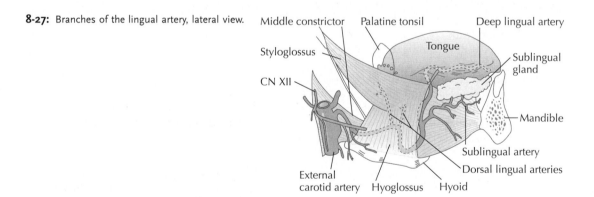

b. **Deep lingual artery**
   - **Terminal branch** from **third part** passing into **tip of tongue**
c. **Sublingual artery**
   - Other **terminal branch** supplying **sublingual salivary gland** and **floor of mouth**
6. **Lingual vein**
   a. Passes **superficial to hyoglossus** muscle with hypoglossal nerve
   b. **Deep lingual tributaries** rapidly **absorb drugs** (e.g., the vasodilator nitroglycerin taken for angina pectoris)
E. **Sublingual Sulcus Region**
   1. **Sublingual gland**
      a. Numerous small ducts open onto floor of mouth on sublingual fold or into submandibular duct
      b. **Postganglionic parasympathetic** innervation from **submandibular ganglion** traveling with lingual nerve

Deep lingual veins rapidly absorb drugs placed under the tongue.

Postganglionic parasympathetic fibers from the submandibular ganglion supply sublingual and submandibular glands.

2. **Submandibular gland**
   a. Wraps around posterior free border of mylohyoid muscle with larger **superficial portion** in submandibular triangle of neck and smaller **deep portion** in floor of mouth
   b. **Submandibular (Wharton's) duct** opens onto **sublingual caruncle** at base of lingual frenulum
   c. **Postganglionic parasympathetic** innervation via direct branches from **submandibular ganglion**

A **salivary gland stone** (salivary calculus) may form in the **submandibular duct,** obstructing the duct and causing the **gland** to be **tense, swollen,** and **painful** when eating. Lymphatic drainage from the lateral part of the anterior two-thirds of the tongue, upper lip, and lateral part of lower lip is to **submandibular lymph nodes,** which overlie the submandibular gland. These nodes may be sites of **metastases** in **carcinoma** or may enlarge due **infection.**

Carcinoma from the upper lip or the side of the anterior tongue metastasizes to the submandibular lymph nodes.

---

3. **Lingual nerve**
   a. Branches from **mandibular nerve** (V_3) and is joined by **chorda tympani (VII)** carrying **preganglionic parasympathetic** and **taste** fibers
   b. Descends from infratemporal fossa to reach **anterior two-thirds of tongue**
   c. Suspends **submandibular ganglion** containing **postganglionic parasympathetic** neuron cell bodies for **submandibular** and **sublingual glands**
4. **Hypoglossal nerve (CN XII)**
   • Lies inferior to lingual nerve and submandibular duct lateral to hyoglossus and deep to mylohyoid

---

Infection of the **sublingual region** may spread rapidly through the floor of the mouth to produce **pain and swelling** in the **submental and submandibular regions (Ludwig angina). Progressive development** is **life-threatening** and is characterized by hardness of the floor of the mouth and posterior superior displacement of the tongue. **Rapid respiratory obstruction** can occur. Most cases originate from **infections of the mandibular molars,** but other sources include **tongue piercing** and **intravenous injections into neck veins.**

Ludwig angina is a life-threatening infection in the floor of the mouth.

X. **Ear (Figure 8-28)**
   A. **External Ear**
      1. **Auricle**
         a. Elastic cartilage covered by skin and anchored to skull by ligaments
         b. Innervated by **great auricular (C2, C3), auriculotemporal** (V_3), and **lesser occipital (C2) nerves**
      2. **External acoustic (auditory) meatus**
         a. Extends from auricle to tympanic membrane, about 2.5 cm
         b. **Outer third** is **cartilaginous** and **inner two-thirds** is **bony**

8-28: External, middle, and inner right ear.

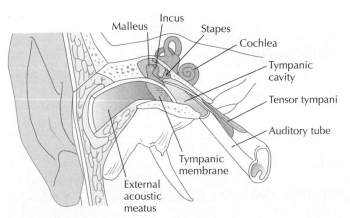

Malleus — Incus — Stapes — Cochlea — Tympanic cavity — Tensor tympani — Auditory tube — Tympanic membrane — External acoustic meatus

Pain may be referred to the ear from pharyngeal or laryngeal cancer via cranial nerves IX and X.

Increased pain from pulling on the ear distinguishes otitis externa from otitis media.

c. Lined by skin containing **ceruminous glands,** which secrete **earwax**
d. Innervated by **auriculotemporal nerve** and **auricular branch of vagus nerve** joined by branches of **facial** and **glossopharyngeal nerves**

External otitis is an inflammation of the auditory canal, usually from moisture in the canal leading to bacterial or fungal infection **(swimmer's ear)** or to an infected hair follicle **(boil).** The condition can be painful because of the tightness of the skin lining the canal that is abundantly innervated. Increased pain from traction on the auricle or opening the jaw helps distinguish otitis externa from otitis media.

Ear pain (otalgia) may be **referred** from the **nasal cavity and paranasal sinuses** via the trigeminal nerve, from the **pharynx and larynx** via the glossopharyngeal and vagus nerves, and from the **cervical spine** via spinal nerves. Causes include **pharyngeal and laryngeal cancer.** Otalgia may be associated with **nausea and vomiting,** a response mediated through the **vagus nerve** and its innervation of the upper gastrointestinal tract.

Temporal bone fracture causes CSF otorrhea.

Communications allow infection to spread from the nasopharynx to the tympanic cavity to the mastoid air cells.

B. **Middle Ear (Tympanic Cavity) (Figure 8-29)**
   • Air-filled cavity within **temporal bone** containing **auditory ossicles**
   1. **Tympanic membrane** (eardrum) **(Figure 8-30)**
      a. Separates external acoustic meatus and tympanic cavity; covered by **skin externally** and **mucosa internally**
      b. Transfers sound vibrations from air to **auditory ossicles**
   2. **Features of tympanic cavity**
      a. **Promontory**
         • Rounded bulge formed on medial wall by **basal turn of cochlea** and covered by **tympanic plexus** derived from **tympanic branch of glossopharyngeal nerve**
      b. **Round window** (fenestra cochleae)
         • Between tympanic cavity and cochlea (scala tympani), closed by **secondary tympanic membrane** that bulges outward to accommodate pressure waves in perilymph

Medial wall of tympanic cavity: lateral view

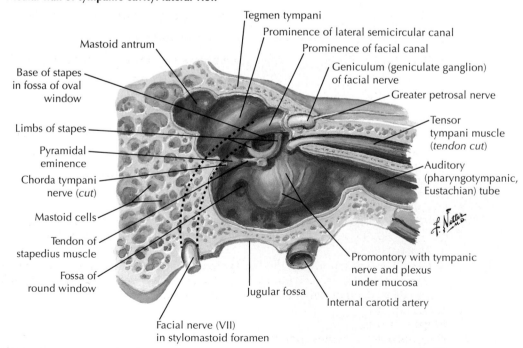

8-29: Medial wall of right middle ear, lateral view. *(From Netter, F H: Atlas of Human Anatomy, 4th ed. Philadelphia, Saunders, 2006, Plate 94.)*

Lateral wall of tympanic cavity: medial (internal) view

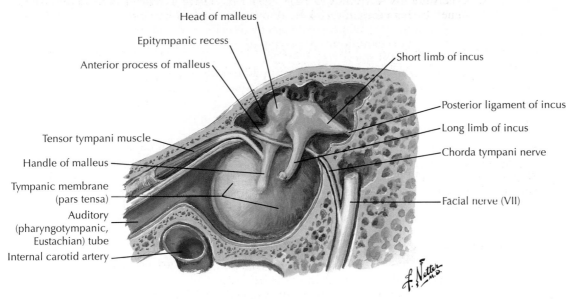

8-30: Lateral wall of right middle ear, medial view. *(From Netter, F H: Atlas of Human Anatomy, 4th ed. Philadelphia, Saunders, 2006, Plate 94.)*

c. **Oval window** (fenestra vestibuli)
  • Between tympanic cavity and vestibule of inner ear closed by **stapes,** which transduces vibrations of auditory ossicles into pressure waves in perilymph of inner ear

> Hearing loss may be mechanical/conductive or due to nerve damage.

> **Otosclerosis** is abnormal bone growth with **fixation** of the footplate of the **stapes** in the oval window, preventing movement and resulting in **conduction deafness.** It is usually inherited as an autosomal dominant condition. Hearing loss may also be **sensorineural** from damage to the spiral organ, cochlear nerve, or brain pathways.

> Otosclerosis is abnormal bone growth fixing stapes in the oval window.

d. **Prominence of facial canal**
  • Ridge above promontory formed by **facial nerve** passing posteriorly from **geniculate ganglion**
e. **Aditus ad antrum**
  • Opens posteriorly from **epitympanic recess** into **mastoid antrum,** providing communication with **mastoid air cells**
f. **Pyramidal eminence**
  • On posterior wall contains **stapedius** muscle
g. **Tegmen tympani**
  • Roof of tympanic cavity separating tympanic cavity from **middle cranial fossa** with temporal lobe of brain
h. **Auditory (pharyngotympanic, Eustachian) tube**
  • Connects anterior wall of tympanic cavity with **nasopharynx**
3. **Auditory ossicles**
  a. Overview
    (1) Transmit vibrations of tympanic membrane to perilymph of inner ear
    (2) Articulate by **synovial joints,** which may be damaged by **arthritis**
  b. **Malleus** (hammer)
    • **Handle** (manubrium) attached to **tympanic membrane** and receives tendon of **tensor tympani** (innervated by V_3), which reflexly contracts in response to loud sounds to dampen vibrations of tympanic membrane
  c. **Incus** (anvil)
  d. **Stapes** (stirrup)
    (1) **Footplate** occupies oval window
    (2) **Neck** receives insertion of **stapedius** (innervated by CN VII), which reflexly contracts to dampen vibrations of stapes at oval window

> Sound waves → eardrum vibrations → auditory ossicle vibrations → perilymph pressure waves → organ of Corti receptors

4. **Nerves related to middle ear**
   a. **Tympanic nerve** (from CN IX)
      (1) Traverses **tympanic canaliculus** to join **tympanic plexus,** supplying **GSA fibers** to tympanic cavity, mastoid air cells, and auditory tube
      (2) Carries **preganglionic parasympathetic** fibers for **parotid gland**
   b. **Lesser petrosal nerve**
      (1) From tympanic plexus enters **middle cranial fossa** and descends through **foramen ovale** or **innominate foramen**
      (2) **Preganglionic parasympathetic** fibers synapse in **otic ganglion,** with **postganglionic parasympathetic** fibers supplying parotid gland
   c. **Facial nerve (CN VII)**
      (1) Enters **internal acoustic meatus** to traverse **facial canal** of temporal bone
      (2) Large **motor root** joined proximally by slender **nervus intermedius** carrying **preganglionic parasympathetic** and **taste fibers**
      (3) Bends sharply backward at **geniculate ganglion** and runs above promontory to reach **posterior wall of tympanic cavity** and descend
      (4) Within **facial canal** gives rise to **greater petrosal nerve, nerve to stapedius,** and **chorda tympani**
   d. **Chorda tympani**
      (1) Branches from **facial nerve** in tympanic cavity just proximal to stylomastoid foramen
      (2) Passes forward lateral to handle of malleus and exits **petrotympanic fissure** to reach infratemporal fossa
      (3) Carries **preganglionic parasympathetic** fibers to **submandibular ganglion** and **SVA taste fibers** from anterior two-thirds of tongue

CN VII traverses the temporal bone via the internal acoustic meatus, facial canal, and stylomastoid foramen.

Fracture of the petrous temporal bone may injure VII to cause facial paralysis and VIII to cause hearing loss and equilibrium disorders.

Facial nerve lesion that paralyzes stapedius causes excessively acute hearing (hyperacusis).

Chorda tympani conveys taste and parasympathetic fibers from facial nerve to lingual nerve.

An upper-respiratory infection often causes otitis media in children because of the shorter, more horizontal auditory tube.

An acute otitis media infection may cause mastoiditis, resulting in life-threatening meningitis and sigmoid sinus thrombosis.

A **red, bulging eardrum** and **fluid in the middle ear** cavity characterize **otitis media,** which is primarily a disease of children because **pharyngeal infection** can more easily reach the middle ear through their shorter, more horizontally oriented auditory tube. Hearing is diminished because of pressure on the eardrum and reduced movement of the **ossicles. Taste** may be **altered** because the **chorda tympani** is affected. **Infection** spreading **posteriorly** from the tympanic cavity can cause **mastoiditis. Infection** that spreads to the **middle cranial fossa** can cause **meningitis** or temporal lobe abscess, and mastoid infection moving into the posterior cranial fossa may produce **sigmoid sinus thrombosis.**

C. **Inner Ear (Figure 8-31)**
   1. Overview
      a. Contains organs of **hearing** and **equilibrium** in **petrous temporal bone** between middle ear and posterior cranial fossa
      b. Consists of communicating chambers of **bony labyrinth** containing corresponding **membranous labyrinth** suspended in fluid **perilymph**
   2. **Cochlea**
      a. Contains membranous **cochlear duct** filled with **endolymph** between **scala vestibuli** and **scala tympani** filled with **perilymph**
      b. Contains spiral **organ of Corti** for hearing in cochlear duct

Cochlea in the inner ear contains receptors for hearing in the organ of Corti.

Meniere disease is characterized by increased endolymph in the inner ear and loss of cochlear hair cells. Clinical findings include dizziness, vertigo (room spinning around), tinnitus (ringing in the ears), and sensorineural hearing loss.

   3. **Vestibule**
      a. Contains membranous **utricle** and **saccule** filled with endolymph and receptors **(maculae)** for linear horizontal and vertical movements
      b. Receives opening of **oval window** from tympanic cavity and communicates with scala vestibuli
   4. **Semicircular canals**
      a. Arranged in **three planes** (two vertical, one horizontal) at right angles so that canal on one side of body works with parallel canal of opposite side
      b. Sensory receptors **(cristae)** for angular movements in dilated **ampullae** at one end of each canal

The maculae of the utricle and saccule detect linear movements; the cristae of the semicircular canals detect angular movements.

Bony and membranous labyrinths: schema

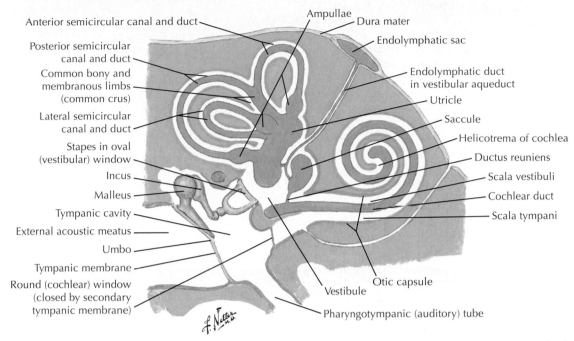

8-31: Middle and inner ear. Note bony and membranous labyrinths. *(From Netter, F H: Atlas of Human Anatomy, 4th ed. Philadelphia, Saunders, 2006, Plate 96.)*

5. **Vestibulocochlear nerve** (CN VIII)
   - Leaves posterior cranial fossa through **internal acoustic meatus** and divides into **vestibular** and **cochlear nerves**

> **Vestibular schwannomas** are benign tumors of the vestibular division of VIII (although referred to as "acoustic neuromas") that usually are located in the cerebellopontine angle. They produce **tinnitus, progressive hearing loss,** and **unsteady gait.** As the tumor enlarges it may compress the facial nerve to produce **ipsilateral facial weakness** and the trigeminal nerve to produce **facial numbness or pain.**

Acoustic neuroma may compress facial and trigeminal nerves to produce facial weakness and pain.

   a. **Vestibular nerve**
      - Innervates **maculae** of utricle and saccule and **cristae ampullares** of semicircular canals with cell bodies in **vestibular ganglion**
   b. **Cochlear nerve**
      - Innervates spiral **organ of Corti** in cochlea with cell bodies in **spiral ganglion**

XI. **Development of Pharyngeal Apparatus**
   A. **Overview**
      1. **Six pairs** of gill-like structures in **4-week-old embryo** from which **face** and **anterior neck** develop; pairs 5-6 not visible externally with **fifth pair 5 often absent**
      2. Consists of **pharyngeal arches** separated externally by **pharyngeal grooves** and internally by **pharyngeal pouches**; double-layered **pharyngeal membranes** of ectoderm-endoderm separate grooves and pouches

The face and the anterior neck of the embryo develop from the pharyngeal arches.

   B. **Pharyngeal (Branchial) Arches (Figure 8-32; Table 8-7)**
      1. Formed by migration of **neural crest cells** around cores of mesoderm; covered externally by ectoderm (skin) and internally by endoderm (mucous membrane)
      2. Each has its own **cartilaginous, muscular, vascular** (aortic arch), and **nervous components.**
      3. Cranial nerve of each arch supplies motor nerve fibers (classified as **special visceral efferent/branchial efferent fibers**) to muscles that develop from that arch.

Neural crest cells form the bones and cartilages of the face.

   C. **Pharyngeal Pouches (Figure 8-33; Table 8-8)**
      - Evaginations of **foregut endoderm** between adjacent arches
   D. **Pharyngeal Grooves (Clefts)**
      1. **Four pairs** of ectoderm-lined depressions between adjacent arches
      2. **First pair** forms **external acoustic meatus** and skin over tympanic membrane

Muscles developing from a pharyngeal arch receive SVE innervation from the cranial nerve of that arch.

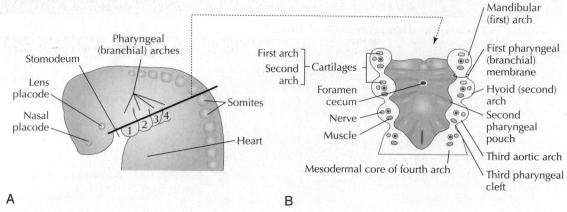

8-32: Pharyngeal arch development at the end of week 4. **A,** Lateral view. *Numbers,* pharyngeal arches. **B,** Section at plane shown in *part A* viewed from above and behind.

TABLE 8-7. HEAD AND NECK DERIVATIVES OF PHARYNGEAL ARCHES

ARCH	BONES AND CARTILAGE	MUSCLES	NERVE	COMMENTS
First arch (mandibular)	Meckel cartilage: malleus, incus, sphenomandibular ligament. Intramembranous: mandible, maxilla, zygomatic bone, squamous temporal bone	Mastication, mylohyoid and anterior belly of digastric, tensor tympani, and tensor veli palatini	CN V	Only mandibular division innervates skeletal muscle (special visceral efferent); first aortic arches contribute to maxillary and external carotid arteries
Second arch (hyoid)	Reichert cartilage: stapes, styloid process, lesser cornu and upper body of hyoid bone, stylohyoid ligament	Facial expression, stapedius, stylohyoid, and posterior belly of digastric	CN VII	Second aortic arches contribute to stapedial arteries
Third arch	Greater cornu and lower body of hyoid bone	Stylopharyngeus	CN IX	Third aortic arches contribute to common and internal carotid arteries
Fourth and sixth arches	Thyroid, cricoid, arytenoid, corniculate, and cuneiform cartilages	Soft palate and pharynx, larynx, striated muscle of esophagus	CN X	Thoracic derivatives of aortic arches
Fifth arch (absent or rudimentary)		No aortic arch derivatives		

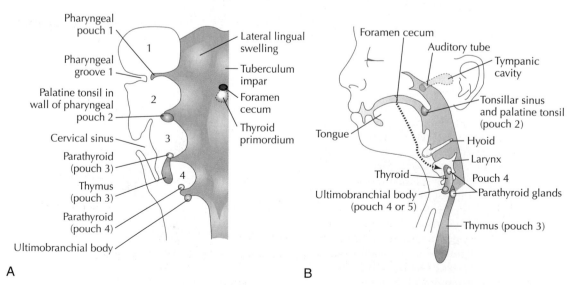

8-33: Derivatives of pharyngeal pouches and floor of pharynx. **A,** Superior view of section through developing pharynx. *Numbers,* pharyngeal arches. **B,** Sagittal section showing derivatives of pharynx. *Arrow,* path of descent of thyroid gland.

TABLE 8-8. DERIVATIVES OF PHARYNGEAL POUCHES

POUCH	POUCH DERIVATIVES	ENDODERM DERIVATIVES	COMMENTS
First pouch	Mastoid antrum, tympanic cavity, and auditory tube	Mucosa of eardrum, tympanic cavity, mastoid antrum, and auditory tube	
Second pouch	Tonsillar fossa	Surface epithelium and crypt lining of palatine tonsil	
Third pouch		Ventral part: thymus Dorsal part: inferior parathyroid gland	Inferior parathyroid gland migrates with thymus; normal thymic development requires neural crest mesenchyme
Fourth pouch		Ventral part: ultimobranchial body Dorsal part: superior parathyroid gland	Ultimobranchial body gives rise to C cells of thyroid gland; superior parathyroid gland migrates with thyroid

3. **Second, third,** and **fourth** grooves lie in **cervical sinus** normally overgrown by second pharyngeal arch

> **Lateral cervical (branchial) cysts** develop in the **neck** from **remnants of the cervical sinus** along the anterior border of the sternocleidomastoid (i.e., laterally). Usually the cysts do not become apparent until late childhood or early adulthood when enlargement, external drainage, or infection may require their removal. The cysts may be connected by a **branchial sinus** externally to the skin along the anterior border of the sternocleidomastoid or internally to mucosa of the tonsillar sinus. A **branchial fistula** connects the skin to the mucous membrane.

A thyroglossal duct cyst occurs in the midline, whereas a branchial cyst occurs in the lateral neck.

E. **Tongue (Figure 8-34)**
   1. Overview
      a. **Mucous membrane of anterior two-thirds** develops from **first pharyngeal arches**
      b. **Mucous membrane of posterior third** develops predominantly from **third pharyngeal arches**
      c. **Muscles** develop from myoblasts that migrate from **occipital somites,** carrying innervation from the **hypoglossal nerve** with them.
   2. **Anterior two-thirds of tongue**
      a. Develops when lateral **distal tongue buds** (lateral lingual swellings) overgrow **median tongue bud** (tuberculum impar)
      b. Receives **general sensation** (GSA) from lingual nerve of first arch (V_3) joined by ingrowth of **chorda tympani** (VII) from second arch for **taste sensation** (SVA)
   3. **Posterior third of tongue**
      a. Develops when tissue of **third arches** in **hypobranchial eminence** overgrows tissue of second and fourth arches
      b. Receives **general** (GVA) and **taste** (SVA) **sensation** (including vallate papillae) from nerve of third arch, **CN IX**

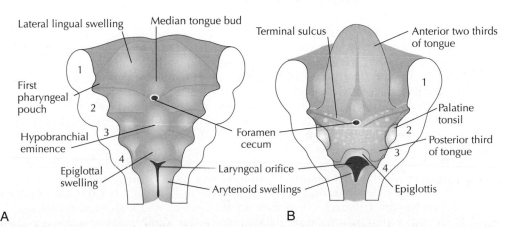

8-34: Development of tongue from pharyngeal floor, viewed from above. *Numbers,* pharyngeal arches.

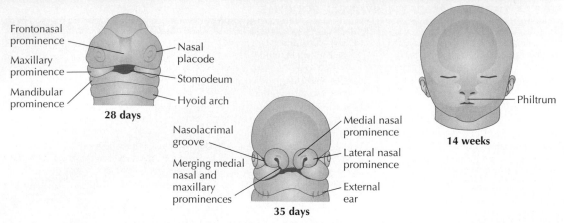

8-35: Three stages in development of the face from the five facial primordia.

F. **Face (Figure 8-35)**
  1. Overview
    a. Formed by merging/fusion of five **facial primordia** that develop around **stomodeum** from migration and proliferation of neural crest ectomesenchyme
    b. Facial primordia receive **sensory innervation** from **trigeminal nerve** with muscles migrating into face from second arch innervated by **facial nerve**
  2. **Frontonasal prominence (V_1)**
    a. Overview
      (1) Forms forehead, rostral boundary of stomodeum, and dorsum of nose
      (2) Inferolaterally on each side, ectoderm thickens as **nasal placode** and sinks into **nasal pit** because of development of **nasal prominences**
    b. **Medial nasal prominences**
      (1) Merge in midline to form **intermaxillary segment,** which gives rise to **philtrum of upper lip, maxillary alveolar process** for four incisor teeth, and **primary palate** (premaxilla)
      (2) Merge with maxillary prominences to complete **upper lip** and **jaw**
    c. **Lateral nasal prominences**
      (1) Merge with maxillary prominences along **nasolacrimal grooves** where **nasolacrimal ducts** later develop
      (2) Form **sides of nose**
  3. **Maxillary prominences (V_2)**
    a. Form **upper cheek** regions and most of **upper lip** and jaw
    b. Merge with medial and lateral nasal prominences and mandibular prominence
  4. **Mandibular prominences (V_3)**
    a. Merge in midline to form **lower jaw** and **lip**
    b. Merge laterally with maxillary prominences at corners of mouth
G. **Nasal Cavities and Paranasal Sinuses**
  1. **Nasal pits** expand as **nasal sacs** as facial primordia enlarge.
  2. Nasal sacs initially separated from oral cavity by **oronasal membranes,** which rupture to form **primitive choanae** posterior to primary palate
  3. Formation of secondary palate completes separation of nasal and oral cavities, leaving **choanae** as communication of nasal cavities with the nasopharynx.
  4. **Paranasal sinuses** develop as outgrowths of nasal mucosa into surrounding bones, retaining their original connection with the nasal cavity for drainage.
  5. **Maxillary sinuses** are present, but small, at birth.
H. **Secondary Palate (Figure 8-36)**
  1. Begins development as **lateral palatine processes** (palatal shelves) that project inferomedially from **maxillary prominences** on each side of tongue
  2. Formed by **reorientation** of **palatal shelves** to horizontal position above tongue and their **fusion** with each other, with primary palate, and with nasal septum
  3. Line of fusion with **primary palate** indicated in skull by **incisive fossa** and **sutures** from it to maxillary alveolar process between lateral incisors and canines

The face develops from five facial primordia around the stomodeum beginning in the fourth week.

Infants with craniofacial malformations often have cardiac defects because truncoconal ridges also develop from neural crest cells.

Paranasal sinuses develop as outgrowths of the lateral nasal wall and retain their connections for drainage.

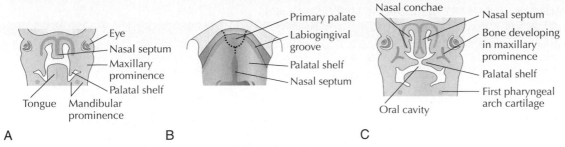

8-36: Development of the secondary palate in coronal sections (**A** and **C**) and inferior view (**B**). Lateral palatal shelves initially oriented vertically (**A**) reorient to horizontal position (**C**) and fuse (**B**).

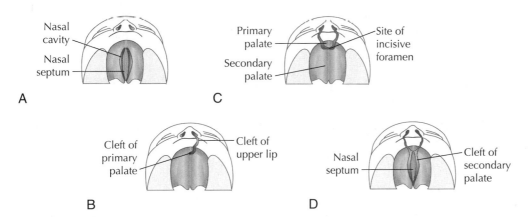

8-37: Cleft lip and cleft palate. **A,** Cleft of secondary palate. **B,** Unilateral cleft of lip and primary palate. **C,** Bilateral cleft of lip and primary palate. **D,** Bilateral cleft lip and cleft palate.

Cleft lip occurs in about 1 in 1000 births when the maxillary and medial nasal prominences fail to merge. It may be **unilateral** or **bilateral** and may occur as an isolated anomaly or with cleft palate. Cleft lip is more common in males. **Cleft palate** occurs in about 1 in 2500 births and is more common in females. Clefts of the secondary palate result from failure of the palatal shelves to fuse in the midline, and clefts of the primary palate occur when the palatal shelves do not fuse with the primary palate. **Multifactorial inheritance** (i.e., a combination of multiple genetic and environmental factors) may be responsible for most cases of cleft lip and palate. **Lateral clefts of the upper lip** and **cleft palate** are among the **most common developmental defects (Figure 8-37).**

Cleft lip results from the failure of maxillary and medial nasal prominences to merge.

XII. Summary of Cranial Nerves (Table 8-9)

TABLE 8-9. SUMMARY OF CRANIAL NERVES

CRANIAL NERVE	FUNCTIONAL COMPONENT	CELLS OF ORIGIN	MAIN FUNCTION
CN I olfactory	SVA	Olfactory mucosa	Smell
CN II optic	SSA	Ganglion cells of retina	Vision
CN III oculomotor	GSE	Oculomotor nucleus	Extraocular muscles: superior rectus, inferior rectus, medial rectus, inferior oblique, levator palpebrae superioris
	GVE	Edinger-Westphal nucleus	Accommodation for near vision: sphincter pupillae and ciliary muscles
CN IV trochlear	GSE	Trochlear nucleus	Extraocular muscle: superior oblique
CN V trigeminal	GSA	Semilunar ganglion	General sensation: scalp, face, upper and lower jaws, oral cavity, nasal cavity, eye

Continued

TABLE 8-9. **SUMMARY OF CRANIAL NERVES—Cont'd**

CRANIAL NERVE	FUNCTIONAL COMPONENT	CELLS OF ORIGIN	MAIN FUNCTION
	SVE	Motor nucleus of CN V (trigeminal nucleus)	Muscles of mastication plus mylohyoid, anterior digastric, tensor tympani, tensor veli palatini
CN VI abducens (abducent)	GSE	Abducens nucleus	Extraocular muscle: lateral rectus
CN VII facial	SVE	Facial nucleus	Muscles of facial expression plus stylohyoid, posterior digastric, stapedius
	GVE	Superior salivatory nucleus	Secretomotor to lacrimal gland, submandibular and sublingual salivary glands, small glands of oral and nasal cavities
	SVA	Geniculate ganglion	Taste from anterior two-thirds of tongue
	GVA	Geniculate ganglion	Visceral sensation: few fibers distributed with GVE
	GSA	Geniculate ganglion	Somatic sensation: external auditory canal and tympanic membrane
CN VIII vestibulocochlear	SSA	Vestibular ganglion Spiral ganglion	Equilibrium (balance) and sense of motion Hearing
CN IX glossopharyngeal	SVE	Nucleus ambiguus	Stylopharyngeus muscle
	GVE	Inferior salivatory nucleus	Secretomotor to parotid salivary gland
	SVA	Inferior ganglion (inferior petrosal)	Taste from posterior third of tongue
	GVA	Inferior ganglion	Visceral sensation: pharynx and posterior third of tongue; visceral reflexes
	GSA	Superior ganglion (superior petrosal)	Somatic sensation: tympanic membrane and middle ear
CN X vagus	SVE	Nucleus ambiguus	Muscles of pharynx, larynx, and soft palate excluding stylopharyngeus and tensor veli palatini but including palatoglossus
	GVE	Dorsal motor nucleus	Cardiac muscle, smooth muscle, and glands of thorax and abdomen
	SVA	Inferior ganglion (nodose ganglion)	Taste over epiglottis
	GVA	Inferior ganglion	Visceral sensation: pharynx and larynx; reflexes: distributed with GVE
	GSA	Superior ganglion (jugular ganglion)	Somatic sensation: external auditory canal and dura
CN XI accessory	SVE	Nucleus ambiguus	Joins vagus to distribute to pharyngeal arch muscles
	GSE	Accessory nucleus	Sternocleidomastoid and trapezius muscles
CN XII hypoglossal	GSE	Hypoglossal nucleus	Intrinsic and extrinsic muscles of tongue except palatoglossus

GSA, General somatic afferent; *GSE*, general somatic efferent; *GVA*, general visceral afferent; *GVE*, general visceral efferent; *SSA*, special somatic afferent; *SVA*, special visceral afferent; *SVE*, special visceral efferent (also called *BE*, branchial efferent).

COMMON LABORATORY VALUES

TEST BLOOD, PLASMA, SERUM	CONVENTIONAL UNITS	SI UNITS
Alanine aminotransferase (ALT, GPT at 30°C)	8-20 U/L	8-20 U/L
Amylase, serum	25-125 U/L	25-125 U/L
Aspartate aminotransferase (AST, GOT at 30°C)	8-20 U/L	8-20 U/L
Bilirubin, serum (adult): total; direct	0.1-1.0 mg/dL; 0.0-0.3 mg/dL	2-17 µmol/L; 0-5 µmol/L
Calcium, serum (Ca^{2+})	8.4-10.2 mg/dL	2.1-2.8 mmol/L
Cholesterol, serum	Rec: <200 mg/dL	<5.2 mmol/L

Cortisol, serum	8:00 AM: 6-23 µg/dL;
	    4:00 PM: 3-15 µg/dL
	8:00 PM: ≤50% of 8:00 AM
		170-630 nmol/L;
		    80-410 nmol/L
		Fraction of 8:00 AM: ≤0.50

Creatine kinase, serum	Male: 25-90 U/L Female: 10-70 U/L	25-90 U/L 10-70 U/L
Creatinine, serum	0.6-1.2 mg/dL	53-106 µmol/L
Electrolytes, serum		
Sodium (Na$^+$)	136-145 mEq/L	135-145 mmol/L
Chloride (Cl$^-$)	95-105 mEq/L	95-105 mmol/L
Potassium (K$^+$)	3.5-5.0 mEq/L	3.5-5.0 mmol/L
Bicarbonate (HCO$_3$)	22-28 mEq/L	22-28 mmol/L
Magnesium (Mg^{2+})	1.5-2.0 mEq/L	1.5-2.0 mmol/L
Estriol, total, serum (in pregnancy)		
24-28 wk; 32-36 wk	30-170 ng/mL; 60-280 ng/mL	104-590 nmol/L; 208-970 nmol/L
28-32 wk; 36-40 wk	40-220 ng/mL; 80-350 ng/mL	140-760 nmol/L; 280-1210 nmol/L
Ferritin, serum	Male: 15-200 ng/ml Female: 12-150 ng/mL	15-200 µg/L 12-150 µg/l

Follicle-stimulating hormone, serum/plasma (FSH)	Male: 4-25 mIU/mL
	Female:
	  Premenopause, 4-30 mIU/mL
	  Midcycle peak, 10-90 mIU/mL
	  Postmenopause, 40-250 mIU/mL
		4-25 U/L
		
		4-30 U/L
		10-90 U/L
		40-250 U/L

Gases, arterial blood (room air)		
pH	7.35-7.45	[H$^+$] 36-44 nmol/L
P$_{CO_2}$	33-45 mmHg	4.4-5.9 kPa
P$_{O_2}$	75-105 mmHg	10.0-14.0 kPa
Glucose, serum	Fasting: 70-110 mg/dL 2 hr postprandial: <120 mg/dL	3.8-6.1 mmol/L <6.6 mmol/L
Growth hormone-arginine stimulation	Fasting: <5 ng/mL Provocative stimuli: >7 ng/mL	<5 µg/L >7 µg/L
Immunoglobulins, serum		
IgA	76-390 mg/dL	0.76-3.90 g/L
IgE	0-380 IU/mL	0-380 kIU/L
IgG	650-1500 mg/dL	6.5-15 g/L

(Continued)

TEST BLOOD, PLASMA, SERUM	CONVENTIONAL UNITS	SI UNITS
IgM	40-345 mg/dL	0.4-3.45 g/L
Iron	50-170 µg/dL	9-30 µmol/L
Lactate dehydrogenase, serum	45-90 U/L	45-90 U/L
Luteinizing hormone, serum/plasma (LH)	Male: 6-23 mIU/mL	6-23 U/L
	Female:	
	Follicular phase, 5-30 mIU/mL	5-30 U/L
	Midcycle, 75-150 mIU/mL	75-150 U/L
	Postmenopause, 30-200 mIU/mL	30-200 U/L
Osmolality, serum	275-295 mOsm/kg	275-295 mOsm/kg
Parathyroid hormone, serum, N-terminal	230-630 pg/mL	230-630 ng/L
Phosphatase (alkaline), serum (p-NPP at 30°C)	20-70 U/L	20-70 U/L
Phosphorus (inorganic), serum	3.0-4.5 mg/dL	1.0-1.5 mmol/L
Prolactin, serum (hPRL)	<20 ng/mL	<20 µg/L
Proteins, serum		
Total (recumbent)	6.0-8.0 g/dL	60-80 g/L
Albumin	3.5-5.5 g/dL	35-55 g/L
Globulin	2.3-3.5 g/dL	23-35 g/L
Thyroid-stimulating hormone, serum or plasma (TSH)	0.5-5.0 µU/mL	0.5-5.0 mU/L
Thyroidal iodine (^{123}I) uptake	8-30% of administered dose/24 hr	0.08-0.30/24 hr
Thyroxine (T_4), serum	4.5-12 µg/dL	58-154 nmol/L
Triglycerides, serum	35-160 mg/dL	0.4-1.81 mmol/L
Triiodothyronine (T_3), serum (RIA)	115-190 ng/dL	1.8-2.9 nmol/L
Triiodothyronine (T_3) resin uptake	25-38%	0.25-0.38
Urea nitrogen, serum (BUN)	7-18 mg/dL	1.2-3.0 mmolurea/L
Uric acid, serum	3.0-8.2 mg/dL	0.18-0.48 mmol/L
Cerebrospinal Fluid		
Cell count	0-5 cells/mm^3	0-5 × 10^6/L
Chloride	118-132 mEq/L	118-132 mmol/L
Gamma globulin	3-12% total proteins	0.03-0.12
Glucose	50-75 mg/dL	2.8-4.2 mmol/L
Pressure	70-180 mmH$_2$O	70-180 mmH$_2$O
Proteins, total	<40 mg/dL	<0.40 g/L
Hematology		
Bleeding time (template)	2-7 min	2-7 min
Erythrocyte count	Male: 4.3-5.9 million/mm^3	4.3-5.9 × 10^{12}/L
	Female: 3.5-5.5 million/mm^3	3.5-5.5 × 10^{12}/L
Erythrocyte sedimentation rate (Westergren)	Male: 0-15 mm/hr	0-15 mm/hr
	Female: 0-20 mm/hr	0-20 mm/hr
Hematocrit (Hct)	Male: 40-54%	0.40-0.54
	Female: 37-47%	0.37-0.47
Hemoglobin A$_{1C}$	≤6%	≤0.06%
Hemoglobin, blood (Hb)	Male: 13.5-17.5 g/dL	2.09-2.71 mmol/L
	Female: 12.0-16.0 g/dL	1.86-2.48 mmol/L
Hemoglobin, plasma	1-4 mg/dL	0.16-0.62 mmol/L
Leukocyte count and differential		
Leukocyte count	4500-11,000/mm^3	4.5-11.0 × 10^9/L
Segmented neutrophils	54-62%	0.54-0.62
Bands	3-5%	0.03-0.05
Eosinophils	1-3%	0.01-0.03
Basophils	0-0.75%	0-0.0075
Lymphocytes	25-33%	0.25-0.33
Monocytes	3-7%	0.03-0.07
Mean corpuscular hemoglobin (MCH)	25.4-34.6 pg/cell	0.39-0.54 fmol/cell
Mean corpuscular hemoglobin concentration (MCHC)	31-37% Hb/cell	4.81-5.74 mmolHb/L

Mean corpuscular volume (MCV)	80-100 μm³	80-100 fl
Partial thromboplastin time (activated) (aPTT)	25-40 sec	25-40 sec
Platelet count	150,000-400,000/mm³	150-400 × 10⁹/L
Prothrombin time (PT)	12-14 sec	12-14 sec
Reticulocyte count	0.5-1.5% of red cells	0.005-0.015
Thrombin time	<2 sec deviation from control	<2 sec deviation from control
Volume		
Plasma	Male: 25-43 mL/kg	0.025-0.043 L/kg
	Female: 28-45 mL/kg	0.028-0.045 L/kg
Red cell	Male: 20-36 mL/kg	0.020-0.036 L/kg
	Female: 19-31 mL/kg	0.019-0.031 L/kg
Sweat		
Chloride	0-35 mmol/L	0-35 mmol/L
Urine		
Calcium	100-300 mg/24 hr	2.5-7.5 mmol/24 hr
Creatinine clearance	Male: 97-137 mL/min	
	Female: 88-128 mL/min	
Estriol, total (in pregnancy)		
30 wk	6-18 mg/24 hr	21-62 μmol/24 hr
35 wk	9-28 mg/24 hr	31-97 μmol/24 hr
40 wk	13-42 mg/24 hr	45-146 μmol/24 hr
17-Hydroxycorticosteroids	Male: 3.0-9.0 mg/24 hr	8.2-25.0 μmol/24 hr
	Female: 2.0-8.0 mg/24 hr	5.5-22.0 μmol/24 hr
17-Ketosteroids, total	Male: 8-22 mg/24 hr	28-76 μmol/24 hr
	Female: 6-15 mg/24 hr	21-52 μmol/24 hr
Osmolality	50-1400 mOsm/kg	
Oxalate	8-40 μg/mL	90-445 μmol/L
Proteins, total	<150 mg/24 hr	<0.15 g/24 hr

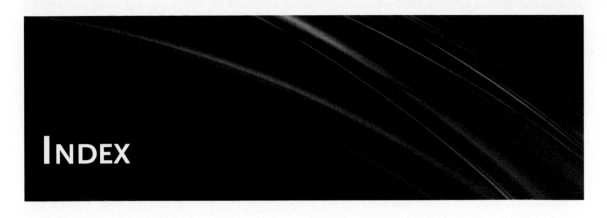

INDEX

Note: Page numbers followed by *b* indicate boxes (margin notes), *f* indicate figures and *t* indicate tables.